Current Topics in Musculoskeletal Medicine

A CASE STUDY APPROACH

Edited by

Mark DeCarlo, MHA, MS, PT, SCS, ATC
Methodist Sports Medicine Center
Indianapolis, Indiana

Kathy Oneacre, MA, ATC
Methodist Sports Medicine Center
Indianapolis, Indiana

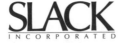

SLACK
INCORPORATED

An innovative information, education and management company

6900 Grove Road • Thorofare, NJ 08086

Publisher: John H. Bond
Editorial Director: Amy E. Drummond
Editorial Assistant: William J. Green

The procedures and practices described in this book should be implemented in a manner consistent with the professional standards set for the circumstances that apply in each specific situation. Every effort has been made to confirm the accuracy of the information presented and to correctly relate generally accepted practices. The author, editor, and publisher cannot accept responsibility for errors or exclusions or for the outcome of the application of the material presented herein. There is no expressed or implied warranty of this book or information imparted by it.

The work SLACK publishes is peer reviewed. Prior to publication, recognized leaders in the field, educators, and clinicians provide important feedback on the concepts and content that we publish. We welcome feedback on this work.

Current topics in musculoskeletal medicine: a case study approach / [edited by] Mark
DeCarlo, Kathy Oneacre
        p. ; cm. -- (Athletic training library)
    Includes bibliographical references and index.
    ISBN 1-55642-434-5 (alk. paper)
    1. Sports injuries--Case studies. 2. Sports injuries--Physical therapy--Case studies. I.
DeCarlo, Mark. II. Oneacre, Kathy. III. Series.
    [DNLM: 1. Athletic Injuries--therapy--Case Report. 2. Bone and Bones--injuries--Case
Report. 3. Muscles--injuries--Case Report. 4. Physical Therapy--Case Report. QT 261
C976 2001]
    RD97 .C87 2001
    617.1'027--dc21

                                                                    00-068784
Printed in the United States of America.
Published by: SLACK Incorporated
                6900 Grove Road
                Thorofare, NJ 08086 USA
                Telephone: 856-848-1000
                Fax: 856-853-5991
                www.slackbooks.com

Contact SLACK Incorporated for more information about other books in this field or about the availability of our books from distributors outside the United States.

Last digit is print number: 10   9   8   7   6   5   4   3   2   1

DEDICATION

I dedicate this book to my parents, Marilyn and Tom.
Kathy Oneacre

To my children Christian and Sarah, whose love and patience have allowed me to pursue so much. Their presence in my life is truly the greatest gift of all.
Mark DeCarlo

CONTENTS

ABOUT THE EDITORS

Mark DeCarlo is the chief operating officer of Methodist Sports Medicine Center, Indianapolis, Indiana; the president of the American Physical Therapy Association, Sports Physical Therapy Section; the vice president of the *Journal of Orthopaedic and Sports Physical Therapy* Board of Directors; and a representative-at-large of the International Federation of Sports Physical Therapists.

Kathy Oneacre received her bachelor's degree in athletic training from Otterbein College and her master's degree from the University of Alabama. She is Director of Research at Methodist Sports Medicine Center where she coordinates research and education activity for the physical therapy department and the staff of orthopedic surgeons and primary care physicians. In addition, she provides outreach athletic training coverage to a local high school.

Contributing Authors

Cheri Alexy, OTR, CHT
Methodist Sports Medicine Center
Indianapolis, Indiana

Jeromy M. Alt, MS, ATC
West Virginia University
Morgantown, West Virginia

James R. Andrews, MD
Alabama Sports Medicine and Orthopaedic
     Center
Birmingham, Alabama

Stephen L. Antonopulos, MS, ATC
Denver Broncos
Englewood, Colorado

Harold G. Baker, MD
St. Francis Hospital
Indianapolis, Indiana

Erin Barill, PT, ATC
Methodist Sports Medicine Center
Indianapolis, Indiana

Tab Blackburn, PT, ATC
Tulane Institute of Sports Medicine
New Orleans, Louisiana

Martin Boutblik, MD
Steadman Hawkins Clinic
Englewood, Colorado

Stephen J. Burns, MD
Medical Group of Michigan City
Michigan City, Indiana

David G. Carfagno, DO
Southwest Sports Medicine and Orthopaedic
     Surgery Clinic
Scottsdale, Arizona

Bruce E. Dall, MD
K Valley Orthopaedics
Kalamazoo, Michigan

John Darmelio, MS, ATC
Methodist Sports Medicine Center
Indianapolis, Indiana

George J. Davies, MEd, PT, SCS, ATC, CSCS
University of Wisconsin-LaCrosse
LaCrosse, Wisconsin

Todd S. Ellenbecker, MS, PT, SCS, CSCS
Physiotherapy Associates
Scottsdale, Arizona

Charles Giangarra, MD
Gunderson Lutheran Sports Medicine
Onalaska, Wisconsin

Thomas V. Gocke III, MS, ATC/L, PA/C
Raleigh Orthopaedic Clinic
Raleigh, North Carolina

Robert S. Gray, MS, ATC
The Cleveland Clinic
West Lake, Ohio

Tinker Gray, MA, ELS
Methodist Sports Medicine Center
Indianapolis, Indiana

Thomas A. Greenwald, MD
Iowa State University
Ames, Iowa

Mike J. Hanley, MS, ATC/L
East Carolina University
Greenville, North Carolina

David F. Hubbard, MD
West Virginia University
Morgantown, West Virginia

Mike Hunker, ATC/L, CSCS
Cathedral High School
Indianapolis, Indiana

Wendy J. Hurd, PT
Health South Rehabilitation
Birmingham, Alabama

Walter L. Jenkins, MS, PT, ATC
East Carolina University
Greenville, North Carolina

Robert G. Jones, MD
Raleigh Orthopaedic Clinic
Raleigh, North Carolina

Geoff Kaplan, PT, ATC
Tennessee Titans
Nashville, Tennessee

Martin J. Kelly, MS, PT, OCS
University of Pennsylvania Health System
Philadelphia, Pennsylvania

Tim Koberna, MA, ATC
Albion College
Albion, Michigan

Tally Lassiter Jr, MD
Orthopaedics East, Incorporated
Greenville, North Carolina

Joseph S. Lueken, MS, ATC
Indiana University
Bloomington, Indiana

Mike Matheny, PT, ATC
Ithaca College
Ithaca, New York

John R. McCarroll, MD
Methodist Sports Medicine Center
Indianapolis, Indiana

Mary Meier, MS, ATC
Iowa State University
Ames, Iowa

Keith Meister, MD
University of Florida
Gainesville, Florida

Andrea J. Michael, ATC
West Virginia Wesleyan College
Buckhannon, West Virginia

Paul Mieling, MS, OTR, ATC
Methodist Sports Medicine Center
Indianapolis, Indiana

Gary Misamore, MD
Methodist Sports Medicine Center
Indianapolis, Indiana

Brian Pease, PT, ATC
University of Indianapolis
Indianapolis, Indiana

David A. Porter, MD, PhD
Methodist Sports Medicine Center
Indianapolis, Indiana

Christopher Price, MD
Indiana University Medical Center
Indianapolis, Indiana

Ralph Reiff, ATC
St. Vincent Sports Medicine
Carmel, Indiana

Arthur C. Rettig, MD
Methodist Sports Medicine Center
Indianapolis, Indiana

Paul Reuteman, MHS, PT, ATC
Gundersen Lutheran Sports Medicine
Onalaska, Wisconsin

Kecia E. Sell, MS, PT, ATC
Fairview Rehab Services
Robbinsdale, Minnesota

Michael A. Shaffer, MSPT, ATC
Iowa State University
Ames, Iowa

Ned Shannon, ATC
University of Indianapolis
Indianapolis, Indiana

K. Donald Shelbourne, MD
Methodist Sports Medicine Center
Indianapolis, Indiana

Hunter Smith, ATC
Indianapolis Colts
Indianapolis, Indiana

Bernie Stento, MS, ATC/L
Chesterton High School
Chesterton, Indiana

Vincent G. Stilger, HSD, ATC
West Virginia University
Morgantown, West Virginia

Adam Swain, PT, OCS, ATC
K Valley Orthopaedics
Kalamazoo, Michigan

James E. Tracy, MS, PT, ATC
East Carolina University
Greenville, North Carolina

Michael L. Voight, DPT, OCS, SCS, ATC
Belmont University
Nashville, Tennessee

Kevin E. Wilk, PT
Health South Rehabilitation
Birmingham, Alabama

J. Scott Woodward, MS, PT, SCS, ATC
Physiotherapy Associates
Englewood, Colorado

FOREWORD

Inherent in the preparation of medical and allied medical professionals is a period of clinical training under the tutelage of experienced, qualified clinicians in their field. The aspiring professional learns through observation and then supervised application of newly acquired skills. Each case is a new learning opportunity, and over time the student gains experience in evaluating a wide variety of problems. The experiences gained in some cases last the span of a career. I can clearly remember the pertinent facts about a few unique cases from my experiences as a student athletic trainer more than 25 years ago.

Unfortunately, only a few students usually benefit from the lessons learned through the management of an individual case. Unique cases and the lessons learned, however, are shared through lectures and published reports. In many situations the standards of practice are defined by an accumulation of case reports. Case reports, though, are scattered through the literature, making it difficult for students and clinicians to review them in a systematic manner.

Current Topics in Musculoskeletal Medicine: A Case Study Approach, edited by Mark DeCarlo and Kathy Oneacre, brings together a respected and experienced group of physicians, athletic trainers, physical therapists, and physician assistants who teach through case studies. This collection of case studies provides a regional progression addressing many of the most common challenges faced in musculoskeletal medicine in a single volume. Most case presentations are preceded by a brief overview of a musculoskeletal injury. The evaluation, including history, physical examination procedures, diagnostic testing, and medical management, is then described in detail. This is a truly unique text that will be a valued reference for the practicing clinicians who care for injured athletes and an important adjunct to clinical training of their students.

Craig R. Denegar, PhD, ATC, PT

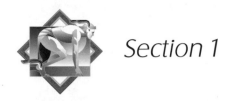

Section 1

Head, Neck, and Spine

Chapter One

Chronic Burner Syndrome in a High School Football Player

Bernie Stento, MS, ATC/L, Stephen J. Burns, MD

INTRODUCTION

The incidence and mechanism of brachial plexus injuries, also known as burners or stingers, in the sport of football has been well documented.[1-9,10] Three predominant mechanisms of injury are reported: traction to the upper roots when the ipsilateral shoulder is depressed and the head is forcefully laterally flexed to the contralateral side, compression of the nerve roots in the neural foramina on the ipsilateral side due to an extension and ipsilateral rotation of the neck (Figure 1-1), and a direct blow in the region superior to the clavicle (Erb's point).[1,2,4,6-9,11-13]

The athlete typically describes a burning paresthesia radiating down the arm from the neck/shoulder region. The C5-C6 nerve roots are the most frequently injured areas.[2,7,9,13] Clancy, et al[2] classified burners into three categories. Burners exhibiting a reversal defect in axonal function lasting from a few minutes to 2 weeks were considered a neurapraxia. Most burners fall into this category with symptoms lasting only minutes. Symptoms lasting longer than 2 weeks resulted in an axonotmesis[11] and a permanent deficit in nerve function was described as a neurotmesis.[3]

Meyer, et al described the relationship between cervical spinal stenosis and the incidence of burners in collegiate football players.[7] They found that the group of players that experienced a burner contained a greater number of athletes with cervical stenosis (47.5%) compared to a group with neck pain (32.2%) or the asymptomatic group (25.2%). They also concluded that players with cervical stenosis had a three times greater risk of suffering a burner via the extension-compression mechanism than players without stenosis, and that linebackers and defensive linemen were found to be at the greatest risk for having a burner. Levitz, et al[6] described the pathomechanics of chronic, recurrent cervical nerve root neurapraxia. They found that extension combined with ipsilateral neck deviation accounted for 83% of these types of injuries. Seventy percent of their patients displayed a positive Spurling's sign (extension and rotation of the head toward the involved arm), 72% had persistent weakness in the deltoid and spinatus groups, 53% had cervical stenosis, and 85% had evidence of degenerative disc disease, as shown in a magnetic resonance imaging (MRI) scan. They also reported that three of seven players without disc disease were 23 years old or younger and had narrowing of the neural foramina due to bony hypertrophy. Both studies clarified that the chronic burner syndrome was not due to a traction type mechanism, but rather an extension-compression mechanism. In a study of fresh frozen cervical spine cadavers, Yoo, et al[10] found that ipsilateral rotation of the head had an additive effect on the extension-induced narrowing of the neuroforamen. This data supports the idea that extension with compression could be one cause of burner injuries.

The objective of this case study is to outline the subjective history, clinical findings, and return to play criteria for a high school athlete with chronic burner symptoms. As has been reported, many football players do not report their symptoms to a health care provider and the injury goes undetected until the symptoms impede participation.[1,2,6-9,12]

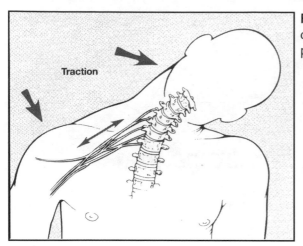

Figure 1-1. Extension with lateral deviation/rotation of the head to the involved side causing the compression mechanism of chronic burners.

Subjective History

The patient was a 17-year-old senior high school football player who played middle linebacker. He first reported his injury during the first half of a game on September 4, 1998. The athlete came off the field complaining of vague tingling and pain radiating from the right side of his neck down to his shoulder region. The athlete reported that pain in and around his right shoulder made his whole arm feel "dead." He reported no symptoms down the right arm or into the hand. The athlete reported that he experienced a minor episode 5 days before the game during practice and continued to have more episodes, each greater in intensity, during the week. He reported that the first burner he experienced was during a preseason scrimmage on August 15, 1998, and he also related that he had one or two burners the previous season but did not report them. The first burner that he can remember having was in the eighth grade. He reported that the symptoms would last only 3 to 4 minutes and would dissipate while he was on the field or shortly after he came off.

Injury Mechanism

The athlete reported that his head snapped back when he tried to tackle someone face mask to face mask. He went on to describe that he felt the hit was off-center and came from his left side. Once the episode resolved, he had no residual weakness or sensation loss. We determined that the mechanism was not one of traction but rather extension, with rotation of the head to the involved side when the athlete was attempting to tackle an opponent.

Clinical Examination

The on-field evaluation revealed weakness of the right trapezius and deltoid areas, decreased sensation over the right trapezius and lateral deltoid area, and point tenderness in the posterior lateral aspect of the upper neck region. Ice was applied to the posterior cervical region and the athlete was not allowed to participate for the rest of the half. During halftime of the game, the athlete was re-evaluated and found to have normal strength and sensation. There was also no area of point tenderness in the posterior cervical region. The athlete warmed up with the team before the second half and had no problems simulating tackling drills. He returned to the game during the second half of play, when he again experienced an episode similar to the one in the first half. At that time, the on-field evaluation was also similar to the one from the first half, however, the athlete was not allowed to return for the remainder of the game. The athlete was referred to the team physician the next day for further evaluation.

Physical findings by the physician revealed equal cervical range of motion (ROM) and strength bilaterally. Spurling's sign revealed only minimal tenderness in the cervical region, as reported by the athlete. Neurologic testing of the right upper extremity was also normal. Because the athlete was a minor and his parents did not accompany him to this evaluation, no radiological testing was performed. The athlete was asked to have his parents accompany him to a physician's appointment on September 8, 1998.

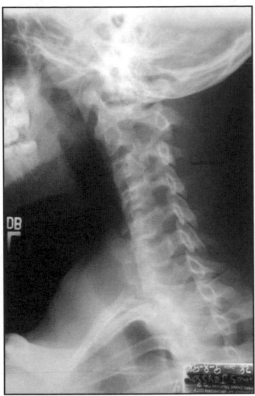

Figure 1-2. X-ray showing a small spur in the neuroforamina between C3 and C4.

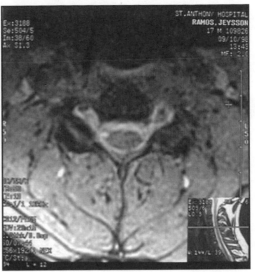

Figure 1-3. The MRI revealed some foraminal stenosis at the level of C3-C4.

DIAGNOSTIC IMAGING

The physician's evaluation was unchanged from 3 days prior. Cervical spine roentgenograms, including flexion/extension and oblique views, were obtained. There was no evidence of instability on the lateral flexion views, and disc spacing was well maintained. However, on one oblique view a small spur in the neuroforamina between C3 and C4 was noted, causing the stenosis in the foramina (Figure 1-2). These findings were explained to the athlete and his parent. An MRI of his cervical spine was ordered before a final decision about return to play was made.

The MRI was conducted on September 10, 1998, and during a follow-up visit on September 11, the results were reviewed with the athlete and his parents. The MRI revealed some foraminal stenosis at the level of C3 and C4 (Figure 1-3), and a Torg ratio (the distance from the midpoint of the posterior aspect of the vertebral body to the nearest point on the corresponding spinolaminar line divided by the anteroposterior width of the vertebral body measured through the midpoint of the body) of .77 was noted at that level. It was explained preliminarily that these findings should not preclude the athlete from participation; however, a second opinion from a spine specialist was recommended.

A spine specialist evaluated the athlete on September 16, 1998 and reviewed the roentgenograms and MRI with him. The physical evaluation showed normal ROM for the cervical spine and shoulder, normal strength in the upper extremity, and normal reflexes in the upper and lower extremities. The spine specialist confirmed the radiographic results and agreed that the athlete was at no increased risk of permanent neck injury.

RETURN TO PLAY CRITERIA

Both physicians believed it was safe for the athlete to resume contact sports with the worse case scenario being a recurrence of the transient neurapraxia in the right arm. The rationale was that the symptoms were transient in nature and resolved without any permanent neurologic or motor deficits. Watkins[13] classified foraminal stenosis as a minimal risk to permanent nerve root damage and reported that most injuries were temporary. The clinical examination has been recommended to be the determining factor in return to play criteria. An athlete should be able to demonstrate normal strength bilaterally in the upper extremities, normal bilateral cervical ROM, and no neurologic symptoms at the time of return.[1-3,9,12]

REHABILITATION/TREATMENT

In the case of this athlete, he was able to return to football practice on September 16, 1998 after receiving clearance from the physicians. We allowed him to practice for 2 days in shoulder pads and helmet using a McDavid Cowboy Collar (McDavid Sports Products, Chicago, Ill) with a back plate. Hovis and Limbird[4] found that the McDavid Cowboy Collar was as effective as a neck roll in preventing excessive neck extension. We secured the Cowboy Collar to the shoulder pads by interlacing it to the front of the shoulder pads to prevent slippage and tried to position the Cowboy Collar so as to limit extreme neck extension when the athlete would tackle. We explained to the athlete and his position coach that the proper tackling technique was essential to preventing recurrences of this condition. We encouraged the athlete to practice tackling without trying to have face mask to face mask contact and lateral deviation/rotation of the head to the right side.

CLINICAL OUTCOMES

After returning to football, the athlete had only one more episode where he had to be removed from a game due to the symptomology. When his symptoms cleared, he was allowed to continue. He worked his way back into the starting rotation and played in six games after returning. At the conclusion of the season, the athlete indicated to us that he frequently "let-up" during the games and did not try to hit and tackle as hard.

DISCUSSION

The question of why a small spur would form in the neuroforamina of the cervical spine has been addressed in the literature. Meyer, et al[7] described the effects of cumulative trauma to the cervical spine, especially in those players who were linemen or linebackers. They hypothesized that the repetitive contact these athletes encountered while blocking or tackling caused repeated sprains that made the facet joint capsules inflamed and developed adhesions around the facets and spinal foramen. This inflammatory process may have lead to a functional narrowing of the foramen, thus compressing the nerve root more easily when the neck was in extension.

Levitz, et al[6] reported that the high incidence of disc disease in their subjects strongly suggested that an alteration in disc mechanics resulted in compression on the nerve root or dorsal ganglion in the neural foramina. This predominantly occurred in older athletes at higher levels of competition.

Meyer, et al[7] also documented the incidence of spinal stenosis in athletes experiencing burners caused by an extension-compression mechanism. They found that 47% of the burner group had spinal stenosis with a Torg ratio of less than 0.8 at one or more levels compared with 32% of the neck pain group and 25% of the asymptomatic group. They were able to conclude that a football player with spinal stenosis had a three times greater chance of having a burner than a player without stenosis. Levitz, et al[6] reported a 53% incidence of spinal stenosis and an 85% incidence of degenerative disc disease (defined as a disc bulging, protrusion, or herniation). Of the 15% (seven players) without disk disease, three had bony hypertrophy of the neuroforamina, and all were 23 years or younger. Kelly, et al[5] found that scholastic football players and wrestlers who experienced at least one burner had significantly narrower spinal canals than age-matched controls. They also stated that the narrow foramina would be the result of narrower cervical canals, thus increasing the likelihood of a "pinch" on the nerve roots. The athlete in this case study did not demonstrate spinal stenosis or degenerative disc disease on roentgenograms or MRI. However, the athlete is in the age category in which osteophyte formation has been reported.

The use of Spurling's sign has been described in the literature as a way to reproduce symptoms during a physical examination.[6,7,13] Levitz, et al[6] found that 70% of their patient population showed a positive Spurling's sign. The athlete was unable to experience a reproduction of all the symptoms with this test but was able to experience some minimal tenderness in the posterior region of the neck. We considered him as having a negative Spurling's sign. We could only hypothesize that the spur was not large enough to reproduce symptoms and, because there was no evidence of degenerative disc disease, there may not have been a significant narrowing of the foramen. Also, the forces we imposed on the athlete during the test were not similar to what he experienced when he tried to tackle someone.

CONCLUSION

The athlete in this case study demonstrated the symptoms of a chronic burner syndrome due to a small spur in the C3 and C4 foramen. Our athlete had a Torg ratio of .77, but there was no evidence of degenerative disc disease. The mechanism of traction to the cervical spine with contralateral deviation is not the prime mechanism of chronic burners, but rather more prevalent as the mechanism of acute brachial plexus injuries. Chronic burners, similar to the athlete in this case study, are more often caused by a forceful extension and rotation of the head toward the involved arm. The athlete should be completely asymptomatic upon return to athletic activity and followed closely if symptoms persist. The history and physical examination, along with proper radiographic testing, will accurately diagnose this pathology and better allow health care providers to make an accurate decision regarding return to play.

REFERENCES

1. Bergfeld JA, Hershman EB, Wilbourne A. Brachial plexus injury in sports: Five-year follow-up. *Orthopaedic Transactions.* 1988;12:743-744.

2. Clancy WG Jr, Brand RL, Bergfeld JA. Upper trunk brachial plexus injuries in contact sports. *Am J Sports Med.* 1977;5:209-216.

3. Hershman EB. Brachial plexus injuries. *Clin Sports Med.* 1990;9:311-329.

4. Hovis WD, Limbird TJ. An evaluation of cervical orthoses in limiting hyperextension and lateral flexion in football. *Med Sci Sports Exerc.* 1994;26:872-876.

5. Kelly JD, Clancy M, Marchetto PA, et al. The relationship of transient upper extremity paresthesias and cervical stenosis. *Orthopaedic Transactions.* 1992-1993;16:732.

6. Levitz CL, Reilly PJ, Torg JS. The pathomechanics of chronic, recurrent cervical nerve root neurapraxia: the chronic burner syndrome. *Am J Sports Med.* 1997;25:73-76.

7. Meyer SA, Schulte KR, Callaghan JJ, et al. Cervical spinal stenosis and burners in collegiate football players. *Am J Sports Med.* 1994;22:158-166.

8. Robertson WC Jr, Eichman PL, Clancy WG. Upper trunk brachial plexopathy in football players. *JAMA.* 1979;241:1480-1482.

9. Sallis RE, Jones K, Knopp W. Burners: offensive strategy for an underreported injury. *The Physician and Sportsmedicine.* 1992;20:47-55.

10. Yoo JU, Zou D, Edwards WT, et al. Effect of cervical spine motion on the non-dominant dimensions of the human cervical spine. *Spine.* 1992;17:1131-1136.

11. Seddon H. *Surgical Disorders of the Peripheral Nerves.* Edinburgh: Churchill Livingstone; 1992.

12. Speer KP, Bassett FJ III. The prolonged burner syndrome. *Am J Sports Med.* 1990;18:591-594.

13. Watkins RG. Neck injuries in football players. *Clin Sports Med.* 1986;5:215-246.

Chapter Two

C6 Fracture/Dislocation in a High School Football Player

John Darmelio, MS, ATC, Harold G. Baker, MD

SUBJECT

The athlete was a 14-year-old high school quarterback who was 6 feet tall and weighed 170 pounds. The injury occurred in an away game near the end of the season. The athletic trainer was present, but the team physician was not.

The athlete was running the ball up the field and lowered his head as he was about to be tackled. He hit helmet to helmet with his opponent and fell to the ground. He was slow to get up and was a little dazed, but returned to the huddle. Before another play could be run, however, he jogged to the sideline and took himself out of the game.

INITIAL CLINICAL EXAM

The athlete reported no loss of consciousness, headache, dizziness, or nausea to the athletic trainer. He stated that his neck was sore and that he had pain high in his right shoulder. He denied numbness and weakness in the affected extremity. His pupils were equal and reactive to light with normal extra-ocular movements. His mental status was normal and the concussion checklist was negative. Palpation of the cervical spine was initially negative for pain. Active flexion and extension of the neck were slightly limited by pain. Rotation to the left was normal but, to the right, elicited significant pain in the neck and a marked decrease in ROM.

Due to the abnormal cervical spine exam and his high index of suspicion for significant neck injury based on the mechanism of injury, the athletic trainer removed the athlete from the game. Ice packs were applied to the right side of the neck and to the right trapezius muscle. The athlete's parents were told of the abnormal exam and reason for removing their son from the game. They were told to monitor the neck pain and if there was any progression of pain, numbness, or weakness in the affected arm or hand they were to go immediately to the nearest emergency room. They were otherwise instructed to contact their family physician (who was also the team physician) for a follow-up examination in 24 hours. The athlete was instructed to continue ice packs, employ light cervical ROM exercises, and was warned not to participate in any conditioning exercises until cleared by the team physician.

The athlete was fairly compliant with his instructions, even though he continued to have some pain in his right trapezius. He went to conditioning the next day where he did some light jogging and watched game films. As the weekend progressed, he continued to have increased pain and stiffness in his neck. He also became aware of some weakness and paresthesias in his right arm. The family doctor immediately ordered a cervical spine x-ray, which was negative for cervical fracture. The parents were then given instructions to change the therapy from ice packs to moist heat and were instructed to bring the athlete and his x-rays to the office on the following morning.

In the physician's office, the athlete had marked tenderness with pressure over the spinous process of C6. Active ROM of the neck to the right was diminished. Passive ROM to the right was limited secondary to

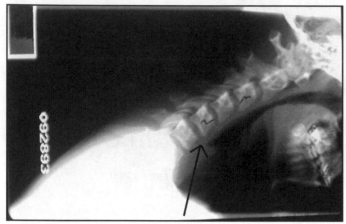

Figure 2-1. X-ray of the cervical spine.

pain. He was not able to shrug the right shoulder, and abduction of the right arm was weak. Reflexes were normal but there was mild C6 paresthesias.

On review of the cervical spine films, the team physician observed a 2 to 3 millimeter (mm) offset in the posterior alignment of the vertebral bodies between C5 and C6 (Figure 2-1) and requested that the athlete return to the hospital for a CT scan of the cervical spine. Over the objections of the radiologist the study was completed. The CT scan revealed a fracture of the C6 facet superiorly where it articulated with the inferior facet of C5 and a 2.5 mm subluxation of C5 on C6. The following morning a consultation was obtained with a spinal surgeon who ordered full flexion and extension lateral cervical spine views, which further confirmed the subluxation.

TREATMENT

The athlete was placed in a cervical collar for 4 weeks. After 4 weeks, pain, weakness, and paresthesias disappeared, the collar was changed to a soft cervical collar, and he was permitted to begin rehabilitation with easy active ROM exercises. He was also allowed to resume cardiovascular conditioning and begin shooting a basketball. After 4 weeks, the soft cervical collar was discontinued and he began functional progression back to basketball drills and scrimmaging.

The athlete played a full season of basketball without difficulty at the end of which he was cleared for all activity, including football. X-rays 9 months postinjury were read as normal, but there still was an appearance of some posterior subluxation. The parents expressed reservations about allowing their son to return to football and the athlete was referred to a neurosurgeon experienced with football. He examined the athlete's x-rays, ordered new films, and upon review, excluded the athlete from further contact sports. The neurosurgeon was concerned that even though the fracture had healed, the risk of playing high school football with a slight posterior subluxation was not acceptable. He excluded the athlete from football and wrestling, but cleared him for basketball and track.

CONCLUSION

Neck injuries account for a large percentage of all serious injuries to football players each year. Many of these have devastating results. Had this athlete been allowed to return to full contact, one more blow to the head and neck could have been disastrous. When the index of suspicion for a serious injury is high, as in this case, the athletic trainer and team physician must work together to definitively exclude occult injury. Guidelines should be established for return to play after spinal injuries. Athletic trainers and physicians should meet each preseason with coaches and athletes to discuss catastrophic injuries and how they occur. Coaches should teach and reinforce safe methods of contact. Effective training for prevention of injury and proper evaluation and treatment must occur; only then will these injuries be prevented.

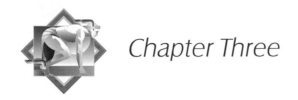

Chapter Three

High School Track Athlete with Confirmed Diagnosis of Spondylolysis

Paul Reuteman, MHS, PT, ATC

Low back pain is a common complaint of adolescent athletes. It is especially prevalent in sports that require repetitive extension and rotation of the trunk combined with compressive forces. The prevalence of low back pain in 11- to 17-year-old athletes is 30.4%.[1] A majority of these symptoms are self- limiting and will likely resolve in a given period of time. If the symptoms do not resolve, however, the athlete must be screened to rule out possible disruption to the pars interarticularis of the lumbar spine, otherwise known as a spondylolysis. Spondylolysis is defined as a stress fracture through the pars interarticularis, which is a narrow part of bone lying between the superior and inferior articular facets on the vertebral arch (Figure 3-1).[2] The frequency of spondylolysis in adolescents who complain of low back pain ranges from 44% to 47%.[3,4] The stress fracture may be unilateral or bilateral and most often involves one vertebral level. Eighty-eight percent of spondylolytic injuries in adolescent athletes occur at the L5 level and 96% occur at either L4 or L5.[5,6,7]

The biomechanics of the lumbar spine predispose it to be susceptible to stress-related injury. Stresses placed on the spine during athletics create a convergence of the athlete's body weight and ground reaction forces on the lower lumbar segments. This repetitive stress of the lower lumbar segments leads to a stress reaction and eventually failure of the pars interarticularis.[2,8,9] In young people, the pars interarticularis is thin, and the neural arch has not yet reached maximal strength. Also, the disc is less resistant to shear forces. Therefore, the pars is very susceptible to injury due to repetitive stresses.[10] Motions that increase the anterior shear forces on the lumbar spine, such as extension and rotation, are most responsible for the pathogenesis of spondylolysis in adolescent athletes.[2,5,6,8,10-12]

There are three stages to disruption of the pars interarticularis:
1. Acute spondylolysis defined as a stress reaction
2. Chronic spondylolysis defined as stress fracture
3. Anterior displacement of the vertebral body defined as a spondylolisthesis[12]

Early detection and diagnosis is critical to enhance healing, minimize the progression of injury to the vertebrae, and improve the athlete's chances of returning to pain-free competition.[5,11,13-16] The following is a report of a high school athlete who was diagnosed with spondylolysis, and the treatment progression that was followed allowed her to continue participation in sports.

SUBJECT

The subject is a female high school track athlete who specialized in running the 100 and 300 meter (m) hurdles. She was a 16-year-old sophomore in high school with the fastest time in the state in the 300 m hurdles when she first complained of back pain to her high school certified athletic trainer. She reported experimenting with her form on hurdles by changing her lead leg during practice approximately 2 days prior, using her right leg as lead leg instead of her left. Since that time, she had experienced muscle spasms in her right

Figure 3-1. Diagram depicting a stress fracture of L5 pars interarticularis.

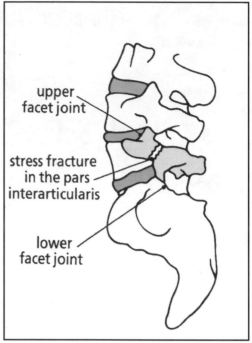

upper facet joint

stress fracture in the pars interarticularis

lower facet joint

lumbosacral region, which radiated down to her right buttock region and occasionally down the posterior thigh, ending at the knee. Pain was especially noted with backward bending of the lumbar spine and with return from end-range flexion.

The patient had a history of low back pain that dated back to the previous track season, when she was a freshman. She reported experiencing some discomfort while participating in the triple jump. This was exacerbated by a hyperextension injury of the lumbar spine during a fall on the hurdles during the state track meet. She continued to have pain intermittently but nothing that limited her ability to participate in athletics during the summer or fall seasons. She did see a chiropractor occasionally for treatments, which provided temporary relief from her intermittent back pain.

The athletic trainer performed a screening on the athlete and referred her to an orthopedic surgeon for consultation. The results of the evaluation by the orthopedic surgeon are given in Table 3-1. The x-rays revealed a lucent cleft in the L5 pars on the left, compatible with a chronic spondylolysis. Because the athlete's symptoms were all on the right side, the physician had a suspicion of a possible acute spondylolysis because the symptoms with which she presented are consistent with this diagnosis.[8,11,14] The physician had ordered a single-photon emission computed tomography (SPECT) scan to help elucidate the diagnosis. This has been shown to be the most sensitive diagnostic test to pick up disruption of the pars interarticularis.[2,7,8,12,13,15-17]

The SPECT scan clearly revealed increased uptake at the right pars interarticularis of L5, which corresponds with an acute spondylolysis (Figure 3-2). The nature of the diagnosis had been discussed with the patient and her parents, and the optimal treatment option was determined to be a course of bracing and restriction from track activity. A modified Boston brace (Figure 3-3) was sized for the patient. This brace has been shown to be an effective tool to immobilize the lumbar spine in order to enhance healing.[5,6,8,10,12] It places the lumbar spine in an antilordotic posture, which decreases the shear forces on the lumbar spine and minimizes the compressive loads on the posterior structures of the lumbar vertebrae. She was to wear it full-time through the day (23 hours on, 1 hour off) for a period of 3 months.[6] During the 3 months she was advised on home exercises, which consisted of general flexibility and abdominal bracing exercises.

Table 3-1

INITIAL ASSESSMENT

Gait	Antalgic gait noticed with decreased weightbearing time over R lower extremity.
Standing Assessment	All pelvic levels are symmetrical. Leg lengths are equal. Increased lumbar muscle tone.
Trunk AROM	Flex: 75% with pain from return. Ext: 50% with right-sided LBP. SB right and left: 75% with right sided LBP. Rot right and left: WNL with pain during rot L
Lower Extremity	All graded a 5/5. Right LBP noted with resisted right hip flexion and knee extension.
Strength	Pain with deep pressure over L5 and L4 spinous process and sacral sulcus on right. Increased resting tone noted in lumbar paraspinal muscles right > left.
Palpation	Sensation is intact bilaterally. Quad reflex is 1+ and Achilles' reflex is 2+ bilaterally. Straight leg raise and slump test are negative.
Neurological	SI joint provocation tests are negative.[44] Faber's test negative,[45] Gaenslen's test negative.[45]
Special Tests	Single leg stance with lumbar hyperextension positive on right,[11] lumbar quadrant sign positive bilaterally.
X-ray and SPECT	Oblique views reveal lucent cleft in the left L5 pars. SPECT reveals increased uptake in the right L5 pars.

LBP = low back pain; WNL = within normal limits; SPECT = single photon emission computed tomography; SI = sacroiliac; SB = slow bend.

At 3 months, the patient was re-evaluated. She exhibited full, pain-free trunk range of motion (ROM), no palpable tenderness, and normal strength. She was instructed to wean off the brace by increasing the time she could take the brace off during the day by 2 hours per week. Her home exercise program was reviewed. She was performing it adequately enough that formalized therapy was not prescribed at that time. She was allowed to return to sporting activities but was required to wear the brace during all practices and game situations for the next 3 months. During the time that she was weaning out of the brace, she was allowed to participate in high school soccer. She was advised to check in with her athletic trainer on a weekly basis to update her status. The patient was able to participate in soccer quite successfully. She wore the brace through the rest of the season for fear of re-injuring the back, even though she had exceeded the necessary 3-month time frame.

She then participated in the basketball season. She was given a lumbar corset brace with a moldable insert that was placed in the lumbar region to limit hyperextension (Figure 3-4). She was able to compete effectively and pain-free for the entire regular season but began experiencing some recurrent symptoms in her back during the state tournament. She began track practice the Monday immediately following the last week of basketball. After 3 days of track practice she experienced back pain significant enough for her to go back to the orthopedic surgeon. She had feared the symptoms that inhibited her from participating in track last year were returning.

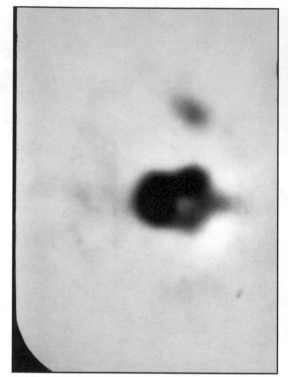

Figure 3-2. SPECT scan revealing a stress reaction of right pars interarticularis at L5.

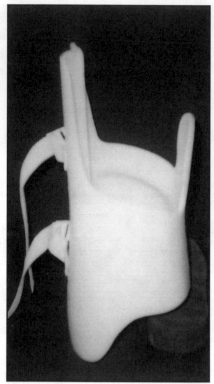

Figure 3-3. Modified Boston brace.

Objectively, she presented with similar signs and symptoms as she did less than a year ago. The orthopedic surgeon ordered a CT scan. This is the recommended test for assessing the amount of healing of the pars interarticularis stress fracture that occurred, and the level of chronicity of the fracture.[10,16,18] The CT scan revealed evidence of a chronic spondylolysis of the left pars interarticularis as displayed previously on the x-rays, and a lucent line through the right pars interarticularis also indicated a nonhealing stress fracture (Figure 3-5). The results of the CT scan were discussed with the patient. Obviously, she was disappointed that full healing of the stress fracture on the right did not occur. She was informed that inadequate healing of the pars is not uncommon and that return to competition is still a feasible goal.[3,4,10,15] It was recommended that formalized physical therapy be initiated to improve muscle balance around the lumbopelvic-hip complex and enhance overall trunk strength during competition to allow the athlete to return to competition.

REHABILITATION

Clinical Evaluation

The patient presented to the physical therapist with primary complaints of right low back pain aggravated by extension, running, and performing hurdles. Lumbar ROM was limited by 50% in extension due to pain. She had full ROM in all other directions with pain at the end range of right sidebending and rotation. Strength assessment of the lower extremities revealed normal strength, but pain was experienced with resisted hip extension in prone and resisted hip flexion in sitting. Palpation revealed minimal tenderness over the spinous processes of L3 to L5. Normal resting muscle tone of the lumbar paravertebral muscles was noted. Further assessment revealed very poor lower abdominal recruitment, poor multifidus recruitment, tight hamstrings and hip flexors, and a tight anterior hip capsule. Her track season had begun 2 weeks prior and she was anxious to return but was frustrated because the pain in her back was significantly inhibiting her per-

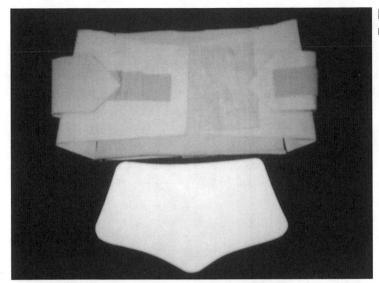

Figure 3-4. Lumbar corset with moldable thermoplastic insert.

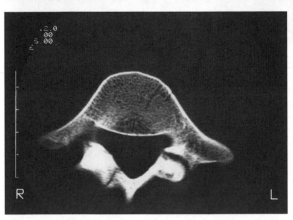

Figure 3-5. CT scan revealing bilateral spondylolysis at L5.

formance. The goals of rehabilitation were discussed with the patient (Table 3-2). We anticipated a time frame of 4 to 6 weeks to achieve these goals. This would allow the patient to compete in the last half of her season.

Conditioning and Flexibility

Flexibility and conditioning exercises are an important part of any rehabilitation program, specifically for those with spondylogenic disorders.[11,19] The flexibility exercises for a patient with a diagnosis of spondylolysis are of significant importance because they target the tissues that play a critical role in the mechanics of the lumbopelvic unit. The hip flexor, with specific regard to the psoas major, is one such muscle. The psoas major originates off the anterolateral aspect of the bodies of T12 to L4 and their respective transverse processes and intervertebral discs, and attaches inferiorly with the iliacus to the lesser trochanter of the femur. The psoas major exerts massive compressive forces on the lumbar spine to provide stability.[20] It has been found to be selectively involved with contralateral loading situations of the spine during activities that require stabilization of the pelvis and spine in the frontal plane.[21] This is very important for a hurdler who requires a significant amount of muscle force to maintain frontal plane stability of the lumbar spine when landing on the lead leg after jumping over a hurdle. However, the psoas has also been thought to create a large amount of anterior shear forces on the lumbar spine as the hip approaches end range extension.[21] An increase in anterior shear forces will likely create an unhealthy amount of stress to the pars interarticularis of the lower lumbar region. For that reason, stretching of the psoas is critical.

Table 3-2

REHABILITATION GOALS AND CORRESPONDING PHASES OF TRUNK STABILIZATION

Facilitation Phase

Abdominal drawing in maneuver[42] with co-contraction of lumbar multifidus muscle with lumbar spine in neutral position. Perform 10 contractions for 10 second holds frequently throughout the day in sitting, standing, or lying down.

Goal One	Improve hip flexor, hamstring, and anterior hip capsule flexibility.
Goal Two	Maintain general conditioning without placing undue compressive forces on lumbar spine.
Goal Three	Improve lower abdominal and multifidus facilitation with lumbopelvic region in a neutral alignment.

Static Stabilization Phase

Supine lower abdominal progression,[46] prone and quadruped alternate arm and leg raise, bridging progression, kneeling exercises,[43] standing resisted hip and shoulder strengthening, swiss ball activities, lunges and squat activity, pulley exercises[22] and medicine ball toss stressing neutral spine posture.

Goal Four — Maintain neutral alignment of lumbopelvic region during upper and lower extremity dynamic movements.

Dynamic Stabilization Phase

Pulley exercises and medicine ball tossing with trunk motion, upper and lower abdominal crunches, resisted hip flexion with use of tubing around ankle to mimic running mechanics, plyometric lunges, resisted upper extremity motions (PNF diagonals).

Goal Five — Pain-free motion of lumbar spine during high level trunk strengthening activities.

Return to Sport Activity Phase

Resisted running with tubing, track running, and track running with hurdling drills.

Goal Six — Return to running.

Goal Seven — Return to running hurdles.

For similar reasons, attention must be directed toward the extensibility of the anterior hip. The geometry of the modified Boston brace creates a posterior tilt of the pelvis, placing the anterior structures of the hip in a shortened position. Over an extended period of time, this may lead to anterior hip capsular tightness. For the general population, this would be insignificant. However, a hurdler relies on the flexibility of the hip to clear the hurdles with his or her trail leg. If tightness is present, compensations will be made that require increased anterior tilting of the pelvis and further compressive forces on the posterior lumbar structures. The ideal way of stretching the anterior hip is to have the patient lie prone with one hip in a figure four position (flexion, abduction, external rotation [FABER] position). The clinician lifts the knee of the extremity in the FABER position while stabilizing at the posterior pelvis. This position mimics the position that the trail leg assumes when jumping a hurdle.

Finally, it is well documented that the hamstrings are often tight in patients with chronic spondylolysis.[8,11,14] It is believed that the hamstrings tighten in attempts to enhance a posterior pelvic tilt and decrease the lordotic posture of the individual. Hamstring flexibility is critical, however, for any athlete who takes part in jumping activities. Effective hamstring stretching was performed with the patient's lumbar spine in a neutral position to isolate the stretch in the hamstrings and minimize end-range spinal motions.

Because the patient wished to compete in the current track season, it was critical she take part in a conditioning program that would maintain her cardiovascular conditioning but would limit compressive forces on the lumbar spine. Activities she took part in were aqua jogging, biking, stair machine, the slide board, the elliptical runner, and roller blading. It was during this time that she was instructed to work on her abdominal facilitation activities, which will be discussed in the next section.

Strengthening of the Lumbopelvic Unit

Strengthening of the trunk muscles is a critical part of rehabilitation of any athlete who has suffered from back pain. It has been well documented that the recruitment of trunk muscles occurs when low back pain is present.[22-28] There are four phases of strengthening that every patient must achieve to ensure successful rehabilitation. The four phases are listed with their corresponding goals in Table 3-2. They are:
1) The facilitation phase
2) The static stabilization phase
3) The dynamic stabilization phase
4) Return to sport activity phase. Progression to the next phase is only accomplished by performing all exercises in the previous phase adequately and pain-free.

THE FACILITATION PHASE

In the first phase is strengthening the deep abdominal muscles (transversus abdominus and internal obliques) and the lumbar multifidus (LM) are specifically targeted. The internal obliques (IO) have a strong attachment to the posterior layer of the thoracolumbar fascia; therefore, they play a significant role in providing stabilization to the lumbopelvic unit.[29,30] The transversus abdominus (TA) lies deep to the internal obliques and also shares a common attachment into the thoracolumbar fascia. The TA and IO impart tension throughout the thoracolumbar fascia, which creates increased stability through the lumbar vertebrae during functional activity.[29,31,32] Contraction of the deep abdominals also increases the intraabdominal pressure by creating a pressurized visceral cavity anterior to the spine. This results in a production of force anterior to the apex of the lumbar lordosis, minimizing anterior shear forces and stabilizing the trunk against excessive rotational forces that accompany upper and lower extremity motion.[25,33,34]

The IO and TR have been found to exhibit varying disruptions in their patterns of recruitment associated with low back pain. O'Sullivan, et al,[31,32,35] revealed that healthy individuals were effectively able to preferentially activate the IO and TA over the rectus abdominus during an isometric contraction. The patients suffering from back pain, however, were unable to preferentially activate the IO from the rectus abdominus. Other studies have found a delayed onset of TA recruitment during upper extremity motions in people with back pain.[25]

The lumbar multifidus muscle is the most medial of the lumbar back multisegmental muscles and has been found to play a major role in providing dynamic stability to the lumbopelvic unit.[25, 36-39] Compared to other stabilizing muscles in close proximity, LM imparts the greatest amount of stability, or "stiffness," to the lumbar spinal unit by increasing compressive loads on the lumbar spine.[28,39,40] The orientation of the LM also allows the muscle to impart a posterior shear force on the lower lumbar segments.[7] The LM works synergistically with the oblique abdominals to stabilize the spine and counteract the flexion component that the obliques impart on the spine. It also works synergistically with the psoas major to counteract the anterior shear force it exerts on the L4-L5 and L5-S1 spinal segments.[33,41] All these muscles work together to square the vertebral segments in the sagittal plane.

Like the deep abdominals, the LM is disrupted in the presence of back pain. The LM undergoes a significant amount of atrophy in response to low back pain.[23] The severity of pain correlates with the amount of muscle atrophy. The greatest amount of atrophy appears to occur at the clinically determined level of involvement. After resolution of low back pain, the LM does not spontaneously return to preinjury status unless it is effectively rehabilitated.[25] This may explain the high rate of reoccurrence of symptoms in individuals with back pain. Several studies have also reported electromyogram (EMG) disturbances of the LM in subjects with low back pain.[26-28]

For this patient, who has a confirmed diagnosis of chronic spondylolysis, it is imperative that she exhibit proper recruitment of the trunk muscles while maintaining a neutral spine before we begin any high-level trunk strengthening activities. The exercises given were directed primarily at the deep abdominal muscles, with coactivation of the LM as described by Richardson and Jull.[42]

STATIC STABILIZATION PHASE

Once an accurate and sustained co-contraction of the deep abdominals and LM had been achieved with the spine in neutral, the exercises were progressed by applying varying loads on the muscles by means of adding leverage through the limbs. Contraction of the TA and LM have been found to precede upper and lower extremity motion in healthy individuals. This suggests that the central nervous system contracts the deep abdominal and LM in anticipation of reactive forces produced by limb movement.[25,34] This reflex loop, however, has been found to be affected by pain. As stated previously, individuals suffering from low back pain exhibited a delay in contraction of the TA and LM during extremity motion. This delayed onset of muscle contraction indicates a deficit in motor control that likely results in inefficient muscular stabilization of the lumbar spine.[25]

Training of these muscle groups has been found to be an effective tool in reducing low back pain suffered due to par interarticularis defects. Lindgren, et al[26] discovered EMG disturbances of the LM had resolved after a rehabilitation program in individuals with confirmed instability in the lower lumbar regions. Interestingly, the patients continued to exhibit the instability radiographically after the symptoms resolved. Therefore, increased LM activity denotes increased functional stability to hypermobile lumbar segments during normal daily activities.

O'Sullivan, et al[32] reported similar results in individuals with a confirmed diagnosis of spondylolysis and who suffered from chronic back pain. Following exercise training with these patients, a decrease in pain levels and functional disability levels was maintained over a 3-year period. This highlights the importance of training the muscles to control trunk stability during functional tasks involving upper and lower extremity motions.

The patient was encouraged to maintain neutral positioning of the lumbar spine with an adequate co-contraction of the deep abdominals and the lumbar multifidus muscles as resistive demands were placed on the upper and lower extremities. A wide variety of training positions must be used to teach the patient control in multiple positions.[11,19,43] By no means does this exhaust all the possible exercises that may be performed. It does highlight the ones that are specific to this patient, whose goal was to return to competition in hurdles.

DYNAMIC STABILIZATION PHASE

Training of the lumbar muscles with the pelvis in a neutral alignment is ideal to minimize the shearing forces that occur at the lower lumbar region. However, in a high-level athlete such as a high school hurdler, it is not realistic to think that the spine can be maintained in neutral alignment during competition. Therefore, strengthening exercises must be progressed to involve spinal motions while still maintaining adequate recruitment of the deep abdominals and multifidus muscles. It must be stressed to the patient that all exercises are to be pain-free. The exercises are only advanced when abdominal and paraspinal control are fully achieved in a neutral position. At first, the athlete required close supervision with verbal and tactile cueing to maintain proper stabilization. As her strength and body awareness improved during the higher-level exercises, less supervision was needed. Special consideration needed to be made to minimize hyperextension of the spine. A list of exercises specific to this athlete is reported in Table 3-2.

RETURN TO ACTIVITY STAGE

This stage was completed at practice with the track team. The athlete was able to successfully return to running activities in 5 weeks. It was very important to communicate openly with the coach and athletic trainer to progress the athlete according to the symptoms she reported. At the time she returned, she was able to perform all higher-level strengthening activities without low back pain. She exhibited significant improvement in facilitation of the trunk muscles and improved lower extremity flexibility. The major fear was the athlete's endurance. It was likely that as she fatigued, her form would suffer and possibly increase the stress on her low back. This was monitored closely by the coaching staff. Her first competition in a meet took place 6 weeks after the initial therapy visit. She did compete with a simple lumbar corset designed for sports patients. She was able to finish the rest of the season relatively pain-free and posted good results during her competition. The following year, she competed at a Division 1 school in the 300 m hurdles.

DISCUSSION

An adolescent athlete often tries to train through pain to maintain competitive status. It is critical, however, for a timely diagnosis of spondylolysis to be made for initiation of early treatment. Unfortunately, with spondylogenic disorders, it is not uncommon to achieve incomplete healing of the pars interarticularis at the affected sight. Micheli, et al[6] reported 88% of patients treated with a modified Boston brace were symptom free and able to return to preinjury status in their sport even though only 32% of them demonstrated adequate bone healing. Congeni, et al,[10] with the use of CT scans, diagnosed chronic nonhealing fractures in 45% of adolescent patients with chronic low back pain. The sports-related lesion to the pars interarticularis is thought to be essentially stable with no risk for further slippage despite continued activity.[2,6,8,10,11]

An accurate and timely diagnosis of spondylolysis is dependent on the effectiveness of a SPECT scan to depict early bony lesions. Bellah, et al[4] studied 162 adolescents with low back pain and found 71 (44%) of those patients had a positive SPECT scan. In 39 of the cases, an abnormality of the par interarticularis was not revealed with an x-ray. The other 32 revealed positive x-rays as well. Because management of spondylolysis is conducted much differently from other lumbar dysfunctions, SPECT scanning should be a common diagnostic examination for any adolescent with extension-related back pain.

If return to athletic competition is a significant goal, a comprehensive rehabilitation program including conditioning, flexibility, and progression of trunk strengthening is recommended. It is imperative that the athlete be trained in proper stabilization activities of the lumbar spine so that he or she gets adequate recruitment of the trunk musculature during competition. This has been found to greatly decrease symptoms and allow individuals to return to their previous level of activity.[19,32,35,43] Each athlete should be progressed through the phases of rehabilitation as described above, letting pain and performance be the guide for progression.

SUMMARY

This case presentation focused on making the diagnosis and providing treatment of a high-level high school track athlete with a confirmed diagnosis of chronic, bilateral L5 pars interarticularis stress fracture. To improve the athlete's ability to participate in track, a progressive rehabilitation program was implemented focusing on minimizing shear forces on the spine by enhancing the recruitment of the deep abdominal and back muscles. Flexibility around the lumbopelvic complex was addressed and the patient was encouraged to maintain her cardiovascular conditioning. Proper care of an acute spondylolysis is early bracing and activity restriction in an attempt to achieve healing of the pars defect. If healing does not occur, the athlete must undergo a strenuous rehabilitation program to improve his or her chance of returning to competition.

REFERENCES

1. Olsen TL, Anderson RL, Dearwater SR, et al. The epidemiology of low back pain in adolescent population. *Am J Public Health*. 1992;82:606-608.

2. Stinson JT. Spondylolysis and spondylolisthesis in the athlete. *Clin Sport Med*. 1993;12(3):517-528.

3. Micheli LJ, Wood R. Back pain in young athletes. *Arch Pediatr Adolesc Med*. 1995;149:15-18.

4. Bellah RD, Summerville DA, Treves ST, et al. Low back pain in adolescent athletes: detection of stress injury to the pars interarticularis with SPECT. *Radiology*. 1991;180:509-512.

5. Steiner ME, Micheli LJ. Treatment of symptomatic spondylolysis and spondylolisthesis with the modified Boston brace. *Spine*. 1985;10(10):93-99.

6. Micheli LJ, Hall JE, Miller ME. Use of modified Boston brace for back injuries in athletes. *Am J Sport Med*. 1980;8(5):351-355.

7. Morita T, Ikata T, Katoh S, Miyake R. Lumbar spondylolysis in children and adolescents. *JBJS*. 1995;77B(4):620-625.

8. Garry JP, McShane J. Lumbar spondylolysis in adolescent athletes. *J Family Pract*. 1998;47(2):145-149.

9. Newell R. Historical perspective spondylolysis. *Spine*. 1995;20(17):1950-1956.

10. Congeni J, McCulloch J, Swanson K. Lumbar spondylolysis. A study of natural progression in athletes. *Am J Sport Med*. 1997;25(2):248-253.

11. Weber MD, Woodall WR. Spondylogenic disorders in gymnasts. *J Orthop Sports Phys Ther*. 1991;14(1):6-13.

12. Johnson RJ. Low back pain in sports. Managing spondylolysis in young patients. *Phys Sp Med*. 1993;21(4):53-59.

13. Ralston S, Weir M. Suspecting lumbar spondylolysis in adolescent low back pain. *Clin Pediatrics*. 1998;37:287-294.

14. Jackson DW, Wiltse LL, Dingeman RD, et al. Stress reactions involving pars interarticularis in young athletes. *Am J Sport Med*. 1981;9(5):304-312.

15. Lusins JO, Elting JJ, Cicoria AD, et al. SPECT evaluation of lumbar spondylolysis and spondylolisthesis. *Spine*. 1994;19(5):608-612.

16. Renshaw TS. Managing spondylolysis. When to immobilize. *Phys Sportsmed*. 1995;23(10):75-80.

17. Read MT. SPECT scanning for adolescent back pain. A sine qua non? *Br J Sports Med*. 1994;28(1):56-57.

18. Raby N, Mathews S. Symptomatic spondylolysis: correlation of CT and SPECT with clinical outcomes. *Clin Radiol*. 1993;48:97-99.

19. Saal JA. Rehabilitation of sport related spine injuries. *Phys Med and Rehabil*. 1987;1:613-638.

20. Bogduk N, Pearcy M, Hadfield G. Anatomy and biomechanics of psoas major. *Clin Biomech*. 1992;7:109-119.

21. Anderson E, Oddsson L, Grundstrom H, et al. The role of the psoas and iliacus muscles for stability and movement of the lumbar spine, pelvis and hip. *Scand J Med Sci Sports*. 1995;5:10-16.

22. Bellow J. Lumbar facets: an anatomic framework for low back pain. *J Manipulative Physiol Ther*. 1996;4(4):149-156.

23. Hides J, Stokes M, Saide M, Jull G, Cooper D. Evidence of lumbar multifidus muscle wasting ipsilateral to symptoms in patients with acute/subacute low back pain. *Spine*. 1994;19(2):165-172.

24. Hides J, Richardson C, Jull G. Multifidus muscle recovery is not automatic after resolution of acute, first episode low back pain. *Spine*. 1996;21(23):2763-2769.

25. Hodges PW, Richardson C. Inefficient muscular stabilization of the lumbar spine associated with low back pain. *Spine*. 1996;21(22):2640-2650.

26. Lindgren KA, Sihoven T, Leino E, et al. Exercise therapy effects on functional radiographic findings and segmental electromyographic activity in lumber spine stability. *Arch Phys Med Rehabil*. 1993;74(9):933-939.

27. Roy SH, Deluca C, Emley M, et al. Spectral electromyographic assessment of back muscles in patients with low back pain undergoing rehabilitation. *Spine*. 1995;20(1):38-48.

28. Roy SH, Deluca C, Emley M, et al. Classification of back muscle impairment based on the surface EMG signal. *J Rehabil Res Dev*. 1997;34(4):405-415.

29. DeRosa C. The morphology of the abdominal muscles: implications of function from structure. *J Orthop Sports Phys Ther*. 1999;29(1):A-22.

30. Vleeming A. The posterior layer of thoracolumbar fascia. Its function in load transfer from spine to legs. *Spine.* 1995;20(7):753-758.

31. O'Sullivan P, Twomey L, Allison G. Altered patterns of abdominal muscle activation in chronic back patients. *Australian Journal of Physiotherapy.* 1997;43(2):91-98.

32. O'Sullivan P, Twomey L, Allison G. Evaluation of specific stabilizing exercise in the treatment of chronic low back pain with radiologic diagnosis of spondylolysis or spondylolisthesis. *Spine.* 1997;22(24):2959-2967.

33. Porterfield J, DeRosa C. *Mechanical Low Back Pain. Perspectives in Functional Anatomy.* Philadelphia, Pa: WB Saunders Company; 1991.

34. Hodges PW, Richardson C. Contraction of the abdominal muscles associated with movement of the lower limb. *Phys Ther.* 1997;77(2):132-144.

35. O'Sullivan P, Twomey L, Allison G. Dysfunction of the neuro-muscular system in the presence of low back pain— implications for physical therapy management. *J Manipulative Physiol Ther.* 1997;5(1):20-26.

36. Cholewicki J, Khachatryan A, Panjabi MM, et al. Stabilizing function of trunk flexor-extensor muscles around a neutral spine posture. *Spine.* 1997;22(19):2207-2212.

37. Crisco JJ, Panjabi MM. The intersegmental and multisegmental muscles of the lumber spine. *Spine.* 1991;16(7):793-799.

38. Panjabi M. Spinal stability and intersegmental muscle forces. *Spine.* 1989;14(2):194-199.

39. Wilke HJ, Wolf S, Claes LE, et al. Stability increase of the lumber spine with different muscle groups. *Spine.* 1995;20(2):192-198.

40. Bogduk N. *Clinical Anatomy of the Lumbar Spine and Sacrum.* 3rd ed. New York, NY: Churchill Livingston;1997.

41. Macintosh JE, Bogduk N. The biomechanics of the lumbar multifidus. *Clin Biomech.* 1986;1:205-213.

42. Richardson C, Jull G. Muscle control-pain control. What exercises would you prescribe? *Manual Therapy.* 1995;1:2-10.

43. Saal JA, Saal JS. Nonoperative treatment of herniated lumbar intervertebral disc with radiculapathy. An outcome study. *Spine.* 1989;14(4):431-437.

44. Laslett M, Williams M. The reliability of selected pain provocation tests for sacroiliac joint pathology. 1994;19(11):1243-1249.

45. Magee DJ. *Orthopedic Physical Assessment.* Philadelphia, Pa: WB Saunders Company; 1987.

46. Sahrmann SA. *Diagnosis and treatment of movement impairment syndromes.* Course notes. 1999.

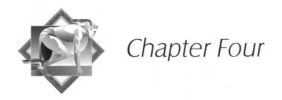

Chapter Four

A Protocol for Conservative Treatment in Athletes with Lumbar Scheuermann's Disease

Adam Swain, PT, OCS, ATC, Tim Koberna, MA, ATC,
Bruce E. Dall, MD

INTRODUCTION

This case report involves a Division 1 collegiate football player who presented with the complaint of low back pain. He was subsequently diagnosed as having lumbar Scheuermann's disease (LSD). An association has been made between trauma to adolescents' skeletally immature spine from weight training and high-risk sports such as football, and the development of symptomatic LSD.[1-3] Although it is common in the adolescent, the actual onset is currently unknown.

LSD is part of a spectrum of Scheuermann's disease (SD) or Scheuermann's juvenile kyphosis (SJK), which was first described by Scheuermann in 1920—shortly after the development of radiography.[4] SJK is the most common cause of structural kyphotic deformity in the adolescent.[5] SJK can be divided into two distinct groups: thoracic (most common) and lumbar (atypical or pseudo-Scheuermann), predicated on the natural history and location of the kyphosis.[3] Approximately two-thirds of cases are thoracic and one-third thoracolumbar and lumbar.[6] Until the mid 1980s, most of the literature centered on thoracic SD. Recently, more study has been directed toward lumbar SD.[3,7] Table 4-1 provides a thorough comparison of the similarities and differences in presentation between thoracic and lumbar SD.

Another common error with SD is confusing it with postural kyphosis. Parents, teachers, and even primary care physicians often mistake SD for postural kyphosis.[4,8] Table 4-2 presents a comparison between SD and postural kyphosis.

SUBJECT

The athlete was a 22-year-old Division 1 collegiate football player who presented with a diagnosis of lumbar SD and associated low back pain. He reported a gradual onset of pain for over 4 years, beginning when he was a freshman in high school. He experienced constant pain that increased with activity. Pain increased significantly during the first "two-a-day" football practice in the fall of 1998 (5 to 6/10 with 10 being the worst pain). Pain was constant during the season, reaching a level of 7/10 during activity. During football practice in the spring of 1999, a spine surgeon identified LSD via physical exam and radiological studies, including magnetic resonance imaging (MRI). The MRI showed vertebral end plate irregularities, Schmorl's nodes, anterior vertebral body wedging, and the loss of normal lumbar lordosis (Figure 4-1). The athlete was then referred to physical therapy for evaluation.

Table 4-1

COMPARATIVE STUDY OF LUMBAR VERSUS THORACIC SCHEUERMANN'S DISEASE

Lumbar	Thoracic
Epidemiology	
Incidence unknown[2]	0.4% to 8% of the general population[1]
Males more commonly affected, especially those involved in competitive sports from rural communities[2]	Prevalence approximately equal in males and females.[10] Females may present more frequently because of concerns with cosmesis[6]
Onset unknown, but common in adolescents[2]	Onset unknown, believed to occur in puberty ages 10 to 12, before appearance of radiological changes[4]
Etiology	
Recent studies show a significant relationship between lumbar SD and mechanical factors, including repeated trauma and heavy lifting[4,14]	True etiology may not be known, but there are theories that exist that have not been proven false
	Mechanical factors increasing pressure on an abnormally round back causing disruption of endochondral ossification at the anterior end plate[3]
	Abnormalities in the matrix of the cartilage and growth plate tissue at the end plate[4,14,9]
	Familial pattern discovered with possible genetic component from an inherited autosomal dominant mode[4,14,9]
	Possible endocrine causes include relationship between SD and increased growth hormone; patients are taller than average with skeletal age greater than chronological age[4,14]
Signs	
Typical patient: adolescent with low back pain of several months' duration with a recent exacerbation due to intense physical activity or injury[2]	Typical patient: adolescent with rigid thoracic kyphosis not reducible with hyperextension.[4] Adolescent presents due to teacher or parental concern with cosmesis; adults present secondary to pain[9]

Table 4-1 continued	
Lumbar	**Thoracic**

Signs

Loss of normal lumbar lordosis/lumbar kyphosis.[2] Flat thoracic spine also noted, giving the impression of a straight back[6]	Increased cervical lordosis, protuberant abdomen, increased lumbar lordosis (associated with spondylolysis/spondylolisthesis)[4]
Associated mild to moderate scoliosis and/or spondylolistheses can be found[2]	Mild associated scoliosis (10 to 20 degrees) involved in 1/3 of cases[4]
	Rounded shoulders and pectoral tightness[4]
Tight hamstrings[2]	Tight hamstrings, hip flexors, and increased anterior pelvic tilt[1]

Radiological Findings

T10 to L4 segments can be involved[2,14]	Apex typically T7 to T9
Loss of normal lumbar lordosis.[2]	Thoracic kyphosis >40 degrees (normal 20 to 40 degrees)[9]
Thoracolumbar kyphosis >30 degrees; thoracolumbar spine normally straight[2]	
More than one vertebra involved but not always consecutively.[2] Possibly anterior vertebral body wedging, but there is disagreement in the literature[2,6,14]	Three or more vertebrae wedged 5 degrees or more, posterior to anterior (recent studies modify the criteria to one vertebra because of the possibility of emerging disease)[4,6]
Schmorl's nodes (herniation of disc material through the end plate).[2] Associated with highest incidence of herniated disc into the spinal canal[6]	Schmorl's nodes[4]
Disc space narrowing[2,6]	Disc space narrowing[2,4,14]
Vertebral end plate irregularities[2]	Vertebral end plate irregularities[4,9,14]

Symptoms

Local intermittent thoracolumbar or upper lumbar pain with radiation to the buttock, thigh, and leg[2]	Pain may or may not be present. If present, usually in the area of the kyphosis with intermittent achy pain and fatigue.[4,6,14] Usually diminishes with spinal maturity.[1,6,8,13] Adults with severe deformity can still have pain.[4,9] Pain can be aggravated by activity and present in the lumbar spine[4]
Palpation tenderness in the mid to upper kyphosis[2]	Palpation shows significant stiffness in the area of lumbar paraspinals[6]
Visual spinal deformity uncommon[2]	Visual spinal deformity commonly noted with sharply increased kyphosis[4,6,9]

Treatment

Bracing to stabilize the lumbar area if patient has significant pain and has failed conservative treatment[2]	Bracing, typically Milwaukee brace (3-point mold aids in extending thoracic spine) if thoracic kyphosis is >45 to 50 degrees and

Table 4-1 continued	
Lumbar	**Thoracic**

Symptoms

	<70 degrees.[4,6] More successful if applied prior to skeletal maturity at approximately age 25.[4,7] Partial reversal of anterior vertebral wedging noted if brace worn during active stage of SD.[13] thoracolumbosacral orthosis (TLSO) bracing for curves below T8 [7]
Stretching hamstrings	Stretching pectorals, hip flexors, and hamstrings[4,6]
Strengthening exercises for the core area, especially the lumbar area[14]	Strengthening exercises for posture and the core area, especially the back extensors and pelvic musculature, to decrease lumbar lordosis[4,6,9,14]
Rest, activity modification (avoid heavy lifting), nonsteroidal anti-inflammatory medication[2,14]	Aerobic exercise[6,14]
Surgery not indicated unless pain cannot be controlled conservatively, then fusion is warranted. This is a rare occasion[2]	Surgery indicated if thoracic kyphosis is controlled >70 to 75 degrees and patient is symptomatic. Anterior and/or posterior fusion typically performed.[4,6,14] Surgery also used when, on rare occasions, paraparesis occurs because the spinal cord is "bow-strung" over the posterior aspect of the vertebrae forming the apex of kyphosis.[4,6,14] This occurs when the apex of the kyphosis is over 2 to 3 vertebrae and exceeds 60 degrees[4,6,14]

Subjective Physical Therapy Evaluation

At rest, the athlete experienced intermittent sharp discomfort at 6/10 in the low back, on the left side greater than the right. With activity, there was constant sharp pain (7 to 9/10), again more on the left side. Intermittent radiating pain to both posterior thighs and buttocks was noted. He had decreased tolerance to supine to sit and sit to stand transfers, and also standing, walking, and running. He had great difficulty participating in agility drills and weight training, especially squatting, lunging, and the leg press.

Objective Physical Therapy Evaluation

Postural position showed decreased thoracic kyphosis and lumbar lordosis with mild moderate/low thoracic left scoliosis. The right leg was noted to be longer than the left. Thoracic range was limited to 20 degrees flexion and extension. Normal ROM for the thoracic spine is 40 degrees flexion and 30 degrees extension. Lumbar ROM was within normal limits. Lower extremity flexibility showed significant tightness in the hamstrings, hip flexors, iliotibial band, and gastrocnemius/soleus group bilaterally. Lower extremity strength was

Table 4-2

COMPARISON BETWEEN SCHEUERMANN'S DISEASE AND POSTURAL KYPHOSIS

Scheuermann's Disease	Postural Kyphosis
Well muscled[14]	Thin, underdeveloped[4,14]
Rigid, does reduce with hyperextension[4,14]	Kyphosis reduces with hyperextension[4,14]
Hyperextension x-ray shows structural kyphosis remains with wedging[4,14]	Hyperextension x-ray shows absence of structural kyphosis and wedging[4,14]
In prone, kyphosis remains fixed and stiff[6]	In prone, kyphosis is correctable without muscle contraction[6]
Conservative treatment may or may not manage pain and deformity depending on progression[1,4]	Postural exercises usually manage pain and deformity[1,4]

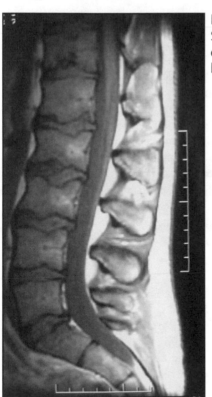

Figure 4-1. The athlete's MRI shows classic signs of lumbar Scheuermann's disease, including Schmorl's nodes, irregular end plates, and slight wedging of the vertebrae to cause a kyphotic alignment in the upper three lumbar vertebrae.

within normal limits, except the hip extensors and abductors, which were 4/5 bilaterally on manual muscle testing. Neural tension and sacroiliac provocation tests were negative. Functional testing showed that the patient had poor dynamic balance in the anteromedial and medial vectors, on the right side greater than the left. To walk relatively pain-free, the patient had to be unweighted on the treadmill 100 lbs.

Physical Therapy Plan

In consultation with the football athletic trainer, an exercise program was recommended that stressed core strengthening that targeted the abdominals, obliques, back extensors, and hip girdle. Lower extremity and quadratus lumborum stretching was also discussed. A heel lift was put in the left shoe on a trial basis. We also recommended continued work on the unweighted treadmill or "aquacizer" in the training room.[9]

REHABILITATION PROTOCOL FOR SCHEUERMANN'S DISEASE

The referral from physical therapy recommended a program stressing core strengthening that targeted the abdominals, obliques, back extensors, and hip girdle. Complete lower extremity stretching was implemented (Table 4-3).

Phase I

The initial phase of rehabilitation emphasized increasing flexibility and initiating strengthening exercises while maintaining cardiovascular fitness. The athlete exercised four times per week for 2 weeks. The flexibility program consisted of a prone back extension stretching exercise and the use of a bar to increase flexibility for the trunk rotators and obliques. The athlete used the bar as an assistive device to stretch rotationally. Other exercises included side bending and rotation. All stretches were performed for 30 seconds and repeated four times each.

The strengthening program in this phase consisted of prone press-ups to isolate the hip girdle and abdominal region and a modified step-up to isolate the quadratus lumborum. For the step-up, the athlete was instructed to step onto a 6-inch step with the involved side unweighted and hip hike the involved side utilizing the quadratus lumborum musculature. Physioball exercises were also introduced and included lateral side bending for flexibility and lateral leg lifting for strengthening. The medicine ball was used for increasing strength of the trunk. Specific exercises included trunk rotation from sitting, kneeling, and standing positions; each exercise was performed 20 times on each side for three sets.

Cardiovascular conditioning was a very important component of this athlete's training, thus unweighting the athlete was incorporated to maintain fitness. The Z-Lift unweighting system (Z-Lift Corporation, Austin, Tex) was used in conjunction with a treadmill. The athlete was supported and 28% of his body weight was removed for the initial session. The amount of weight taken off the athlete was determined by the recommendations of the Z-Lift system. The athlete was instructed to perform a jogging activity for 30 minutes at a speed of 6.0 miles per hour on the treadmill.

Phase II

Flexibility of the lower extremity and strengthening of the hip girdle and abdominals were targets during phase II, which was approximately 2 weeks in length. Proprioceptive training was introduced during this phase as well. Unweighted running with 18% of the athlete's weight taken off was continued. Stretching of the gastrocnemius/soleus complex, the hamstrings group, the iliopsoas musculature, and the hip rotators was added to the flexibility program. Exercises were performed four times holding each stretch for 30 seconds. Strengthening of the hip girdle was achieved using the four-way hip machine. This isotonic exercise incorporates exercises for the abductors, adductors, hip flexor and hip extensor musculature. All groups of muscles were isolated for a three set, 10 repetition exercise bout. Additionally, a prone hop abduction exercise was performed to fatigue, as well as a hip extension exercise to fatigue. Abdominal strengthening was performed dur-

Table 4-3

SUMMARY OF REHABILITATION PROGRAM FOR SCHEUERMANN'S DISEASE
Phase I (1 to 14 Days)

Clinical Goals

Decrease low back pain during activity, increased trunk flexibility, increased trunk strength, and maintenance of cardiovascular fitness.

Exercises

Prone back extension: athlete lies prone on the table and raises arm and leg simultaneously, working toward raising both arms and legs simultaneously. Bar exercises: trunk rotation, sitting; lateral bending, sitting; forward bending and rotating, sitting. Physioball stretches: lateral bending (Figure 4-2). Strength: prone press-ups, step-ups—hip hikes, lateral leg lifting (physioball), trunk rotations with medicine ball (sitting, kneeling, standing). Cardiovascular conditioning: unweighted running.

Phase II (14 to 28 Days)

Exercises

Flexibility: gastrocnemius/soleus group, hamstrings, iliopsoas, gluteus group. Hip strengthening—Isotonic 4-way hip machine: abduction/adduction and flexion/extension. Prone hip abduction performed to fatigue. Prone hip extension performed to fatigue. Abdominal strengthening: supine lower abdominal curl and supine abdominal curl with twist. Physioball strengthening. Prone hip extension. Proprioception: single leg balance, forward reach, diagonal reach (Figure 4-3), and lateral reach. Cardiovascular fitness: unweighted running—18% body weight removed, 6mph for 30 minutes.

Phase III (From 28 days)

Exercises

Step-ups on 10-inch box: anterior and lateral. Medicine ball with rebounder: chest pass and chest pass with lateral stepping. Medicine ball: anterior chops and lateral chops (Figure 4-4). Proprioception: foam roller balance (Figure 4-5) and balance and pickups.

Agility Activity

Carioca, stance and step, lock and move (Figure 4-6), medicine ball push (Figure 4-7), and dip and flip movement (Figure 4-8).

Clinical Follow-Up

Athlete integrated himself into team activities with minimal discomfort. Continued exercises on his own in the weight room.

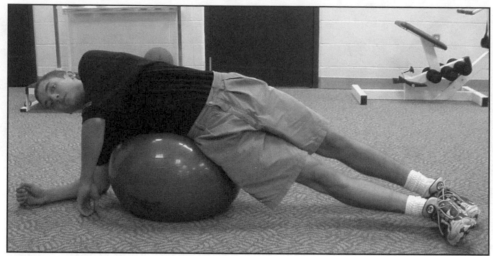

Figure 4-2. Physioball stretching for the obliques and erector spinae musculature.

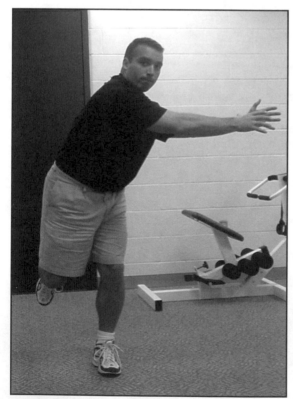

Figure 4-3. Proprioception exercise: single leg balance reaching diagonally. The athlete is using total body stability.

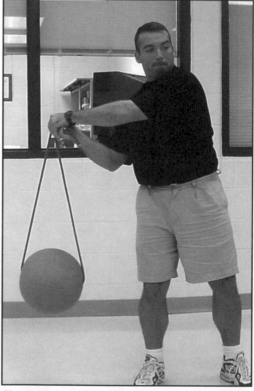

Figure 4-4. Athlete positioning to execute a lateral chop activity with the medicine ball.

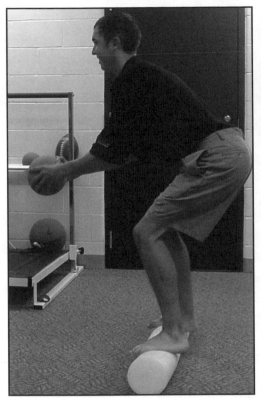

Figure 4-5. Use of foam rollers for proprioception exercise using total body stability.

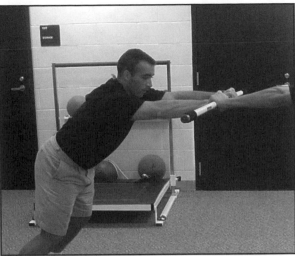

Figure 4-6. Starting position for lock and move exercise. Exercise continues laterally for a designated distance. Athletes resist one another while performing the lateral movement.

ing this phase with exercises including lower abdominal curl-ups. An abdominal curl with a rotational twist was performed to incorporate the oblique muscles. All exercises were performed for a three-set, 20-repetition count. Finally, the athlete laid prone on the Physioball, balanced with the upper extremity, and lifted the legs simultaneously for back extension strengthening. Proprioception training included single leg balancing with simultaneous reach forward and then laterally.

Phase III

The third and final phase of exercise included more sport-specific exercises as they related to this athlete's activity. The athlete performed repetitive anterior and lateral step-ups on a 10-inch plyometric box. Medicine ball training using a rebounder was also used. A chest pass exercise and chest pass with lateral stepping was performed. This exercise was speed based and emphasized strength and agility. Medicine ball training also continued with chopping activities performed anteriorly and laterally. Proprioception training increased in difficulty, using foam rollers for balancing while having the athlete bend forward and perform a reaching activity. Football agility exercises were incorporated into this phase.

The duration of phase III was approximately 3 weeks. The athlete was instructed to use pain as his guide during activity. This athlete integrated himself back into normal team activities and continues to be monitored for symptoms.

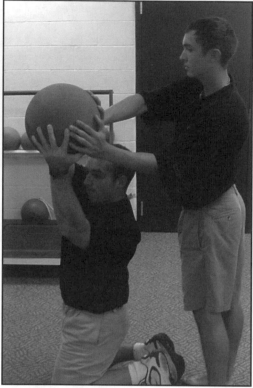 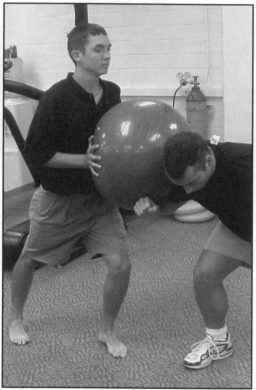

Figure 4-7. Medicine ball push: athlete brings ball up and therapist pushes ball in opposite position. Athlete maintains good posture while controlling the ball down.

Figure 4-8. Dip and flip: athlete dips shoulder and delivers a blow with the arm to the Physioball, recreating a football type activity.

RESULTS

The patient was able to return to full contact without difficulty after 4 weeks of rehabilitation. He continues to participate in Division 1 collegiate football, with intermittent symptoms that are manageable in the training room. The patient understood that this is a chronic condition, necessitating a change in lifestyle—not just a brief period of rehabilitation. We made it clear to him that pain and dysfunction could return if he did not maintain his exercise program.

DISCUSSION

Lumbar Scheuermann's disease is a subset of SD delineated by its location, painful presentation, and decreased responsiveness to treatment. There is significant support in the literature, some circumstantial, relating signs and symptoms of LSD with excessive loading of the immature spine.[1,2,3] The vertebral body is less resistant to vertical compression than the intact intervertebral disc.[1] Roaf[10] was able to show that vertebrae loaded vertically in the adolescent spine would distort significantly at the end plate with no changes in the shape of the nucleus pulposus and only a minimal alteration of the annulus. Jayson, et al[6] had similar results in terms of intervertebral disc pressure and end plate damage. They related heavy lifting in a forward bent position (preflexed) in a skeletally immature individual, especially in sitting, with pressure on the intervertebral disc substantial enough to cause an end plate fracture. Greene, et al[1] surmised that activities that put athletes in a preflexed position, such as football, gymnastics, rowing, and weightlifting, decrease the shock absorbing properties of the vertebrae.[1] This occurs when blood is squeezed from the vertebrae in the forward bent position, thus increasing the load on the disc, causing it to rupture through the end plate.[1] The theory that LSD changes are caused by adverse mechanical pressures on the immature spine is further supported by the positive effect of bracing these patients and the presence of spondylolysis and spondylolisthesis.[1] The athlete in our case study admitted to beginning early unsupervised weight training, along with participation in tackle football at the age of 8 years.

CONCLUSION

Scheuermann's disease is an entity that presents in either the midthoracic or upper thoracolumbar/upper lumbar area; however clinically, LSD appears to be more painful and difficult to treat. A standard of care has not been established for LSD treatment, although many authors allude to rehabilitation activities.[2,3] We feel that our rehabilitation program addressed the need to provide trunk strength, lower extremity strength/flexibility/balance, and aerobic conditioning, all in a functional manner. It is important to note the use of unweighted activities[11] in the early phases of rehabilitation, allowing the athlete to participate in functional exercises without exacerbating the load-bearing pathology.

It is also essential to be cognizant of emergent neurological signs with LSD patients. Thoracolumbar and upper lumbar disc herniations can put pressure on neurological structures, possibly causing clonus, a positive Babinski sign, numbness and/or tingling in the lower extremities, saddle numbness, and spasticity. These symptoms can be intermittent and are usually worsened with back hyperextension. Any hint of these symptoms requires immediate referral to a physician for further evaluation and testing.

REFERENCES

1. Greene TL, Hensinger RN, Hunter LY. Back pain and vertebral changes simulating Scheuermann's disease. *J Pediatr Orthop*. 1985;5:1.

2. Micheli LJ. Low back pain in the adolescent: differential diagnosis. *Am J Sports Med*. 1979;7:362.

3. Myer JJ, Herman MJ, MacEwen GD. Radiologic case study: lumbar Scheuermann's disease. *Orthopedics*. 1998;21:484.

4. Ali RM, Green DW, Patel TC. Scheuermann's kyphosis. *Curr Opin Pediatr*. 1999;11(1):70-5.

5. Lemire JJ, Mierau DR, Crawfore CM, et al. Scheuermann's juvenile kyphosis. *J Manipulative Physiol Ther*. 1996;19:195.

6. Jayson MIV, Herbert CM, Barks JS. Intervertebral discs nuclear morphology and bursting pressure. *Ann Rheum Dis*. 1973;32:308.

7. Blumenthal SL, Roach J, Herring JA. Lumbar Scheuermann's: A clinical series and classification. *Spine*. 1987;12:929.

8. Lowe TG. Current concepts review: Scheuermann's disease. *J Bone Joint Surg Am*. 1990:72:940.

9. Scoles PV, Latimer BM, Digiovanni BF, et al. Vertebral alterations in Scheuermann's kyphosis. *Spine*. 1991;16:509.

10. Roaf R. A study of the mechanics of spinal injuries. *J Bone Joint Surg*. 1960;42B:810.

11. Tribus CB. Scheuermann's kyphosis in adolescents and adults: diagnosis and management. *J Am Acad Orthop Surg*. 1998;6:36.

12. Bradford D. *Juvenile Kyphosis Textbook of Scoliosis and Other Spinal Deformities*. 3rd ed. Philadelphia, Pa: WB Saunders Company; 1994:349-367.

13. Chiu KY, Luk KD. Cord compression by multiple disc herniations and intraspinal cyst in Scheuermann's Disease. *Spine*. 1995;20:1075.

14. Liebenson C. *Rehabilitation of the Spine*. Baltimore, Md: Williams & Wilkins; 1996.

Chapter Five

Acute Subdural Hematoma in a High School Football Player

Mike Hunker, MS, ATC/L, CSCS

INTRODUCTION

The athlete was a 17-year-old high school football player who was 70 inches tall and weighed 170 lbs. His past medical history included two concussions sustained while playing football the previous season, his junior year. He and his family consulted with a neurosurgeon after both episodes. Computerized tomography (CT) scans were normal. Headaches subsided approximately 1 week after the second concussion. His ability to concentrate and his memory returned shortly thereafter. The athlete did not return to play after the second episode because his team was eliminated from post-season play shortly after the injury.

Before his senior season, the athlete was fitted for a custom helmet as a precaution against further injury. He passed his pre-participation physical exam just before the start of the football season and 1 month prior to the injury. A mild sternoclavicular joint sprain kept the athlete out of the first 2 weeks of football practice. The athlete related no injuries during the 2 weeks of practice leading up to the injury.

SUBJECTIVE HISTORY

Symptoms began during the second half of a football game on August 28, 1998, however the athlete did not report these to a coach, athletic trainer, or team physician. He came out of the game during the second half because all starters were removed due to a big lead over the opposing team. The athlete related that initial symptoms during the second half of the game. The symptoms were partial loss of hearing in his right ear and intense headaches. He could not recall any events from that point on in the game. He did not recall a specific mechanism of injury. Coaches, teammates, and the athlete's parents also could not recall a specific mechanism. Those around the athlete at the end of the game said that he appeared normal as he departed the field and returned to school. His friends said that he complained of intensifying headaches and began vomiting after he left the school. They took him to a restaurant where his parents were. His parents noted that he appeared to remain conscious, but he was unresponsive to any of their questions and they immediately summoned an ambulance.

The athlete was taken to a nearby hospital where he underwent a CT scan that showed a very small-slit and right acute hematoma with no shift (the hematoma was not large enough to push the midbrain over) (Figure 5-1). Physical examination revealed a Glasgow coma score of 12 (out of a possible 15). An initial score greater than 11 is associated with a more than 90% chance of complete recovery. Surgery was not indicated, but he was admitted to the hospital. The athlete regained memory approximately 5 to 6 hours after the onset of memory loss in the restaurant. Dizziness and headache were his chief complaints. Vicodin (Knoll Pharmaceutical Co, Whippany, NJ) was prescribed for pain relief.

Figure 5-1. CT scan showing small-slit acute hematoma on the right with no shift.

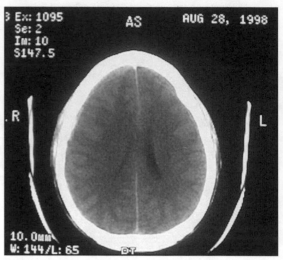

The athlete was kept in the hospital for 5 days secondary to continuous severe headaches. He was awake and alert during this time and was discharged once the headaches subsided. He had normal gait and could tolerate a regular diet. Written and verbal discharge instructions were given to the athlete and his parents and included instructions to call or return to the hospital if headaches returned, or if he developed lethargy, weakness, nausea, or fever.

Headaches intensified the week after being discharged from the hospital. The athlete felt that this corresponded with his returning to classes. Follow-up CT scan showed a thin subdural hematoma. Pain medication was prescribed and the patient's headaches lessened slightly. Difficulty with immediate recall and concentration lapses was still common when the patient returned for follow-up with the neurologist 2 weeks after the injury. The athlete stated that he did not become symptom free until approximately 1 month after his injury.

The athlete, his parents, and the neurologist agreed that he should not resume participation in football. He remained a vital member of his team by attending every practice and game for the remainder of the season. He successfully completed his senior year of high school and is currently attending college.

DISCUSSION

Head injuries account for 4.5% of all high school sports injuries.[1] Estimates of traumatic head injuries per year range from 200,000 to 300,000.[2] Football players are inherently at risk for concussions due to the nature of the sport.

Subdural hematoma is the most common cause of death among athletes with traumatic head injuries. Typically, blood collects in the space between the inner and outer membranes of the brain. The pressure from the hematoma can damage brain tissue and cause loss of brain function. Because there is little or no cortical atrophy, the space available for blood collection is small. The symptoms from the hematoma may be more related to the underlying brain injury than to the clot.[3] The delay in symptoms after injury is due to the slow formation of the hematoma and subsequent increase in intracranial pressure.

The athlete is usually rendered unconscious and may exhibit decerebrate posturing. Treatment at a trauma facility with a neurosurgeon present is critical for proper care. CT scans can confirm the diagnosis and help determine the location and magnitude of the injury. Surgery is dictated by the size of the hematoma.

SUMMARY

This case presented the recognition and treatment of an acute subdural hematoma in a high school football player. His symptoms did not present immediately after an identifiable injury. Instead, his condition began to deteriorate several hours after playing in a game. The symptoms he eventually developed were consistent with an acute subdural hematoma.

Treatment included transport and admittance to a trauma center, CT scan, and observation. The athlete was discharged after 5 days of observation. His symptoms were absent approximately 1 month after his injury, and a follow-up CT scan at 4 weeks post-injury was normal. He successfully completed high school and is currently attending college.

REFERENCES

1.   Garrick SG, Requa R. Medical care and injury surveillance in the high school setting. *Phys Sports Med.* 1981;9(2):115-120.

2.   Centers for Disease Control and Prevention. Sports related recurrent brain injuries. *Morbidity and Mortality Weekly Report.* 1997;10:22-227.

3.   Torg JS, ed. *Athletic Injuries to the Head, Neck, and Face.* 2nd ed. St. Louis: Mosby–Year Book; 1991.

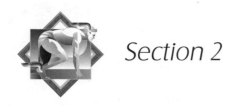

Section 2

Shoulder

Chapter Six

Rehabilitation of the Overhead Athlete Following Thermal-Assisted Anterior Capsulorrhaphy

Kevin E. Wilk, PT, Wendy J. Hurd, PT, Keith Meister, MD,

James R. Andrews, MD

HISTORY

The patient was a 20-year-old, right-hand dominant sophomore who played quarterback for a Division I football program. He also played third base for a minor league professional baseball team. The athlete was injured on January 1, 1998, during a football bowl game when he was tackled from behind. His right arm was carrying the ball, and as he fell his body rolled over the football, pulling his entire shoulder girdle anteriorly and stretching the anterior aspect of his shoulder. The athlete began experiencing posterior shoulder pain after this hard tackle, which worsened with throwing.

The team physicians performed a thorough physical examination immediately following the game and ordered radiographs. No fractures or bony abnormalities were noted. Magnetic resonance imaging (MRI) was performed a week later secondary to persistent pain complaints. The MRI showed a humeral head cyst, fraying of the posterior labrum, a partial undersurface rotator cuff tear, and evidence of internal impingement. Previous history revealed several episodes of posterior impingement and rotator cuff tendonitis sustained during his high school career. These episodes were successfully treated with nonoperative rehabilitation. He reported no previous dislocations or sensations of his shoulder being unstable. Based on the physical examination and diagnostic imaging results, a diagnosis of rotator cuff strain with possible anterior subluxation was made. Initial rehabilitation began in the athletic training room and consisted primarily of ROM exercises, modalities (electrical stimulation, ultrasound, and cryotherapy), and a gradual strengthening program for the shoulder musculature. The athlete did not throw until February when he reported to baseball's spring training. At that time he was able to hit and perform some light throwing without pain, but did no hard (long distance or high intensity) throwing secondary to the recent injury and ongoing posterior shoulder soreness. Until spring football practice began in mid-March, rehabilitation exercises and reduced throwing activities continued to be the treatment plan. Posterior shoulder pain recurred when throwing the football during the second week of practice. Pain was present primarily during late cocking and early acceleration. The remaining portion of the acceleration phase was pain-free, but there was slight discomfort present with follow-through. Posterior shoulder pain worsened with increased throwing activities and as the number of throws increased. The athlete managed to continue with practice and played in the spring scrimmage game with minimal to moderate pain. Following the game, he noted significant soreness posteriorly. Upon completion of spring football he returned to his professional baseball team but was unable to throw with maximal effort. Again, the pain was located posteriorly during late cocking and early acceleration. At this time, the team physician recommended further orthopedic testing and examination.

Secondary to persistent pain that was limiting full sports participation, the athlete was referred to our facility on May 5, 1998 for consultation. During the examination, the patient demonstrated a mild muscular weakness of the supraspinatus muscle and external rotators. The patient exhibited increased external rotation ROM (145 degrees) with a corresponding decrease in internal rotation (45 degrees) compared to the opposite shoulder. Upon palpation, tenderness was noted at the infraspinatus insertion and posterior capsule. Detailed findings of the physical examination are in Table 6-1. Follow-up radiographs and MRI were consistent with initial imaging tests performed earlier in the year. Based on the physical examination and imaging test results, a diagnosis of internal impingement with probable partial thickness tearing of the posterior rotator cuff and probable fraying of the posterior labrum was made.

The team physician, patient, and family discussed possible plans of action. After the patient expressed concerns over the possibility of missing the fall football season if further conservative rehabilitation failed, the decision was made to proceed with surgical intervention.

Surgery

Arthroscopic surgery was performed on May 5, 1998 on the patient's right shoulder. Prior to surgery, examination under anesthesia revealed 2+ laxity anteriorly and 1+ laxity posteriorly and inferiorly. Under direct visualization, all structures appeared normal and intact with the exception of the infraspinatus muscle and the posterior labrum. As expected, both of these structures demonstrated pathological fraying—the posterior-superior labrum exhibited fraying near the 10 to 11 o'clock position and the rotator cuff exhibited a 20% thickness tear. Fraying of the posterior labrum and undersurface rotator cuff were debrided. Based on the laxity assessment of the anterior capsule, a thermal capsular shrinkage procedure was then performed starting at the posterior band of the inferior glenohumeral ligament and extending anteriorly all the way up to the biceps tendon (Figure 6-1). Thermal shrinkage of the tissue was seen and the humeral head appeared to sit more centrally in the glenoid cavity. The surgical procedure was completed and the laxity assessment indicated improved stability. The patient's arm was taken through an arc of motion—external rotation to 85 to 90 degrees, internal rotation to 60 degrees, and flexion to 175 degrees.

Rationale

Internal impingement is a clinical condition first described by Walch et al[1] in 1992. In their series that involved 17 athletes (most were tennis players), all complained of posterior shoulder pain when their arms were in full external rotation at 90 degrees abduction, and none demonstrated excessive anterior laxity with ligamentous testing. With arthroscopic examination, all patients exhibited impingement between the posterosuperior edge of the glenoid and the insertion of the rotator cuff when the arm was placed in the throwing position.

Since Walch et al's original description of internal impingement in 1992, further investigation has revealed that this physiologic contact occurs consistently and is common in overhead athletes when abduction with extreme external rotation is performed.[2,3] Repetitive, forceful impingement of the posterosuperior glenoid against the undersurface of the rotator cuff, which occurs during throwing, leads to pathologic changes.

It has been our experience that patients with posterior impingement typically present with the following clinical signs and symptoms:[4]

- Pain with excessive external rotation in 90 degrees abduction during functional activities (late cocking and deceleration phases of throwing).
- Positive internal impingement sign (Figure 6-2).[5]
- Excessive external rotation (120 to 165 degrees).
- Limitation of internal rotation (40 to 60 degrees).

Table 6-1		
PREOPERATIVE OBJECTIVE FINDINGS		
Range of Motion	Right	Left
Flexion	180 degrees	180 degrees
Abduction	180 degrees	180 degrees
External rotation (at 0 degrees)	90 degrees	90 degrees
External rotation (at 90 degrees)	145 degrees	110 degrees
Internal rotation (at 90 degrees)	45 degrees	60 degrees
Strength		
Supraspinatus	4+/5	5/5
External rotation	4+/5	5/5
Internal rotation	5/5	5/5
Special Tests		
Sulcus	--	--
Anterior drawer	1+	1+
Anterior fulcrum	1+	1+
Apprehension	--	--
Posterior drawer	1+	1+
Clunk test	+	--
Posterior impingement	+	--

- Tenderness upon palpation posteriorly.
- Muscular weakness of external rotators.
- Muscular weakness in "empty can" position.
- Scapular weakness.
- History of recurrent symptoms.

We believe the two most significant anatomic factors contributing to the mechanism of internal impingement are glenohumeral joint soft tissue asymmetry and adaptive bone changes. The thrower with glenohumeral joint asymmetry will present with anterior capsular laxity and posterior rotator cuff tightness, allowing increased anterior humeral head translation to occur during the throwing motion. This increased anterior translation, combined with horizontal abduction of the humerus in late cocking, results in undersurface rubbing of the rotator cuff.

Excessive glenohumeral ligament laxity occurs in throwers secondary to either congenital or acquired mechanisms, or a combination of both. This increased anterior laxity is necessary for throwers to achieve extreme amounts of external rotation and properly position the upper extremity during the cocking phase of the throwing motion. Overhead athletes who do not have congenital laxity of the shoulder joint often develop what is referred to as "thrower's laxity."[6] Over time, repetitive throwing creates functional and adaptive changes in the structures surrounding the shoulder joint complex. The glenohumeral ligaments, primarily the anterior band of the inferior glenohumeral ligament (this ligament is the primary restraint to anterior translation with the arm in external rotation at 90 degrees abduction), demonstrate increased laxity to accommodate the necessary increased external rotation seen in the successful thrower.[7]

The posterior tightness a thrower frequently presents with is rarely secondary to posterior capsular restric-

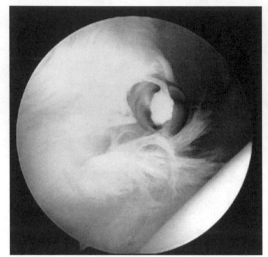

Figure 6-1. Thermal capsular shrinkage of the glenohumeral capsule was performed.

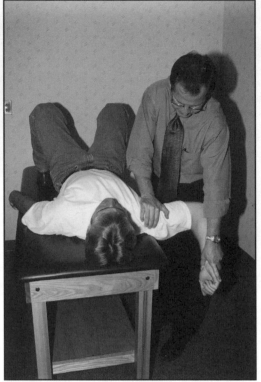

Figure 6-2. Positive internal impingement sign: pain with full external rotation at 90 degrees abduction as impingement occurs between the undersurface of the rotator cuff and the posterosuperior edge of the glenoid.

tions, but is instead most commonly associated with tightness of the posterior rotator cuff. Adaptive osseous changes may also account for the common loss of internal rotation. During arm deceleration of the pitching motion, forces at the glenohumeral joint reach high levels—400 + 90 newtons (N) of posterior sheer force and a compressive force of 1090 + 110 N.[8] During deceleration, the teres minor, posterior deltoid, and the lower trapezius must act eccentrically to decelerate the arm, resist glenohumeral joint distraction, and dissipate the tremendous forces generated during the throwing motion. Electromyographic (EMG) activity of the infraspinatus and teres minor during arm deceleration is 37% and 84%, respectively (based on the percentage of a maximal voluntary isometric contraction). Repetitive high-intensity contractions can result in muscular hypertrophy with secondary musculotendinous tightness. Therefore, following the thermal capsulorrhaphy, it is essential that stretching exercises are performed to ensure not only restoration of motion, but also a proper balance of glenohumeral motion.

If both anterior laxity and posterior tightness can be considered common findings in throwers, the fine balance of functional stability must be achieved in order to maintain effective and pain-free throwing. The neuromuscular system must recognize joint position and initiate the synergistic cocontraction of the surrounding musculature to prevent humeral head subluxation. For this reason, dynamic stability should be emphasized during both operative and nonoperative rehabilitation of the overhead throwing athlete. Thus, dynamic stabilization drills are performed throughout the rehabilitation program.

Rehabilitation

Following surgery, the patient was placed on our accelerated rehabilitation program for thermal-assisted anterior capsulorrhaphy performed on athletes with acquired laxity (overhead throwers). This program structure is based on the location of the thermal treatment on the capsular tissue, tissue status of the patient (ie, the degree of ligamentous laxity), the status of the dynamic stabilizers, the activity level of the individual, and the patient's response to surgery. The first 2 to 4 weeks of rehabilitation are marked by limited activity; this is to prevent overstretching of the capsule. After 4 weeks the patient's ROM is gradually restored, with particular emphasis on restoration of external rotation and abduction. From weeks 6 to 12, restoration of ROM is imperative, again with emphasis placed on external rotation at 90 degrees abduction and shoulder elevation. In the final phases of rehabilitation, once ROM has been nearly normalized, strengthening exercises and proprioception drills are emphasized. The patient is placed on a gradual throwing program once proper ROM, strength, and proprioception are obtained.

Phase I

At the time of hospital discharge (1 day postoperatively), the patient demonstrated passive ROM of the surgical shoulder of flexion—0 to 60 degrees, external rotation in the scapular plane of 10 degrees, and internal rotation in the scapular plane of 35 degrees. The patient complained of diffuse shoulder soreness with motion and exhibited a spasm end feel with motion in all planes. The patient was instructed to apply cryotherapy to his shoulder six to eight times daily to diminish postsurgical pain, muscular spasm, and inflammation.[9,10] Active assistive and passive ROM exercises began immediately following surgery with imposed restrictions to protect the healing tissue. Early motion exercises were performed to nourish articular cartilage, assist in collagen tissue synthesis and organization, and restore proprioception and assist in neuromodulation of pain.[11-18] Performing passive ROM also allowed the clinician to assess the quantity of the motion and the end feel, with the advancement of motion best described as both a patient-and-tissue dependent process. If the end point of motion was soft with significant give, likely due to poor capsular healing, ROM progression was slowed. If the end point became firm or hard with less than desired motion, advancement of ROM was accelerated to prevent excessive scar tissue formation and loss of motion. The guidelines for restoration of motion following thermal capsular shrinkage for the overhead thrower are 60 degrees of external rotation (ER) at 90 degrees abduction at 4 weeks, 75 degrees of ER at 90 degrees abduction at 6 weeks, and 90 degrees of ER at 90 degrees of abduction at 8 weeks. From week 8 to week 12 motion is progressed to 115 to 120 degrees of ER at 90 degrees abduction for the thrower.

The patient's ROM gradually improved after surgery. At 2 weeks postoperatively, the patient exhibited 25 degrees of external rotation and 45 degrees of internal rotation in the scapular plane. The patient continued to demonstrate a spasm end feel. Four weeks after surgery, the patient's motion continued to improve with external rotation in the scapular plane progressing to 55 degrees; the patient's shoulder elevation was approximately 145 degrees. The patient's end feel at week 5 to 6 appeared to change from more of a spasm end feel to a firm end feel.

At week 8, the patient's external rotation at 90 degrees of abduction had progressed to 95 degrees with a firm end feel. Until this time, the treating rehabilitation specialist delayed aggressive stretching to prevent the capsule from stretching out.

Strengthening for the first two postoperative weeks included isometric strengthening of the elbow and shoulder girdle musculature. At 2 weeks the patient began short lever arm strengthening (bicep/tricep, and internal rotation [IR]/ER with tubing), gradually progressing to full-lever arm, light isotonic strengthening at 4 weeks. Active ROM for shoulder flexion and abduction began 3 weeks following surgery. Emphasis throughout the rehabilitation process was placed on rotator cuff and scapular musculature, without neglecting elbow and wrist strengthening of the involved extremity. At week 6, the athlete was placed on our "Thrower's Ten" strengthening program.[19] This is a strengthening program that specifically addresses the vital muscles involved in the throwing motion and is based on the collective research of numerous investigations.[20-24]

Restoring proprioception, neuromuscular control, and functional stability is critical for successful rehabilitation of the overhead athlete. Early neuromuscular re-education goals include restoring neurosensory properties of the micro-traumatically injured shoulder ligaments and enhancing the sensitivity of the afferent mechanoreceptors.[25] Proprioception training was initiated immediately after the thermal procedure to ensure sensory stimulus to the capsular structures. We feel this is critical due to the possible negative effects to the capsule following a thermal capsulorrhaphy. Specific drills used during the early phases of rehabilitation include rhythmic stabilization (RS) and reciprocal isometric (RI) contractions for the internal rotators/external rotators of the shoulder; they are performed at various degrees of shoulder abduction. Additionally, proprioceptive neuromuscular facilitation (PNF) drills are performed midrange, progressing to end range. The PNF pattern we most commonly utilized was the D2 flexion/extension pattern with manual resistance, incorporating RS, slow reversal holds, and RI.[26,27] The PNF technique utilized specific skilled sensory input from the clinician to bring about or facilitate a specific movement pattern. The manual techniques allowed the clinician the opportunity to increase the patient's awareness of specific movement patterns and reinforce or facilitate weak patterns.

Phase II

Entering phase II of the rehabilitation program at week 9, the patient's ROM was progressed emphasizing adequate external rotation to restore proper throwing mechanics. Plyometric training progressed from two-hand drills at week 9 to one-hand drills at week 12 (Figure 6-3).[28]

Twelve weeks postoperatively, the patient exhibited adequate passive ROM of the right shoulder and a firm end feel with both external rotation and flexion. The patient also exhibited excellent stability—1+ laxity to anterior displacement and 1 laxity to inferior and posterior displacement testing. Strength testing indicated excellent strength of all shoulder musculature. Based on clinical assessment, the end feels exhibited into flexion and external rotation, active-assistive L-bar and pulley exercises were continued, and capsular stretching for the inferior capsule and posterior rotator cuff in an effort to normalize motion, were initiated. Due to the patient's tightness in motion with shoulder flexion and external rotation at 90 degrees abduction, an aggressive joint mobilization program was initiated. Grade III and IV inferior glides were initiated to increase shoulder elevation, and anterior glides were initiated to improve external rotation. The thrower's ten strengthening program was continued, with aggressive weight training of the larger muscle groups (pectoralis major, latissimus dorsi, etc) beginning at week 9. Neuromuscular drills focused on enhancing dynamic joint stability. During this phase, the extremity was placed in positions at end ranges and the patient was instructed to dynamically stabilize the joint while manual resistance techniques such as RS and RI were performed. In the overhead athlete, the proprioceptive neuromuscular facilitation (PNFD2) pattern and IR/ER at 90 degrees abduction are frequently utilized positions. Because the scapula provides proximal stability for the upper extremity, enabling greater distal segment mobility, closed chain scapulothoracic neuromuscular control drills were integrated. Enhanced scapulothoracic proprioception and kinesthesia results in more effective force couples surrounding the shoulder complex and enhanced dynamic glenohumeral joint stability.

One of the most significant additions during this phase of rehabilitation was the plyometric drills. Plyometric exercises employ three phases, all intended to utilize the elastic and reactive properties of the muscle to generate maximal force production. The first phase is the setting or eccentric phase, where a rapid prestretch applied to the musculotendinous unit stimulates the muscle spindle. The second phase is the amortization phase, representing the time between eccentric and concentric phases. This phase should be as short as possible so that beneficial neurological effects of the prestretch are not lost. The final concentric phase is the resultant facilitated concentric muscular contraction from the prestretch stimulus. Plyometric drills served to enhance muscular performance and were an excellent transition exercise from traditional dumbbell strengthening to throwing. Plyometric drills were performed for 1 month prior to throwing, with 2 weeks of two-hand drills followed by 2 weeks of one-hand drills. This month of transitional and advanced exercise gave the athlete time to condition the shoulder muscles for the significant stresses of throwing, retrain the neuromuscular system, and gradually restore proper throwing mechanics.

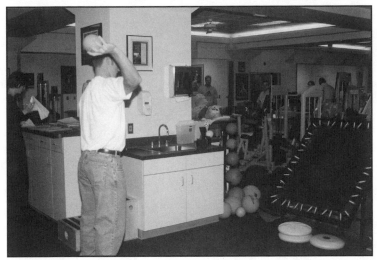

Figure 6-3. The one-hand baseball throw.

At week 12, the patient was allowed to begin an interval football throwing program specifically designed for him. Approximately 2 1/2 weeks into the throwing program, the treating rehabilitation specialist called our center to report that the patient had been experiencing significant shoulder pain during the throwing program, located posteriorly and superiorly at the subacromial space. Pain worsened with throwing and soreness persisted upon completion of the throwing program. The patient's ROM was 109 to 112 degrees external rotation at 90 degrees abduction and 170 degrees elevation (both with a firm end feel). Capsular mobility was 1+ in all directions. Based on the patient's pain complaints and clinical examination findings, the patient was instructed to terminate the throwing program and initiate an aggressive stretching and joint mobilization program. It was determined that the loss of motion was causing the patient's pain complaints and inhibiting his ability to throw. Consequently, joint mobilizations in both the anterior and inferior directions were initiated. During the next 3 weeks, the patient's ROM improved to 125 to 128 degrees of external rotation at 90 degrees abduction and 180 degrees of flexion with a capsular end feel. With the restoration of full ROM, all pain complaints were resolved. At 17 1/2 weeks postoperatively the patient was reinitiated on the interval throwing program and allowed to perform some practice drills with the team.

Frequently, rehabilitation specialists and physicians feel that all patients who undergo a thermal capsular shrinkage will regain motion with little effort, and often the concern is gaining too much motion. We have clinically observed that capsular tightness and loss of motion occurred in approximately 15% of thermal procedures. Generally, the patient exhibits loss of motion with a spasm (painful) end feel. Clinically, these patients exhibit capsular restrictions and resemble an adhesive capsulitis patient. Hayashi, et al[29] reported that 6 of 42 patients (14%) exhibited loss of motion 6 months after a thermal capsulorrhaphy and required a second procedure to achieve full motion. Ellenbecker and Mattalino[30] reported on 20 patients who underwent a thermal capsular shrinkage procedure. Although the authors' protocol emphasized full ROM at 12 weeks, only four patients (20%) exhibited full external ROM, and six patients (30%) exhibited full abduction motion. Thus, the clinical belief that all thermal capsulorrhaphy patients will regain full motion without aggressive stretching is not true. Some patients may experience an adverse reaction to the procedure and require aggressive stretching and joint mobilization to normalize motion. Conversely, we have observed that some patients (14 to 18%) will regain motion with little effort. The clinician must address each patient carefully to determine which patients appear to be healing with excessive capsular scarring opposed to inadequate tightening and which patients appear to be progressing according to schedule. We believe assessing the patient's ROM and end feels at 6, 10, and 12 weeks postoperatively will dictate both the rate of the patient's progress and emphasis of treatment during each phase of the rehabilitation program.

Phase III to IV

Entering phase III 20 weeks after surgery, the patient had full, pain-free ROM with excellent strength and stability. Having met all necessary criteria, the athlete was 2 1/2 weeks into the interval throwing program. As fall was approaching, emphasis was placed on throwing the football, reserving baseball throwing and hitting for the following season. The purpose of an interval program is to progressively and systematically increase the demands placed on the shoulder while the patient is performing sport-specific activities. Using this type of gradual return to sport activities minimizes the risk of reinjury and allows progressive adaptation of the shoulder and other body parts to the repetitive stresses of athletic activities.

At approximately 21 weeks postoperatively the patient began throwing passing routes. At week 23, he was cleared to play. Having successfully completed the interval throwing program, the athlete returned to play on October 3, 1998 and competed in the 1998-1999 college football season asymptomatically with a record of 6-1 as a starting quarterback, including a major college bowl victory.

Follow-Up

The patient chose not to participate in baseball for the 1999 season, focusing instead on his senior year of football. He was the starting quarterback for a Division 1 college football program for the 1999 season, and at the time of this writing is 16 months postoperative. His ROM is 178 degrees of elevation, 128 degrees of external rotation at 90 degrees abduction, and 62 degrees of internal rotation at 90 degrees abduction.

CONCLUSION

For the overhead throwing athlete with internal impingement with acquired instability, nonoperative treatment is often successful at returning the athlete to play. If conservative treatment is unsuccessful, an arthroscopic debridement with a thermal-assisted anterior capsulorrhaphy may provide the surgeon a reasonable surgical option. This arthroscopic procedure appears to have fewer postoperative complications (such as loss of motion) compared to open stabilization procedures. Rehabilitation following thermal capsulorrhaphy is based on the patient's response to surgery, with the rate of progression based on the amount of motion and the end feel at various time frames. Emphasis on posterior rotator cuff and scapular strengthening, as well as proprioceptive and dynamic stability of the glenohumeral joint, are critical components of the exercise regimen as the athlete prepares for return to sport activities.

In a recent study at our institution, 28 overhead athletes who underwent thermal capsulorrhaphy were evaluated at least 24 months following the procedure.[31] Eighty-four percent returned to previous levels of throwing, with the average time frame being 9.2 months. Since May of 1997, over 300 thermal capsulorrhaphies have been performed on overhead throwing athletes. We have clinically noted that approximately 15% appear to struggle with obtaining motion, while approximately 15% appear to gain motion very quickly. It is our recommendation that the postsurgical rehabilitation program following this procedure be based on the patient's response to surgery. Therefore, the rehabilitation specialist must reassess the patient's motion weekly in order to adjust the rate of progression. Careful attention to the recovery of motion is critical to ensuring a successful outcome with this procedure.

REFERENCES

1. Walch G, Boileau P, Noel E, et al. Impingement of the deep surface of the supraspinatus tendon on the glenoid rim: an arthroscopic study. *J Shoulder Elbow Surg.* 1992;1:239-245.

2. Halbrecht J, Tirman P, Atkin D. Internal impingement of the shoulder: comparison of findings between the throwing and non-throwing shoulders of college baseball players. *Arthroscopy.* 1999;15:253-258.

3. Jobe C. Posterior superior glenoid impingement. Expanded spectrum. *Arthroscopy.* 1995;11:530-536.

4. Wilk K. Rehabilitation guidelines for the thrower with internal impingement. Paper presented at the 17th annual Injuries in Baseball Course. January 22, 1999; Birmingham, Ala.

5. Meister K, Bates J, Gilmore M. The posterior impingement sign: evaluation for diagnosis of posterior impingement in the shoulder of the overhead athlete. Paper presented at: AOSSM Meeting. July 14, 1998; Vancouver, BC.

6. Wilk K. The thrower's shoulder: evaluation and common injuries. Paper presented at the 1997 Advances on the Knee and Shoulder Course. May 24, 1997; Hilton Head, SC.

7. O'Brien S, Schwartz R, Warren R, et al. Capsular restraints to anterior-posterior motion of the abducted shoulder: a biomechanical study. *J Shoulder Elbow Surg.* 1995;4:298-308.

8. Fleisig G, Dillman C, Andrews J. Biomechanics of the shoulder during throwing. In: Andrews J, Wilk K, eds. *The Athlete's Shoulder.* New York, NY: Churchill Livingstone; 1994:355-368.

9. Speer K, Warren R, Horowitz L. The efficacy of cryotherapy in the postoperative shoulder. *J Shoulder Elbow Surg.* 1996;5:62-68.

10. Knight K. *Cryotherapy: theory, technique, and physiology.* Chattanooga, Tenn: Chattanooga Corporation; 1995.

11. Coutts R, Rothe C, Kaita J. The role of continuous passive motion in the rehabilitation of the total knee patient. *Clin Orthop.* 1981;159:126-132.

12. Dehne E, Tory R. Treatment of joint injuries by immediate mobilization based upon the spiral adaptation concept. *Clin Orthop.* 1971;77:218-232.

13. Haggmark T, Ericksson E. Cylinder or mobile cast brace after knee ligament surgery: a clinical analysis and morphologic and enzymatic studies of changes in quadriceps muscle. *Am J Sports Med.* 1979;7:48-56.

14. Perkins G. Rest and motion. *J Bone Joint Surg Br.* 1954;35:521-539.

15. Salter R, Simmonds D, Malcolm B, et al. The effects of continuous passive motion on healing of full thickness defects in articular cartilage. *J Bone Joint Surg Am.* 1980;62:1232-1251.

16. Salter R, Hamilton H, Wedge J. Clinical application of basic research on continuos passive motion for disorders and injuries of synovial joints. A preliminary report of a feasability study. *J Orthop Res.* 1984;1:325-342.

17. Tipton C, Mathies R, Martin R. Influence of age and sex on strength of bone-ligament junctions in knee joints of rats. *J Bone Joint Surg Am.* 1978;60:230-236.

18. Noyes F, Mangine R, Barber S. Early knee motion after open and arthroscopic anterior cruciate ligament reconstruction. *Am J Sports Med.* 1987;15:149-160.

19. Wilk K, Andrews J, Arrigo C, et al. *Preventative and Rehabilitative Exercises for the Shoulder and Elbow.* 5th ed. Birmingham, Ala: American Sports Medicine Institute; 1997.

20. Townsend H, Jobe F, Pink M, et al. Electromyographic analysis of the glenohumeral muscles during a baseball rehabilitation program. *Am J Sports Med.* 1991;19:264-269.

21. Moseley J, Jobe F, Pink M, et al. EMG analysis of the scapular muscles during a shoulder rehabilitation program. *Am J Sports Med.* 1992;20:128-134.

22. Blackburn T, McLeod W, White B. EMG analysis of posterior rotator cuff exercises. *J Ath Training.* 1990;25:40-45.

23. Jobe F, Moynes D. Delineation of diagnostic criteria and a rehabilitation program for rotator cuff injuries. *Am J Sports Med.* 1982;10:336-342.

24. Pappas A, Zawacki R. Rehabilitation of the pitching shoulder. *Am J Sports Med.* 1985;13:223-231.

25. Lephart S, Pinciuero D, Giraldo J, et al. The role of proprioception in the management and rehabilitation of athletic injuries. *Am J Sports Med.* 1997;25:130-137.

26. Knott M, Voss D. *Proprioceptive Neuromuscular Facilitation.* New York, NY: Hoeber Medical Division–Harper and Row; 1968.

27. Wilk K, Arrigo C. Current concepts in rehabilitation of the athletic shoulder. *J Orthop Sports Phys Ther.* 1993;18:365-378.

28. Wilk K, Voight M, Keirns M, et al. Stretch shortening drills for the upper extremity: theory and clinical application. *J Orthop Sports Phys Ther.* 1993;17:225-239.

29. Hayashi K, Massa K, Thabit G, et al. Histologic evaluation of the glenohumeral joint capsule after laser-assisted capsular shift procedure for glenohumeral instability. *Am J Sports Med.* 1999;27:162-172.

30. Ellenbecker T, Mattalino A. Glenohumeral range of motion and rotator cuff strength following arthroscopic anterior stabilization with thermal capsulorrhaphy. *J Orthop Sports Phys Ther.* 1999;29:160-167.

31. Levitz C. The use of arthroscopic thermal shrinkage in the management of internal impingement. Paper presented at: the 17th annual Injuries in Baseball Course. January 24,1999; Birmingham, Ala.

Chapter Seven

Posterior Sternoclavicular Joint Dislocation in a Collegiate Football Player

Vincent G. Stilger, HSD, ATC, Jeromy M. Alt, MS, ATC,

Andrea J. Michael, ATC, David F. Hubbard, MD

INTRODUCTION

Sternoclavicular (SC) joint dislocations are relatively uncommon, accounting for less than 1% of all dislocations.[1-4] Posterior SC joint dislocations were first described in 1824.[2,5-8] The injury is difficult to diagnose and often dangerous because it can induce fatal mediastinal complications that may result in death.[4,5]

The primary injury mechanism of a posterior SC joint dislocation is a violent blow to the posterolateral aspect of the shoulder with the arm adducted and flexed.[3] This position is often typical of a football player who is carrying the ball. Often during a tackle, the shoulder is left unprotected and exposed to injury.[3] Typically, individuals with an SC joint dislocation present with the neck flexed toward the injured side, supporting the flexed elbow with the opposite hand, and complaining of local pain.[3] The majority of reported SC joint dislocations occur in males between the ages of 25 and 30, secondary to decreasing mobility and laxity of the SC joint with age.[1,3,9,10]

We are presenting this case to report the immediate acute care, diagnosis, and eventual closed reduction of an SC dislocation in a football player. Rehabilitation is discussed in order to provide a baseline protocol for an athlete or individual who has suffered a posterior SC joint dislocation. Due to the uniqueness of a posterior SC joint dislocation, the certified athletic trainer must be able to evaluate, recognize, and refer the athlete to avoid any potentially serious complications.

ANATOMY

The SC joint is a diarthrodial joint comprising the large medial end of the clavicle, the sternum, and to a lesser extent the first rib.[11] It is the only articulation the upper extremity has to the trunk, and virtually every motion of the upper extremity involves motion of the SC joint.[12] This skeletal arrangement makes the joint particularly weak; however, it is secured by strong ligaments that anchor the clavicle to the sternum. The anterior sternoclavicular ligament and the stronger posterior sternoclavicular ligament stabilize the articulation by preventing upward displacement of the clavicle. These ligaments are actually joint capsular thickenings that anchor the medial end of the clavicle to the sternum.[13] The posterior ligament is much thicker, which may account in part for the infrequency of posterior dislocations.[7] The clavicular notch of the sternum is smaller than the medial end of the clavicle, thus causing the clavicle to rise higher than the sternum.[14,15] In addition, less than half of the medial clavicle articulates with the sternum.[16] The two articulating surfaces are incongruent, and the joint is therefore potentially unstable.[12] A fibrocartilaginous disc, which is interposed between the two articulating surfaces, functions as a shock absorber against medial forces along the axis of the clavicle.[12,15] Just posterior to the SC joint are several major vessels of the superior mediastinum.

CASE STUDY

On September 19, 1998, during a National Collegiate Athletic Association (NCAA) Division 1 football game, a 21-year-old male athlete (6' 2", 180 lbs) was injured while returning a punt late in the second quarter of a game. The injury occurred when the athlete landed on the lateral aspect of his right shoulder while being tackled by two opponents (Figure 7-1).

At the conclusion of the play, the athlete remained down on the artificial surface and was immediately examined on the field by two certified athletic trainers (ATCs). The athlete complained of pain from his sternum halfway to the shoulder but indicated no popping, snapping, or other odd sensations. Evaluation revealed no acute acromioclavicular (AC) pain, no breathing difficulties, and extreme pain from the middle to the medial clavicle. Differential diagnoses included possible clavicular fracture, Salter-Harris-type fracture, sternoclavicular sprain, or costoclavicular sprain. While being escorted from the field to the sidelines, the ATC supported the athlete's involved arm. On the sidelines, the team orthopedist immediately referred the athlete to the athletic training room for x-rays. The athlete was transported to the athletic training room with his elbow at 90 degrees, his upper arm splinted to his body, and the extremity supported by the ATC.

Once the athlete arrived in the athletic training room, his equipment and pads were removed, and he was prepped for x-rays, which were negative for a clavicular fracture. However, the athlete still had extreme pain in the medial one-third of the clavicle toward the SC joint. The athlete's chief complaint was pain aggravated by even the slightest movement or motion. Due to extreme pain, we were unable to thoroughly evaluate the athlete with regard to palpation, range of motion (ROM), neurological assessment, and special tests. However, swelling and a slight depression were noted directly over the SC joint. He also stated he felt as if "something was stuck in his throat."

Acute care consisted of a transcutaneous electrical nerve stimulator (TENS) unit and ice applied to the SC joint. Additionally, the athlete was placed in a sitting position because lying down was too painful.

After further evaluation of the x-rays, the team orthopedist referred the athlete to the emergency room and a trauma surgeon. The trauma surgeon noted that the athlete was stable, with no signs of shortness of breath, no vascular compromise to the right upper extremity, and no pulse irregularities compared to the contralateral side. Additional x-rays were obtained at the emergency room using the Rockwood or "serendipity" view (Figure 7-2). This view is taken while the individual is supine and the x-ray tube is angled superiorly 40 degrees to the head from the vertical and centered on the manubrium.[12,15] Radiographic analysis revealed that the right clavicle shifted posteriorly and the left clavicle was centered and intact. Computed tomography (CT) was obtained to demonstrate the nature of the dislocation. The CT scan also revealed the trachea had shifted to the left, which accounted for the athlete's feeling as if something was stuck in his throat (Figure 7-3). After all examinations were complete, the final diagnosis was a right posterior sternoclavicular (SC) joint dislocation with an accompanying left tracheal shift.

A closed reduction was attempted with the athlete under general anesthesia. With the athlete supine, a rolled up towel was placed between the scapula to retract the shoulders and to force the medial portion of the clavicle anteriorly. The surgeon directed a posterolateral force on the shoulder, immediately relocating the athlete's clavicle. The closed reduction was confirmed under fluoroscopy and clinical examination. Upon retraction of the shoulders, the athlete's trachea shifted back into position with no internal injury or trauma to the trachea. Had the closed reduction not been successful, the physicians were prepared to perform an open reduction surgical technique. After closed reduction, the athlete was placed in a sling and swathe, was still neurovascularly intact, exhibited no signs of shortness of breath or dysphagia, and was hospitalized overnight. He was discharged from the hospital the following morning with strict instructions to return immediately to the emergency room if he experienced any problems. At this time, the course of action was immobilization with a sling and swathe, ice, and medication for pain control.

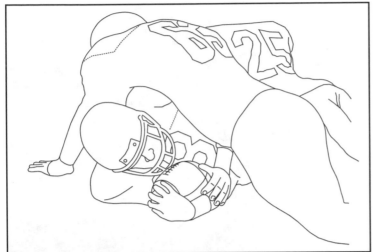

Figure 7-1. Line drawing showing the injury mechanism of a right posterior SC joint dislocation.

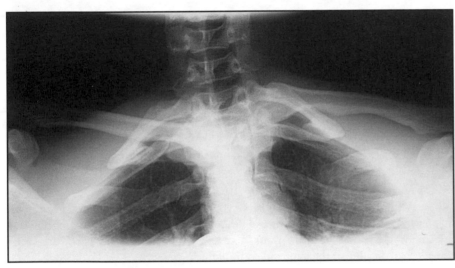

Figure 7-2. Rockwood or "serendipity" view showing the right posterior SC joint dislocation. Note the inferior posterior portion of the right medial clavicle in comparison to the left (arrows).

A physician's visit was scheduled for 10 days after the reduction. The athlete reported no numbness, tingling, or temperature change in his right hand, and he had minimal pain. Physical examination revealed minimal tenderness on palpation over the right SC joint; however, some stiffness was present in the right shoulder during glenohumeral motion. The SC joint was stable, and the athlete was neurovascularly intact. X-ray examination, using the Rockwood view, revealed that the joint was reduced and the joint space appeared symmetrical to the contralateral side. The athlete was instructed to remain in the sling for 2 more weeks, at which time a follow-up visit was scheduled with the trauma surgeon.

Physical examination revealed no tenderness over the SC joint, minimal atrophy in the right arm, and full ROM in the neck and shoulder. Neurovascularly he was intact. No x-rays were taken, and the trauma surgeon planned to examine the athlete again in 4 weeks. He was now allowed to progress to all motions, pain-free. The trauma surgeon examined the athlete 2 months after the injury; full ROM was noted, no prominence of the SC joint was present, and he was neurovascularly intact. Rockwood x-rays revealed callus formation around the right SC joint. The trauma surgeon granted a full release to perform activities as tolerated, except for football contact. A decision had been made to grant the athlete a medical redshirt.

In the ensuing off-season, the athlete participated in all conditioning drills and weight training activities as tolerated. Certain movements, such as the overhead shoulder press, incline bench, and bench press, were closely monitored due to the mechanism of his injury. The athlete was seen by the physician before spring

Figure 7-3. CT scan showing posterior dislocation of the right SC joint. Note the right medial clavicle lies posterior to the sternum.

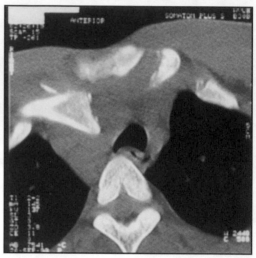

drills and was given clearance to participate in spring football practice with no restrictions, which he did without incident.

POST-REDUCTION REHABILITATION

The team orthopedist and trauma surgeon treated the athlete somewhat conservatively because of the lack of information regarding the treatment and rehabilitation protocol of this rare injury. Therefore, a treatment and rehabilitation protocol was formulated based on discussions with other physicians, athletic trainers, and physical therapists. A perusal of the literature produced minimal information regarding treatment protocol.

Phase I: 0 to 10 Days Post-Reduction

The athlete wore a sling at all times during the first 10 days. No motion of the shoulder was allowed and the athlete iced the SC joint several times a day while immobilized in the sling. Glenohumeral motion was avoided due to the rotation of the clavicle on the manubrium. No rehabilitative exercises were performed during this time to allow for adequate healing of the joint and surrounding ligaments.

Phase II: 10 Days to 3 Weeks Post-Reduction

During phase II, the athlete continued with icing but could take the sling off for showers and treatment in the athletic training room. He began working on wrist flexion and extension, elbow flexion, extension, pronation, supination, and grip strength (Table 7-1). Cardiovascular conditioning using the stationary bike or stair machine was also incorporated.

Phase III: 3 to 6 Weeks

ROM exercises were initiated beginning with Codman/pendulum exercises and progressing to active-assisted ROM (glenohumeral abduction to 60 degrees) in all directions. Because the athlete tolerated these activities with minimal to no discomfort, he was allowed to progress 5 days later to glenohumeral ROM in all directions with no weight. Eventually, the athlete progressed to light resistance (8 lbs or less), carefully avoiding SC joint distraction.

Phase IV: 6 to 12 Weeks

Resistance was increased to all glenohumeral motions. A bench press was simulated using cuff weights and surgical tubing and was progressed to a modified bench press by placing the athlete on an examining table to stop horizontal extension at 90 degrees. After 10 days of these exercises, the athlete was allowed to progress to light weight training activity using the Hammer strength machines.

Hammer strength machines were used initially to encourage proper technique, control, and safety. Once the weight was increased on the Hammer strength machines, the athlete progressed to free weights, using low weight, and gradually increased to heavier weight. The athlete was allowed to participate in noncontact drills with his teammates while they prepared for a bowl game approximately 12 weeks after the injury.

DISCUSSION

Mechanism

Posterior SC joint dislocations occur as a result of direct or indirect trauma to the shoulder particularly during vehicular accidents or athletic injuries.[9] The mechanism most commonly reported in athletics is a blow to the posterolateral aspect of the shoulder.[1,9,15] However, this athlete was injured when he fell to the artificial surface while being tackled, and two opponents landed directly on top of him. This resulted in a lateral compression injury mechanism to the shoulder girdle. During this mechanism, the lateral clavicle is displaced anteriorly, and a taut costoclavicular ligament, acting as a fulcrum, simultaneously displaces the medial end of the clavicle into a retrosternal position.[1,9,12,13,15] A less frequent athletic injury mechanism resulting in a posterior SC joint dislocation is a direct anterior-to-posterior blow to the medial clavicle, causing it to shift posteriorly.[17,18] In any case, should one suspect a posterior sternoclavicular joint dislocation, it is important to understand the exact mechanism in order to identify the extent of the injury and the possible structures involved.

Clinical Presentation

Clinical signs and symptoms associated with a posterior SC joint dislocation often vary from case to case and may include breathing difficulties, dysphagia, cyanosis in the neck or upper extremity due to venous congestion, hoarseness, neurovascular changes such as weakness and numbness in the ipsilateral upper extremity, a less prominent sternocleidomastoid muscle on the ipsilateral side, and shoulder and arm pain.[3,4,7,8,12,13,15,17-19] The clinical signs and symptoms exhibited by this athlete were consistent with those reported in the literature. On initial observation, the medial end of the clavicle will be depressed, thus making the diagnosis even more difficult; however, later swelling may conceal the deformity and mask the anatomical structures of the joint.[1,9,17] An SC joint dislocation should be suspected in any athlete who has pain, swelling, or deformity over the medial clavicle after trauma.[12,15]

Typically an athlete with a suspected SC joint dislocation will flex the neck toward the ipsilateral side while the upper extremity on the injured side is flexed at the elbow and supported by the opposite arm.[1,4,9,17] The individual will also protect the affected arm and may assume a kyphotic posture.[7] Any attempt to straighten the neck is usually met with great discomfort and painful resistance.[1,12,13,17,18]

Differential Diagnosis

An injury that may resemble a posterior SC joint dislocation is a displaced Salter-Harris type I epiphyseal fracture of the medial end of the clavicle. Radiographically, the medial end of the clavicle is the last epiphysis to fuse, but it does not appear before the age of 18 and may not close until the age of 25.[9,12,13,15,18] Therefore, an epiphyseal fracture, rather than a dislocation, should be considered in individuals younger than 25 years of age who have sustained trauma to the medial clavicle.[9,12,13,15,20] A Salter-Harris fracture is often difficult to diagnose even with a CT scan and actually may not be recognized until surgery is performed.[20]

Whether the injury is a Salter-Harris fracture or a posterior SC joint dislocation, it will be treated in a similar manner with a period of 4 to 6 weeks of immobilization.[2,12,13,15]

Table 7-1

REHABILITATION PROTOCOL FOLLOWING A
POSTERIOR STERNOCLAVICULAR DISLOCATION

Phase (Time after injury)	Activity
Phase I (0 to 10 days)	Strict immobilization with ice only while in the sling 2 to 3 x daily
Phase II (10 days to 3 weeks)	Active wrist ROM—flexion, extension, radial and ulnar deviation -4 x 25, 2 x/day Active elbow ROM—flexion, extension, pronation, supination 4 x 25, 2 x/day Cardiovascular conditioning—bike, stair machine Only allowed out of the immobilizer for showering
Phase III (3 to 6 weeks)	Pendulum exercises—forward/backward, side/side, circumduction (cw/ccw) 2 x 20 each UBE (upper body ergometer) Wall walks (flexion and abduction) 2 x 15 each Wrist flexion, extension -3 x 15 Gripping exercises with Power Grip Active assistive exercises—Glenohumeral ROM to 60 degrees abduction progressing to glenohumeral AROM in all directions—flexion, extension, abduction, adduction, internal and external rotation • 3 x 15 with no weight initially but progressing to weight and nothing heavier than 8 lbs • Horizontal flexion and extension were performed supine and the athlete was not allowed past the midline All AROM exercises were performed looking at the mirror in order to avoid shoulder hiking Continue cardiovascular conditioning—bike, stair machine
Phase IV (6 to 12 weeks)	Added weight to all glenohumeral motions—increased weight as tolerated Bicep curls—3 x 10—alternating days with tricep french curls Tricep french curls—3 x 10—alternating days with bicep curls Elbow pronation and supination with weight—1 lb progressing to tubing at 3 x 15 Modified bench press—3 x 10—10 lbs progressing to 25 lbs Progressed to limited weight lifting using the Hammer strength machines (controlled apparatus) Bench press, incline press, shoulder press, shrugs, back shrugs, lateral raises (deltoid) (the only discomfort noted was during overhead motions such as the shoulder and incline presses) Progressed to free weights Participated in drills but no contact

Complications

Complications may occur as a result of a posterior SC joint dislocation. This athlete sustained a lateral shift of the trachea as a result of the posterior SC joint dislocation, causing him to feel as if there was an obstruction in his throat. The displaced medial end of the right clavicle was compressing the trachea, thus causing it to shift left of its normal position. Even though the athlete in this case presented with only minor complications, all signs and symptoms should be noted due to the possible development of more serious complications.

Serious complications from a posterior SC joint dislocation may occur when the medial end of the clavicle suddenly intrudes into the thoracic inlet and compresses vital structures of the superior mediastinum. These vital structures are located just posterior to the SC joint and include the major vessels of the neck (brachiocephalic and subclavian arteries and veins, jugular veins, and carotid arteries), brachial plexus, trachea, esophagus, apex of the lung, and vagus nerve.[4-6,8,9,11,15,19] Providing the only protection between these vital structures and the SC joint are the sternohyoid and sternothyroid muscles.[5] Complications include compression of the trachea and recurrent laryngeal nerve, causing dyspnea and vocal changes, particularly with movement of the ipsilateral arm, hoarseness of the voice, pressure on the brachial plexus leading to thoracic outlet syndrome, pressure on the subclavian vessels leading to thrombus formation, vascular insufficiency, obstruction of the carotid artery causing syncope, pneumothorax, hemothorax, and impingement of the esophagus leading to dysphagia.[18,19,21,22] Possible fatal complications include laceration of the major vessels and of the trachea.[9,23] Worman and Leagus[24] noted that 16 of 60 patients with posterior SC joint dislocations sustained complications involving the trachea, esophagus, and major vessels, with death occurring in two of 16 patients. In addition, late complications such as occlusion of the subclavian vein may occur and have been reported as late as 4.5 years post-injury.[7,25]

Diagnostic Techniques

Plain radiographs of the athlete's clavicle immediately following the injury were of little assistance in making a diagnosis. However, the team orthopedist suspected a more serious problem because the definition of the SC joint was lost on the right side. Typically, plain anteroposterior radiographs are notoriously unreliable in demonstrating clavicular dislocations because the anatomy of the region is confused by overlapping bony shadows.[4,6,26-28] With plain radiographs, the clavicles will be in alignment when a horizontal line is drawn through them. With a posterior SC joint dislocation, the medial end of the dislocated clavicle will be inferior to the horizontal line, thus noting asymmetry between the medial clavicular ends.[12,18]

Additional radiographic imaging using the Rockwood or "serendipity," confirmed the athlete's posterior SC joint dislocation. This view allows for comparison between the injured and uninjured SC joints and is helpful in assisting physicians with an injury diagnosis.[9,12] This is particularly important when an early diagnosis is crucial to a successful outcome, due to the possibility of major vascular complications.[12]

CT scans are ideally suited and the most reliable when diagnosing posterior SC joint dislocations.[4,5,8,12,13,15] CT scans are particularly useful, as they show both the dislocation and the anatomical detail of the major vessels, esophagus, and trachea in relation to the SC joint.[4,8,18]

Reduction Techniques

Closed reduction was the method utilized in this case to reduce the posteriorly displaced portion of the medial clavicle and was chosen because there was no danger of compromise to the mediastinal structures. A rolled-up towel was placed between the scapula to retract the shoulders while manual abduction was performed. The athlete's medial clavicle reduced immediately with little assistance from the physicians. Early closed reduction under general anesthesia is the method of choice as long as it is performed within 24 to 48 hours of the injury. Good results have been achieved as late as 5 days post-injury using a closed reduction technique.[1,2,15,20] However, the sooner the posterior SC dislocation is reduced, the less chance there is of developing long-term complications such as thoracic outlet syndrome.[2] All patients who have a posterior SC joint dislocation should be admitted to the hospital for at least 24 hours of observation after reduction.[18]

Open reduction for an SC joint dislocation is used when the patient is seen 72 hours post-injury, if the diagnosis is initially missed, or if complications arise from a closed reduction.[1,8] However, due to the potential complications from this injury, it is advisable to have a thoracic/vascular surgeon available for both open and closed reductions because the dislocated clavicle may act as a tamponade against a lacerated vessel, with subsequent severe hemorrhage on reduction.[7,24]

Biomechanical Considerations

Immediately following the injury, the supine position caused the athlete the greatest amount of pain due to the posterior sag of the glenohumeral joint, causing the medial end of the clavicle to press anteriorly against the brachial plexus. Therefore, the movement produced in the glenohumeral joint indirectly produced motion in the SC joint, thus increasing the athlete's pain.

During the early treatment phase and later stages of rehabilitation, certain movements were restricted. Abduction was limited because it forced the shoulder to retract, causing the medial end of the clavicle to shift anteriorly on the sternum. Horizontal extension was another limited motion that primarily occurred during the negative phase of the bench press. Also, during the terminal end of the positive phase of the bench press (horizontal flexion), the anterior stress on the clavicle with respect to the sternum causes the clavicle to shift posteriorly, recreating the mechanism of injury. Therefore, these exercises and movements were initially restricted because of the shearing forces they created at the SC joint.

SUMMARY

Posterior SC joint dislocations rarely occur in athletics. Therefore, this case study addressed the injury mechanism, clinical presentation, complications, diagnostic techniques, reduction techniques, and biomechanical considerations associated with a posterior SC joint dislocation. A rehabilitation program was developed and implemented based on recommendations from the trauma and orthopedic surgeons. Additional information was gathered from other physicians, athletic trainers, and physical therapists. Due to the close proximity of the SC joint to vital structures within the superior mediastinum, posterior dislocations may have potential life-threatening complications; therefore, the athletic trainer needs to be able to evaluate the injury, recognize the signs and symptoms, and refer the athlete to more definitive medical care. With proper management and acute care, the general prognosis for a posterior SC joint dislocation is excellent.

REFERENCES

1. Gazak S, Davidson SJ. Posterior sternoclavicular dislocations: Two case reports. *J Trauma*. 1984;24:80-81.
2. Leighton RK, Buhr AJ, Sinclair AM. Posterior sternoclavicular dislocations. *Can J Surg*. 1986;29:104-106.
3. Marker LB, Klareskov B. Posterior sternoclavicular dislocation: an American football injury. *Br J Sports Med*. 1996;30:71-72.
4. Weingarten MJ, Tash R, Klein RM, et al. Posterior dislocation of the sternoclavicular joint. *New York State Journal of Medicine*. 1985;85:225-226.
5. Jougon JB, Lepront DJ, Dromer CE. Posterior dislocation of the sternoclavicular joint leading to mediastinal compression. *Ann Thorac Surg*. 1996;61:711-713.
6. Kiroff GK, McClure DN, Skelley JW. Delayed diagnosis of posterior sternoclavicular joint dislocation. *Med J Aust*. 1996;164:242-243.
7. Martin SD, Altchek D, Erlanger S. Atraumatic posterior dislocation of the sternoclavicular joint. *Clin Orthop*. 1993;292:159-164.
8. Thomas DP, Davies A, Hoddinott HC. Posterior sternoclavicular dislocations a diagnosis easily missed. *Ann R Coll Surg Engl*. 1999;81:201-204.
9. Luhmann JD, Bassett GS. Posterior sternoclavicular epiphyseal separation presenting with hoarseness: A case report and discussion. *Pediatr Emerg Care*. 1998;14:130-132.
10. Noda M, Shiraishi H, Mizuno K. Chronic posterior sternoclavicular dislocation causing compression of a subclavian artery. *J Shoulder Elbow Surg*. 1997;6:564-569.

11. Yang J, Al-Etani H, Letts M. Diagnosis and treatment of posterior sternoclavicular joint dislocations in children. *Am J Orthop.* 1996;25:565-569.

12. Cope R, Riddervold HO, Shore JL, et al. Dislocations of the sternoclavicular joint: anatomical basis, etiologies, and radiologic diagnosis. *J Orthop Trauma.* 1991;5:379-384.

13. Cope R, Riddervold HO. Posterior dislocation of the sternoclavicular joint: report of two cases, with emphasis on radiologic management and early diagnosis. *Skeletal Radiol.* 1988;17:247-250.

14. Arnheim DD, Prentice WE. *Principles of Athletic Training.* 10th ed. Boston, Mass: McGraw-Hill Publishers; 2000.

15. Cope R. Dislocations of the sternoclavicular joint. *Skeletal Radiol.* 1993;22:233-238.

16. Rockwood CA, Green DP, Bucholz RW. *Fractures in Adults.* 3rd ed. Philadelphia, Pa: Lippincott; 1991.

17. Ono K, Inagawa H, Kiyota K, et al. Posterior dislocation of the sternoclavicular joint with obstruction of the innominate vein: case report. *J Trauma.* 1998;44:381-383.

18. Pearson MR, Leonard RB. Posterior sternoclavicular dislocation: a case report. *J Emerg Med.* 1994;12:783-787.

19. Williams CC. Posterior sternoclavicular joint dislocation. *Phys Sportsmed.* 1999;27:105-113.

20. Ferrandez L, Yubero J, Usabiaga L, et al. Sternoclavicular dislocation. Treatment and complications. *Ital J Orthop Traumatol.* 1988;14:349-355.

21. Penn I. The vascular complications of fractures of the clavicle. *J Trauma.* 1964;4:819-831.

22. Howard FM, Shafer SJ. Injuries to the clavicle with neurovascular complications. *J Bone Joint Surg Am.* 1965;47:1335-1346.

23. Greenlee DP. Posterior dislocation of the sternal end of the clavicle. *JAMA.* 1944;125:426-428.

24. Worman LW, Leagus C. Intrathoracic injury following retrosternal dislocation of the clavicle. *J Trauma.* 1967;7:416-423.

25. Stankler L. Posterior dislocation of the clavicle: a report of two cases. *Br J Surg.* 1962:164-168.

26. Abel MS. Symmetrical anteroposterior projections of the sternoclavicular joints with motion studies. *Radiology.* 1979;132:757-759.

27. Hobbs DW. Sternoclavicular joint: a new axial radiographic view. *Radiology.* 1968;90:801.

28. Destouet JM, Gilula LA, Murphy WA, et al. Computed tomography of the sternoclavicular joint and sternum. *Radiology.* 1981;138:123-128.

Chapter Eight

Arthroscopic Capsular Shift in a High School Athlete

Brian Pease, PT, ATC

INTRODUCTION

Multidirectional instability (MDI) is a common problem that occurs with young athletes, especially those involved in throwing activities. Most often these athletes present with pain in the shoulder related to an overuse phenomenon. This can occur with changes in training regimens, such as going from land-based to water activities in swimming, or stepping up training regimens in either throwing or volleyball. Athletes will present with pain, not only during activity, but also at rest and occasionally at night. Multidirectional instability typically presents as what appears to be rotator cuff tendonitis associated with "impingement" type symptoms; but given the patient's age and activity level, this is an unlikely diagnosis. Conservative care for patients with MDI poses a considerable challenge when working with the overhead athlete. This case will describe the presentation, rehabilitation, surgery, and post-operative management of a high school athlete with MDI.

INITIAL EXAMINATION

The subject of this case report was a 16-year-old high school junior who played varsity football and baseball. The young man presented during the football season with an 18-month history of intermittent anterior-lateral pain in his right dominant shoulder, exacerbated with weight training and throwing from the outfield. Rehabilitation focused on rotator cuff strengthening and was successful in decreasing pain, but the athlete was unable to return to unrestricted activity. He complained of occasional numbness and tingling down the arm and into the hand, and a sensation of a "dead arm" after hard throws from the outfield. Associated problems included pain that would wake him at night and a precipitous increase in the perception of shifting and clunking in the shoulder. The athlete did not report problems with short throwing or batting. The athlete was an otherwise happy young man with no other associated physical problems or previous shoulder surgery.

Physical examination revealed a well-developed male with full symmetrical ROM. Mild winging of the scapula was noted with eccentric control of scapular downward rotation when lowering the arm to the side. Resisted testing revealed 4/5 strength of the lower trapezius and serratus anterior. Radiographs and magnetic resonance imaging (MRI) revealed no evidence of degenerative change or rotator cuff pathology.

Cervical motion and upper quadrant testing failed to elicit symptoms, eliminating the cervical spine as a possible contributing factor to the athlete's complaints. Neurological exam of the upper extremities found that motor, sensory, and reflexes were all grossly intact, thus ruling out nerve root or peripheral nerve entrapment or irritation. Tenderness was noted at the supraspinatus, long head of the biceps, and infraspinatus tendon insertion areas. Initial examination findings are summarized in Table 8-1.

Table 8-1

SUMMARY OF INITIAL EXAMINATION FINDINGS

Clinical Test	Outcome
Cervical Spine Clearing	
Active range of motion	Negative
Quadrant test	Negative
Range of Motion	
Elevation	180 degrees
External rotation at 0 degrees	75 degrees
Internal rotation behind back	T6 (T3 uninvolved)
External rotation at 90 degrees	115 degrees (95 uninvolved)
Internal rotation at 90 degrees	85 degrees (90 uninvolved)
Strength	
Base internal rotation	Strong and pain-free
Base external rotation	Strong and pain-free
Abduction at 30 degrees	Strong and pain-free
Abduction with external rotation at 90 degrees	Strong and painful
Empty can test	Strong and painful
Glenohumeral Stability	
Load and shift test	2½+ posterior
Apprehension test	2+ inferior
Relocation Test	1½+ anterior
Sulcus sign	Positive for symptom replication
Tenderness	
Palpation of glenohumeral tissues	Tender supraspinatus, infraspinatus, and LH bicep tendons
Neurological Exam	
Motor, sensory, reflexes	Negative

CONSERVATIVE MANAGEMENT

After the initial examination, the surgeon diagnosed MDI with a possible labral tear, both of which were exacerbated with prolonged and vigorous overhead activities, in particular lifting weights and throwing. Given the timeline of approaching spring baseball and the patient's and family's desire to avoid surgery initially, a conservative course of care was deemed appropriate. We hoped that the athlete would respond to a more specific and comprehensive rehabilitation regimen. Under the guidance of an athletic trainer, the next 4 to 6 weeks of rehabilitation included a specific rotator cuff strengthening program along with application of tape to control abnormal glenohumeral motion. Activity was reduced to include only pain-free weight training and sports-related activity.

The patient began a home exercise program emphasizing anti-inflammatory care, relative rest, scapular stabilization, rotator cuff strengthening and endurance, and taping the glenohumeral joint. We felt that it was imperative to educate the athlete and his parents as to the various components of his rehabilitation program, and to stress his responsibility in performing these activities as prescribed. The patient was given this program based on the assumption that he would adhere to a daily regimen of rehabilitation in order to provide the greatest opportunity for maximal benefit. Notes were sent to the coach and athletic trainer informing them of the suggested treatment progression.

The athlete received a prescription for nonsteroidal anti-inflammatory drugs (NSAIDs) and was instructed to take them regularly and only in the dosage prescribed. The athlete was then educated on the application of ice for pain relief and inflammation control during his first 7 to 10 days of rehabilitation. We stressed the possibility that the initial exercise program might cause some unintended aching in the shoulder, and that the NSAIDs and ice would allow him to continue rehabilitation despite this short-term irritation.

The concept of relative rest, as applied to the athlete's shoulder, implies that we wanted the athlete to perform at a maximal pain-free level. Thus, any painful activities of daily living (ADLs), weight training activities, or recreational activities were stopped or modified as needed. We emphasized that the patient should continue to do what he could in terms of muscular and cardiovascular training.

A final component of the initial approach was to provide stabilization to the shoulder during ADL and exercise during the first 7 to 10 days of rehabilitation. Humeral head stabilization was provided by applying Cover Roll and Leukotape (Beiersdorf, Hamburg, Germany) to the glenohumeral joint for extrinsic stabilization. The tape was applied in a "V," with the apex at the deltoid insertion, the posterior strip anchored to the lateral one-third of the spine of the scapula, and the anterior strip anchored to the distal one-third of the clavicle. With the tape applied in this manner, the athlete was able to approach an active cocking position of the shoulder without pain.

Specific rotator cuff strengthening focused on the supraspinatus and infraspinatus muscles. The patient started with prone horizontal abduction with external rotation at 100 degrees abduction, sidelying external rotation, and standing elevation with neutral rotation (scaption) to 100 degrees elevation.

Scapular stabilization exercises for the lower trapezius and serratus anterior were also prescribed. Lower trapezius stabilization included having the patient lie prone and lift his arm forward and upward approximately 30 degrees from his head. To strengthen the serratus anterior, the athlete performed wall push-ups, which progressed to hands and knees cat/camel exercises, and eventually to modified and full push-ups. A summary of conservative treatment intervention, goals, and parameters is in Table 8-2.

Initial changes in pain, strength, and perceived stability were noted at the follow-up subjective and objective examination. After progressing through conservative rehabilitation for 6 months, it became apparent that nonoperative treatment was not going to return the athlete to his desired level of function. In March of his junior year, the athlete opted to undergo an arthroscopic capsular shift.

Surgical Intervention

The patient was taken to the operating room and, after general anesthesia, was placed in the left lateral decubitous position. Examination of the shoulder under fluoroscopic control revealed frank dislocation posteriorly and anteriorly. The shoulder was taken through a full range of abduction and external rotation, and again revealed a frank anterior dislocation. Full flexion with a posteriorly directed force resulted in posterior dislocation. Following exam under fluoroscopy and sterile preparation of the patient, the arm was placed in a shoulder holder device.

A posterior visualization portal, an anterior transarticular portal (adjacent to the long head of the biceps), and a second anterior portal superior to the subscapularis (midglenoid portal) were established. Inspection of the entire shoulder joint was performed, revealing a posterior-superior SLAP (superior labrum anterior to posterior) lesion and evidence of a small rotator cuff tear of the posterior aspect of the supraspinatus tendon at the confluence with the infraspinatus tendon. Redundancy of the posterior and inferior capsule, as well as the anterior capsular ligaments, was noted. No defects were found on the articular surfaces of the humerus or glenoid, and no lesions were visualized in the subscapularis or anterior supraspinatus tendons. There was

Table 8-2
SUMMARY OF CONSERVATIVE MANAGEMENT

Intervention	Goal	Sets and Repetitions
Activity modification	Allow tissue healing	
Ice application	Inhibit pain and inflammation	20 minutes, 3 x daily
Shoulder taping	Reduce abnormal forces	Applied every 48 hours
Rotator cuff strengthening	Provide dynamic stabilization	Three to five sets of 20 to 30 repetitions; 0 to 2.5 lbs
Scapular strengthening	Provide foundation for glenohumeral function	Three to five sets of 20 repetitions
Proprioceptive exercises	Increase afferent feedback	Three to five sets of 10 to 20 repetitions

no frank Bankart lesion, and though redundant, the anterior capsular ligaments were attached. A positive drive-through sign was noted using the arthroscope. Further anterior visualization revealed no loose bodies in the subscapularis recess, and the tendon attachment was sound. There was no evidence of a SLAP lesion at the location of the biceps anchor.

An arthroscopic trimmer was used to clean up the small partial-thickness tear in the posterior portion of the supraspinatus tendon, and also to debride the posterior-superior labral tear. A slotted shaver blade was used to roughen the synovial lining of the capsular structures. A suture hook was used to pass a nylon-coated wire to plicate the anterior capsular ligaments and eliminate approximately 1 cm of redundancy. This was done at the 5:30 position of the capsulolabral complex, bringing the inferior capsular structures to the glenoid labrum. A suture was passed through the labrum and capsular tissues to the appropriate position, approximating the ligaments to the labrum once the arthroscopic knot was tied. Two more sutures were passed through the anterior structures in similar fashion, eliminating much of the redundancy and providing an anterior soft tissue bumper to the anterior aspect of the shoulder. Similar methods were used to secure the posterior and posterior-inferior portions of the capsulolabral complex. The shoulder was gently taken through full ROM with no evidence of dislocation and was placed in a sling in neutral rotation and 15 degrees abduction.

POSTOPERATIVE MANAGEMENT

Postoperatively, the patient's shoulder was placed in a sling and worn full-time for 6 weeks, removing it only for bathing. The patient began passive shoulder rotation and active elbow, wrist, and hand exercises on postoperative day 1. Passive external rotation was initiated with the elbow resting on the sling at the side. Forward flexion was begun by performing pendulum exercises to avoid undue stress on the posterior capsule, as may occur when passive elevation is performed in supine. No active motion of the shoulder was allowed during this period of rehabilitation.

The patient was evaluated 4 weeks postoperatively. Postoperative clinical findings are in Table 8-3. Passive shoulder flexion from a seated position using over-the-door pulleys was initiated at this time. Passive external rotation was increased to tolerance, and pendulum exercises were increased to 110 to 120 degrees of forward flexion. Pain-free, submaximal isometric exercises in all planes were added with the arm in neutral, elbow at the side position.

Six weeks after surgery no passive assessment of supine external or internal rotation was made. Use of the immobilizer was discontinued and the athlete was allowed to begin active ROM exercises in all available pain-free planes of motion with an emphasis on elevation, external rotation, and horizontal abduction with external rotation. The patient was not allowed to push, pull, or lift anything outside of his rehabilitation program.

Table 8-3					
POSTOPERATIVE CLINICAL FINDINGS					
Postoperative Time					
	4 Weeks	**6 Weeks**	**8 Weeks**	**3 Months**	**4 Months**
<u>Range of Motion</u>					
Flexion	100 degrees	125 degrees	140 degrees	180 degrees	Full active motion as compared to noninvolved side
Abduction	90 degrees	NT	180 degrees	NT	
External rotation	45 degrees	65 degrees	65 degrees	75 degrees	
Internal rotation	NT	L2	Lacked 1 inch	T5	
<u>Strength</u>					
Supraspinatus	NT	4/5	4+/5	5/5	5/5
Infraspinatus	NT	4/5	4+/5	5/5	5/5
Serratus anterior	NT	4/5	4+/5	5/5	5/5
Subscapularis	NT	4+/5	5/5	5/5	5/5

Eight weeks after surgery the patient displayed 80 degrees of external rotation at 90 degrees of abduction. Mild tenderness was noted at the supraspinatus tendon. One to 2 lbs of weight were added to active ROM exercises to strengthen the rotator cuff, working toward five sets of 20 pain-free repetitions.

Three months postoperatively, the patient reported no problems or limitations with activities of daily living and rated his shoulder at 80% of his desired level of function. The patient was encouraged to increase resistance from 2 lbs up to 5 for the rotator cuff program and to begin gentle stretching into external rotation in an abducted position. Scapular stabilization exercises were begun in partial weightbearing for the serratus anterior and in a prone position for the lower trapezius. The patient was instructed to progress toward weightbearing serratus anterior strengthening and plyometric activities with a small Plyoball. He was allowed to begin running and gently swinging a bat as long as these activities were pain-free.

Four and one-half months after surgery, examination revealed that the patient had full passive supine external and internal rotation without apprehension. A load and shift test revealed 1+ anterior, inferior, and posterior translation. The athlete began a light throwing program supervised by the athletic trainer at school and was allowed to play baseball as a designated hitter during a summer baseball league. Both activities were tolerated very well. The throwing regimen advanced from light toss to full, unrestricted throwing from 4 ½ months to 6 months after surgery. Strengthening progressed to an endurance bias, with five sets of 30 to 40 repetitions. Table 8-4 summarizes the rehabilitation activities and timing after surgery.

Reassessment at 6 months revealed the patient had returned to full, unrestricted, pain-free activity. The athlete reported no instability or "dead arm" sensations. ROM was full, pain-free, and symmetrical. The patient reported excellent satisfaction with the result and was released to full, unrestricted activity. On follow-up 9 months after surgery, the patient had a normal physical exam and was involved in an unrestricted weight training and off-season throwing program.

Table 8-4

SUMMARY OF POSTOPERATIVE REHABILITATION PROGRESSION

	Range of Motion	Strength	Activity
Immediate postoperative	Active elbow, wrist, and hand ROM Passive shoulder external rotation to 25 degrees		None (wearing a sling)
2 weeks	Passive external rotation 45 degrees Pendulum to 70 to 90 degrees		None (wearing a sling)
4 weeks	Passive external rotation to tolerance Pendulum to 110 degrees	Submaximal isometrics	None (wearing a sling)
6 weeks	Active ROM in all planes Passive elevation and external rotation at 90 degrees	High repetitions, no-load external rotation, scaption, and Hughston exercises	Activities of daily living
8 weeks	Passive elevation and external rotation at 90 degrees	High repetitions, low-load external rotation, scaption, and Hughston exercises	Activities of daily living
3 months	Passive ROM as needed	Rotator cuff endurance Scapular stabilization exercises	Light toss, swing
4 1/2 months		Rotator cuff endurance Scapular stabilization exercises Plyometrics	Throw and swing
6 months			Full participation

SUMMARY AND CONCLUSION

In summary, this 16-year-old high school baseball player with MDI presented with an 18-month history of shoulder pain and functional limitations, and failed to return to his desired sport activities after 6 months of specific, supervised rehabilitation. Surgical treatment with an arthroscopic capsular plication, followed by

6 months of structured and progressively more independent rehabilitation activities, resulted in an excellent result as measured by ROM restoration, absence of instability signs, and return to full, pain-free throwing and weight training. Coordination of the progression of activity and the monitoring of rehabilitation between the physician, physical therapist, and athletic trainer was critical in the ultimate success of treatment of this throwing athlete with MDI.

MDI can be successfully treated in some cases with rehabilitation alone; however, when conservative management fails to restore full pain-free function, arthroscopic plication of the inferior glenohumeral ligaments performed on the glenoid side can be successful in restoring full functional abilities, even in recalcitrant cases. This is true not only for young athletes, but for any individual for whom capsular laxity is a significant component of clinical presentation and subsequent treatment focus. The athletic trainer, physical therapist, and physician must approach the physical examination and management of MDI with a well coordinated, problem-oriented approach.

REFERENCES

1. Burkhead WZ, Rockwood CA. Treatment of instability of the shoulder with an exercise program. *J Bone Joint Surg Am.* 1992;74:890-896.

2. Forwell LA, Carnahan H. Proprioception during manual aiming in individuals with shoulder instability and controls. *J Orthop Sports Phys Ther.* 1996;23:111-119.

3. Hintermeister RA, Lange GW, Schultheis JM, et al. Electromyographic activity and applied load during shoulder rehabilitation exercises using elastic resistance. *Am J Sports Med.* 1998;26:210-220.

4. Litchfield R, Hawkins R, Dillman CJ, et al. Rehabilitation for the overhead athlete. *J Orthop Sports Phys Ther.* 1993;18:433-441.

5. Wilk KE, Arrigo CA, Andrews JR. Current concepts: the stabilizing structures of the glenohumeral joint. *J Orthop Sports Phys Ther.* 1997;25:364-379.

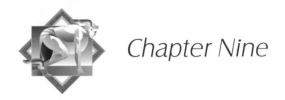

Chapter Nine

Rotator Cuff Tear in a Collegiate Football Player

Gary Misamore, MD, Ralph Reiff, ATC

INTRODUCTION

This case study reviews the evaluation and management of a collegiate football player who sustained a severe partial tear of the rotator cuff. Minor partial tears, overuse tendonitis, strains, and contusions of the rotator cuff are common in young athletes. However, severe partial tears and full-thickness tears of the rotator cuff are relatively rare in young athletes. This report demonstrates that the history and physical examination may not be conclusive in distinguishing between rotator cuff tendonitis and a rotator cuff tear. This case study outlines the progressive rehabilitation program utilized in preparing this athlete for his return to full activity, demonstrating the relatively long time typically needed to achieve full recovery from such major rotator cuff injuries.

HISTORY

The patient was a 21-year-old NCAA Division 1 football player who injured his nondominant left shoulder in late October during a football game. The patient did not recall a single significant precipitating injury, but did have a number of minor injuries to the shoulder during that game, caused by falls directly onto the shoulder and by falls onto the outstretched arm. Despite discomfort in the shoulder, he continued to play through the rest of the game. He experienced increasing discomfort after the game, and by the next morning was hardly able to lift his arm due to the pain. The pain he experienced was localized to the posterior aspect of the shoulder. He had no history of prior shoulder injuries or symptoms.

EXAMINATION

Physical examination by the athletic trainer immediately after the game revealed no obvious site of tenderness about the shoulder. Rotational movements were full, but there was limitation of overhead elevation secondary to discomfort. Physical examination of the shoulder performed by an orthopedic surgeon 6 days after the injury revealed only minimal tenderness over the supraspinatus tendon near its insertion into the greater tuberosity. Active elevation of the arm was limited because of pain at 120 degrees on the affected left side compared with 160 degrees on the right. External rotation remained full at 65 degrees bilaterally. Internal rotation was also full bilaterally. Accurate testing of strength in flexion and abduction could not be performed at that time because of the patient's inability to provide active resistance during manual muscle testing secondary to pain. He did demonstrate normal strength of both internal rotation and external rotation without significant discomfort. There was no palpable crepitus anywhere on the shoulder during examination. There were no signs of impingement and no findings of instability of the glenohumeral joint.

INITIAL MANAGEMENT

Considering the age of the athlete and the absence of a significant identifiable injury event, we felt it was unlikely that he had suffered a major tear of the rotator cuff. A diagnosis of rotator cuff strain was made and an aggressive course of conservative care was initiated by the athletic trainer with the intention of returning the athlete to competition quickly in order to allow him to complete the last 2 weeks of the football season. The patient was treated with over-the-counter analgesics for pain, and he was provided with a sling for support and comfort. He began a course of rehabilitation consisting of electrical stimulation, phonophoresis, and cryotherapy, along with exercises for restoration of shoulder motion. The patient was treated with four therapy sessions per day during the first week post-injury.

Although the patient did have gradual improvement of shoulder symptoms with this treatment regimen, he experienced persistent discomfort and disability that prevented him from returning to competition during the last few weeks of the season. Conservative treatment was continued for approximately 8 weeks from the time of onset. The progression of recovery reached a plateau approximately 4 weeks after the injury. Examination by the physician 8 weeks after the injury again revealed weakness of forward elevation associated with pain. At that time, there was no residual cuff tenderness and there were no signs of rotator cuff impingement. There still was no evidence of instability of the shoulder.

DIAGNOSTIC IMAGING

X-rays taken at 6 days after the injury were normal. Magnetic resonance imaging (MRI), performed 8 weeks post-injury, revealed a severe partial thickness tear of the rotator cuff involving the superficial portion of the supraspinatus tendon. There was no evidence of extension of the tear into the deep portion of the cuff on the joint surface of the tendon. There was a small accumulation of bursal fluid in the subacromial space. There was minimal narrowing of the acromial humeral space and no spur formation or other abnormalities of the acromion.

OPERATIVE TREATMENT

Persistence of significant pain and weakness despite nonsurgical management, combined with the significant MRI findings, led us to recommend surgical treatment. The patient was taken to surgery on January 16, 1997, at which time arthroscopy revealed a minor partial tear of the rotator cuff on the joint surface of the tendon. A limited debridement of the tear on that surface of the tendon was performed. Loose tissue around the tear margins was removed so that all margins of the tendon in the area of tearing were smooth and stable. Arthroscopic inspection of the subacromial space revealed significant tightness of that space but no fraying of the acromion or rotator cuff that would suggest a process of chronic impingement. We found a tear of the superficial portion of the rotator cuff, without extension to the deepest fibers of the tendon where the joint surface partial tear had been identified during arthroscopy of the joint. We determined that this tear affected more that 50% of the thickness of the supraspinatus tendon. Since the tear was relatively large, and the patient had failed to improve with conservative care, surgical repair of the torn rotator cuff was indicated.

The rotator cuff was decompressed by arthroscopic acromioplasty, then an open repair of the tendon was performed. Surgical exposure of the rotator cuff was accomplished through a longitudinal split in the deltoid muscle along the line of the muscle fibers. The deltoid split was extended only 4 cm distally from the lateral edge of the acromion in order to avoid injury to the recurrent axillary nerve. The torn area of the rotator cuff was minimally debrided. The medial aspect of the greater tuberosity at the normal cuff insertion site was abraded to create a bleeding surface of bone in order to enhance healing. Tunnels were created through the tuberosity from the abraded area medially to the cortex of the tuberosity laterally. Multiple sutures were placed through the margin of the torn supraspinatus tendon, and those sutures were passed through the transosseous tunnels, exiting on the lateral side of the greater tuberosity. As those sutures were tied laterally, the torn rotator cuff tendon was securely reapproximated to the prepared bone bed at the normal cuff insertion site.

Immediately postoperatively, cryotherapy was initiated with a Cryo/Cuff. The patient was treated with nonsteroidal anti-inflammatory drugs and narcotic analgesics in order to control pain. The arm was protected in a shoulder immobilizer.

POSTOPERATIVE REHABILITATION

Surgery was performed on an outpatient basis and the patient was released to the athletic training staff for postoperative care. The physician, physical therapist, and athletic training staff established the following rehabilitation protocol.

Week 1

Rehabilitation goals for the first week focused on protection of the limb for early healing and for reduction of pain and swelling. The patient was instructed to wear an immobilizer at all times except when bathing. The athletic trainers assisted the athlete with wound care and pain management during the first week. Therapeutic modalities included electrical stimulation and ice packs twice daily for 20 minutes each. The athlete was instructed and assisted in pendulum exercises. Gentle range of motion (ROM) exercises using a pulley for elevation of the arm and a broom handle for external rotation, were initiated. The athletic trainer assisted the patient with performance of these passive ROM exercises. In addition, the athletic trainer administered massage to the affected arm, upper back, and cervical regions. During this time, the athlete indicated that pain during therapy reached a maximum of 6 on a 0 to 10 scale.

RATIONALE

The experience of the physician, physical therapist, and athletic trainer has demonstrated that aggressive pain management and early initiation of ROM can be very beneficial in achieving successful outcomes. It remains the opinion of the athletic trainer that massage used early after surgery helps to desensitize the affected extremity and allows for the development of a good rapport between the athlete and the athletic trainer, which will prove to be beneficial during later phases of rehabilitation.

Weeks 2 to 6

Rehabilitation goals during this time frame were achievement of full ROM and initiation of early strengthening exercises. Additionally, efforts were continued for reduction of swelling and pain. During this phase, the athlete continued to wear the immobilizer except during bathing. The athletic training staff continued to perform massage to the upper extremity and also initiated gentle massage of the surgical scar in order to desensitize that area. The athlete continued with progressive passive ROM exercises using the pulley for elevation and a broom handle for external rotation. In addition, the athletic trainer performed joint mobilization and joint distraction. Postural exercises for the upper torso were initiated and included head tilts, chin tucks, and scapular squeezes. The athletic trainer also initiated active scapular elevation, depression, protraction and retraction exercises, exercises for scapulothoracic joint mobilization, and stabilization. During the early phases of this time period, the athlete indicated a pain rating of 4 during therapy but little or no pain during daily activities. By the end of this phase, the pain rating decreased to 2/10 during exercise.

RATIONALE

Although early restoration of motion is important for satisfactory outcome from this surgery, all exercises during the early phases of healing must be performed with caution. The rotator cuff repair is relatively fragile and early active use of the arm for exercises can cause disruption of the surgical repair.

Weeks 6 to 12

Objective data for ROM and strength are in Table 9-1. Six weeks after surgery the patient was allowed to discard the arm immobilizer. More aggressive stretching for the end ROM was initiated, active ROM exercises were begun, and the patient was gradually advanced into resistive strengthening as tolerated. Treatment

Table 9-1		
POSTOPERATIVE WEEK 6 PHYSICIAN EVALUATION		
	Left	Right
Tenderness	None	None
Motion:		
• Active elevation	90 degrees	160 degrees
• Passive elevation	115 degrees	160 degrees
• Active external rotation	20 degrees	65 degrees
• Passive external rotation	45 degrees	65 degrees
• Strength	Not tested	Not tested

by the athletic trainers included hot/cold contrast treatments and myofascial pull of the arm to enhance ROM. Theraband (Hygenic Corp, Akron, Ohio) strengthening exercises were initiated in the planes of flexion, extension, external rotation, and internal rotation. Approximately 9 weeks postoperatively, the patient achieved full ROM; rehabilitation now focused on strength development. Early in this phase, the athlete graded pain at 2/10 during exercise and as pain-free during activities of daily living. By the late portions of this phase, the patient graded rehabilitation pain as 0/10.

Weeks 14 to 20

Strength training was advanced under the direction of the athletic trainer and the strength coach. In addition to working on rotator cuff muscles, focus also turned to the development of large muscle groups in the weight room. Strength training on the impulse machine was performed eccentrically and concentrically. The athlete was completely pain-free for all rehabilitation exercises, strength training, and daily activities during this phase. Results of ROM and strength assessment are in Table 9-2.

Functional Progression

Throughout the patient's postoperative recovery there was significant emphasis on maintaining general conditioning of the athlete, as well as maintaining involvement with his peer group of athletes. It has been our impression that injured athletes can suffer psychologically while recovering from a significant injury. Due to withdrawal from sports participation, the athlete may lose his "athlete identity." To alleviate this psychological response, the entire athletic department worked to integrate the athlete into all activities of his peer group in which he was able to participate. Placing the athlete into a leadership role with his teammates, requiring him to maintain the schedule and rules of the team, and holding him accountable for maintaining all requirements of his rehabilitation sessions are a few tactics we used to aid the psychological healing of the injured athlete.

During the first 4 weeks after surgery, the athlete was placed on a cardiovascular conditioning program of low-impact aerobic activity. During that early postoperative phase, the patient did have periods of moderate discomfort in his shoulder due to the shoulder rehabilitation exercises; therefore, it was necessary for us to remain flexible in our demands. By 4 weeks postoperatively, the patient was quite comfortable and from that point on was able to maintain a reasonable level of aerobic activity. He participated in an endurance-based lower extremity and torso weight training program under the direction of the strength coach and the athletic training staff. The athlete remained active on a stationary bike and treadmill. By 8 weeks postoperatively the patient had comfortable motion in his shoulder, allowing him to produce power swings of his arm. At that point he was able to participate in higher intensity cardiovascular training.

Table 9-2		
POSTOPERATIVE WEEK 14 PHYSICIAN EVALUATION		
	Left	Right
Tenderness	None	None
Motion:		
• Active elevation	155 degrees	160 degrees
• Passive elevation	160 degrees	160 degrees
• Active external rotation	60 degrees	65 degrees
• Passive external rotation	65 degrees	65 degrees
Strength (isometric measurements):		
• Flexion	27 lbs	33 lbs
• Abduction	23 lbs	28 lbs
• External rotation	36 lbs	33 lbs

While cardiovascular conditioning and torso and lower extremity strength were maintained, upper extremity activities focused on proprioceptive activities along with the previously described shoulder rehabilitation program.

The athlete performed all rapid response and catch activities while positioned on a minitrampoline to increase coordination and confidence.

Clinical Outcome

Five months postoperatively, the patient stated that subjectively he felt as though he had recovered completely. Objective examination at that time was essentially normal. The patient was released to proceed with normal weightlifting and conditioning in preparation for the next football season. Re-examination immediately before initiation of football practice (7 months postoperatively) again revealed a normal shoulder in all regards. At that point, the patient was released to full contact in football with no residual restrictions. The patient played through the remainder of his collegiate career without further symptoms or problems relative to the shoulder.

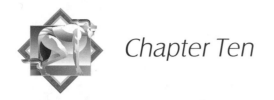

Chapter Ten

Open Anterocapsulolabral Reconstruction in Overhead Athletes

George J. Davies, MEd, PT, SCS, ATC, CSCS, Charles Giangarra, MD

INTRODUCTION

Multiple shoulder disorders have been associated with overhead athletes, including instability, impingement syndrome, tendonitis, and rotator cuff tear. Although most athletes will respond to nonoperative treatment, restoring athletes to their prior competitive level following surgery has been unpredictable. The loss of throwing ability after rotator cuff surgery, acromioplasty, or rotator cuff repair has been documented in the literature.[1] In addition, the loss of motion associated with surgical reconstruction for instability has left the athletes with stable shoulders, but not enough motion to continue to compete in their sport at the same competitive level.[2-4] The anterocapsulolabral reconstruction and its subsequent modifications were developed to restore preinjury level of function in overhead athletes with anterior instability.[5-7]

We will present the cases of two overhead athletes who underwent this procedure, a subsequent rehabilitation program, and returned to their prior level of competitive sports. The first patient was an elite high school swimmer who required surgery after 1 year of nonoperative treatment for shoulder pain. The second athlete was a National Collegiate Athletic Association (NCAA) Division III baseball player who required the procedure secondary to chronic shoulder pain in order to continue to compete at the collegiate level.

PATIENT

The patient was a 13-year-old female who presented to the office with a 1-year history of right dominant shoulder pain. The patient was an accomplished swimmer and had been competing for 4 years prior to the onset of her symptoms.

The patient described an insidious onset of anterior shoulder pain, which progressed to the point where she was unable to participate in practice or competition. She also had pain with activities of daily living. She began a rehabilitation program that included over-the-counter nonsteroidal anti-inflammatory medications without relief. She was then referred to our institution for evaluation.

On physical examination, the patient was noted to be hyperelastic with a thumb to forearm distance of 0 degrees, recurvatum of the elbow, and 125 degrees of glenohumeral external rotation with the arm abducted to 90 degrees. She had posterior tenderness along the infraspinatus muscle, with tenderness over the lateral border of the acromion and the long head of the biceps tendon. She had a positive Neer and Hawkins impingement sign. Rotator cuff strength was excellent against manual muscle testing. Stability examination revealed increased laxity in the anterior/posterior direction with load and shift test. Sulcus sign was graded as 1+ and symmetric. Radiographs were normal for her age.

Prescription nonsteroidal anti-inflammatory medication was prescribed. Swimming activity was discontinued and she restarted physical therapy for anti-inflammatory modalities. She progressed to a scapulothoracic and rotator cuff rehabilitation program.

Four months later, the patient was pain-free, but computerized Cybex (Lunnex Inc, Ronkonkona, NY) isokinetic dynamometer testing still revealed weakness. Rehabilitation was continued; at 6 months post initial presentation she was placed in aquatic therapy and started on a progressive return to swimming program. Eight months after her presentation she returned to swimming competitively without pain and was discharged from acute care. One month later, the patient returned with increased pain and the feeling of her arm going dead with swimming.

The physical examination at this time indicated a return of the positive impingement signs. She was also noted to have mild apprehension and pain with abduction and external rotation and a positive relocation test. Surgery was scheduled shortly thereafter—approximately 1 year following her initial presentation to our office. At arthroscopy, the patient was noted to have a Jobe type III shoulder, with instability and secondary impingement due to hyperlaxity.

POSTOPERATIVE REHABILITATION

The shoulder functions most frequently in athletics as a link in a kinetic chain of sequentially activated body segments, as described by Kibler[8] and Pink, et al.[9] The specific sequence of activation depends on the sport and activity, but all basically go in a proximal to distal direction. The activation sequence is the most biomechanically efficient to allow for generation of large forces and large accelerations to the arm.[10] Studies have shown that 54% of the force and 51% of the kinetic energy delivered to an athletic implement (such as a tennis racquet) through the shoulder is created by the lower legs, hip, and trunk.[8]

POSTURE AWARENESS/TRAINING

Patient education is critical when addressing posture. If the patient's awareness of posture can be internalized with various methods, then perhaps posture can also be permanently improved.

RESTORATION OF NORMAL JOINT ARTHROKINEMATICS

Mobilization techniques, heating and stretching, and self-stretching exercises were used to create a plastic deformation for the areas of the capsule (noncontractile tissue) that were hypomobile. Static stretching and proprioceptive neuromuscular facilitation (PNF) contract-relax techniques were used to increase the flexibility of the muscle/tendon unit (contractile). These treatments were used simultaneously along with the various strengthening exercises. Our philosophy is that as patients gain passive range of motion (ROM), it is necessary to concomitantly improve dynamic stability of the newly acquired motion for it to become functional.

RANGE OF MOTION EXERCISES

The patient performed a home exercise program of self-stretching and ROM exercises. Figures 10-1 through 10-3 demonstrate examples of exercises the patient used in her home exercise programs. When the patient was in the clinic, heating in a stretched position and mobilization techniques were used to create a plastic deformation in the noncontractile and scar tissues to assist the patient in regaining full ROM. Additionally, PNF contract-relax techniques were used to increase the flexibility of the contractile units. The goals were to have the patient achieve full ROM approximately 8 weeks after surgery.

THERAPEUTIC EXERCISE PROGRAM

The design of the therapeutic exercise program followed the exercise progression continuum advocated by Davies.[11] This exercise progression continuum uses the following sequence of exercises and progression:
- Multiple angle isometrics—submaximal intensity
- Multiple angle isometrics—maximal intensity
- Short arc exercises—submaximal intensity
- Short arc exercises—maximal intensity

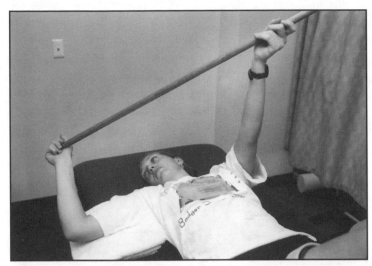

Figure 10-1. Self range of motion stretching exercises to increase external rotation.

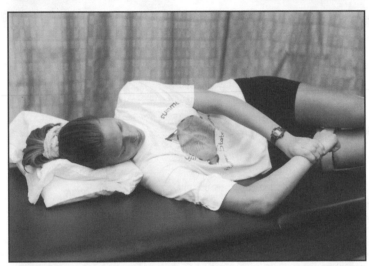

Figure 10-2. Self range of motion stetching exercises to increase internal rotation.

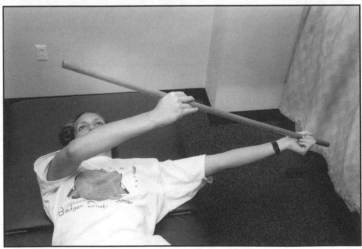

Figure 10-3. Self range of motion stretching exercises to increase horizontal adduction.

Figure 10-4. Concept rower for total body training and muscular endurance and a posterior dominant shoulder.

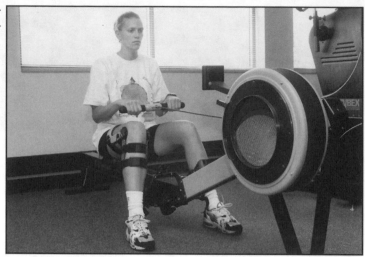

- Full ROM—submaximal intensity
- Full ROM—maximal intensity

Most exercises were performed in a super set fashion, meaning the agonist/antagonistic muscles were exercised in a reciprocal manner to maintain muscle balance in the shoulder complex by working opposing muscles. It also saved time in the clinic because the patient did not have to wait for a muscle's recovery phase, since the muscle that is not exercising is having a relative rest period. The patients' programs used three sets of 10 repetitions at a comfortable working weight based on the pathology and particular patient limitations.

Total Body Strengthening

The patient participated in total body strengthening (TBS) programs beginning with the legs as the foundation.[12] Performing squats or leg press exercises worked the major muscle groups in the legs. Furthermore, specificity of training, such as adductor muscle group training used in the breaststroke for the swimmer, were incorporated. The patient also was encouraged to participate in a total body conditioning program in which she worked on exercises for strengthening her trunk muscles through core stabilization exercises. Total body conditioning was particularly important for this patient because of her interest in returning to competitive sports.

Many exercises can be incorporated to accomplish the total body training. One method of training uses a Versa-Climber (Heart Rate, Inc, Costa Mesa, Calif) in which cardiovascular, lower extremity, and upper extremity exercises occur simultaneously.

Upper body ergometer cycling was also used for 10 minutes with the patients forward cycling and retrocycling. The emphasis of cycling direction is based on the patient's particular pathology. In this case, because of the history of an anterior-inferior subluxation and the surgical stabilization to correct the problem, the emphasis in cycling was on retrocycling to create a posterior dominant shoulder. Using a Concept Rower (Concept2, Inc, Morrisville, Vt) with just the legs also helped emphasize development of posterior power and endurance (the concept of a posterior dominant shoulder will be discussed in more detail later in this chapter) (Figure 10-4). These exercises were used as a warm-up for endurance training of the trunk, scapulothoracic musculature, shoulder area, and distal arm.

Scapulothoracic Exercises

The scapulothoracic joint is a dynamic base of support that provides efficient functioning of the glenohumeral joint. Consequently, exercises were initiated for this area with emphasis specific for the athlete. Concentric contractions were the focus for the athlete. Scapulothoracic stabilization training was performed with emphasis on the four core exercises advocated by Moseley, et al:[14]

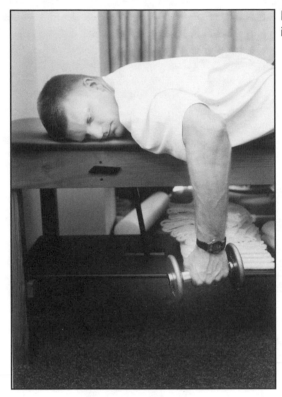

Figure 10-5. Scapulothoracic exercises using a rowing motion for the retractors.

1. Decline bench press with a plus (protraction at the end of the ROM) and a neutral grip or dumbbell presses with a plus. The decline bench position was used to prevent compressing the subacromial space and to strengthen the anterior scapulothoracic muscles.
2. Decline rowing motion with a neutral grip or dumbbells with scapulothoracic retraction against gravity (Figure 10-5). Decline rowing also helped prevent compression of the subacromial space and strengthened the posterior muscles to promote a posterior dominant shoulder.
3. Press-ups. Press-up exercises recruit the most electromyographical (EMG) activity of both the scapulothoracic and glenohumeral joints and were used to strengthen the shoulder girdle depressors.
4. Scaption with the thumb up. This exercise strengthened the superior muscles of the scapulothoracic area. Each of these four exercises was performed in a super set fashion.

Total Arm Strength

Additional exercises using similar principles to those described above were applied for total arm strength (TAS) training response. The muscles of the elbow, forearm, wrist, and hands were also exercised to strengthen the entire kinetic chain of the upper extremity.[15,16]

Glenohumeral Joint Exercises

In our opinion, the rotator cuff muscles are the key to a shoulder rehabilitation program. Based on our recent research and empirically based clinical experiences, developing functional stabilization and a dynamic caudal glide of the glenohumeral joint is critical. Therefore, much of the training that we incorporated used various rotational exercises for the rotator cuff muscles, placing the shoulder and arm in different positions. Furthermore, developing a posterior dominant shoulder is critical for rehabilitation of most patients with shoulder problems, particularly those with anterior instability problems. Our recent research demonstrated that patients with rotator cuff impingement syndromes secondary to anterior instabilities demonstrated a specific external rotator deficit.[12,17-24]

Various therapeutic exercise programs have been advocated for treating dysfunctions of the glenohumeral joint.[12,19,25-37] This is an appropriate clinical decision because weakness of the rotator cuff muscles has been shown to correlate with shoulder impairments.[17,38-45] The various therapeutic exercise programs advanced for strengthening the rotator cuff muscles have included research on EMG analysis,[19,27,39,46-49] cadaveric studies,[50] studies using isokinetics as the primary exercise modality,[43,45,46,51-57] and various methodological training studies to improve performance.[21,51,54,56,58-61]

Glenohumeral joint exercise training was performed with emphasis on the four core exercises recommended by Townsend, et al:[19]

1. Glenohumeral flexion to strengthen the anterior muscles of the glenohumeral joint.
2. Prone external rotation and horizontal extension of the glenohumeral joint to strengthen the posterior structures of the glenohumeral joint.
3. Press-ups were utilized to recruit the scapulothoracic and glenohumeral joints, as well as to strengthen the shoulder girdle depressors.
4. Scaption with the thumb down ("empty can position") because internal rotation of the glenohumeral joint prestretches the supraspinatus and increases the EMG activity. Although this is recommended as one of the four core exercises of the glenohumeral joint, it oftentimes iatrogenically causes increased pain and inflammation, partially because internal rotation of the glenohumeral joint is also the common impingement position of the joint. Therefore, we caution clinicians to be careful with this position. Itoi, et al[62] recently determined that more pain was observed in the "empty can" test position compared to the "full can" test position. The authors recommended that the "full can" position may be more beneficial in the clinical setting for testing. We expand this concept to rehabilitation suggesting that the "full can position" creates fewer iatrogenic complaints of pain when patients isolate the supraspinatus muscle during exercises.

Kinesthetic/Proprioception Exercises

Research indicates that patients with shoulder instabilities have kinesthetic deficits and that appropriate surgery and rehabilitation can change these deficits.[12,54,63-69] Although controversy exists as to the best way to rehabilitate the shoulder for kinesthetic deficits, it is an important aspect of the rehabilitation program that needs to be addressed.[12,69,70] We recently presented a prospective, randomized, controlled clinical trial to try and determine the effectiveness of our rehabilitation intervention.[60] Because of several limitations of a prospective clinical study, there were limitations of the study with patient compliance and follow-ups, which therefore lead to inconclusive results. Definite trends were demonstrated in several areas that were positive for improving pain, function, and objective tests; however, because of the aforementioned limitations, there were no significant differences demonstrated in the study.

KINESTHETIC TRAINING EXERCISES

- Manual rhythm stabilization perturbation training (Figure 10-6)
- Shoulder horn and Body Blade (Body Blade, Playa Del Ray, Calif) training (Figure 10-7)
- Body blade training for glenohumeral rotations (Figure 10-8)
- Closed kinetic chain (CKC) exercises (Figure 10-9)
- Cuff link CKC exercises—two arms (Figure 10-10)
- Cuff link CKC exercises—one arm (Figure 10-11)
- Plyometric training with the Plyoback (Functionally Integrated Technologies, Watsonville, Calif) system (Figure 10-12)

Plyometric training has been advocated as a means of enhancing shoulder complex performance.[12,27,37] However, there are few published research articles on the topic, and most of the information remains anecdotal. We published a prospective study on the effects of plyometrics on training the shoulder complex and found there were no positive training responses in untrained female subjects.[54] However, we recently completed a follow-up study using trained male subjects and found positive training results with an increase in passive glenohumeral external rotation and isokinetic performance at faster speeds as well as increases in func-

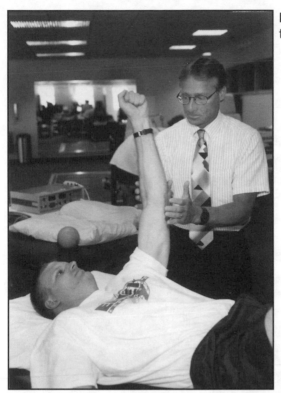

Figure 10-6. Manual rhythm stabilization perturbation training.

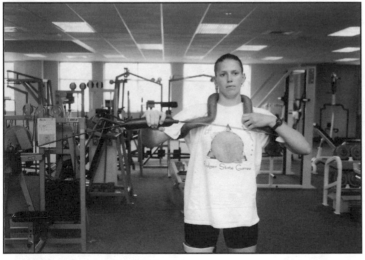

Figure 10-7. Rotator cuff rotational exercises using the shoulder horn to support the supraspinatus and the Body Blade for the rotators.

tional performance testing.[58] Therefore, we feel that using plyometric training with appropriate patients does play a role in the comprehensive rehabilitation of the shoulder complex.

Contra-Coup Concept of Shoulder Stability

Our approach to patients with glenohumeral instability is to use the contra-coup concept of shoulder stability (C3-S2). The emphasis is on developing the muscle's power on the opposite side of the injury to try to develop a dynamic compensation for the underlying static restraint incompetency, or in these cases to provide dynamic stability to the surgical reconstructive procedure.[12,23,24] Therefore, since these patients had an

Figure 10-8. Rotator cuff rotational exercises using the Body Blade.

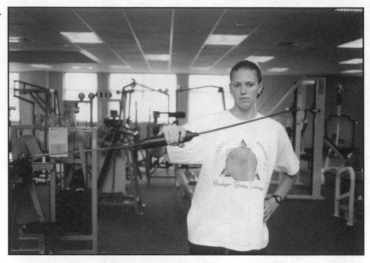

Figure 10-9. Closed kinetic chain exercises.

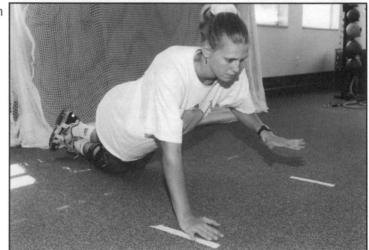

Figure 10-10. Closed kinetic chain exercises using the cuff link with two arms.

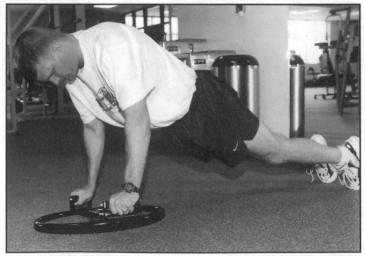

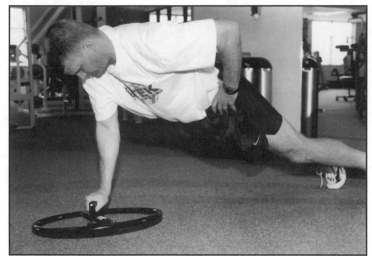

Figure 10-11. Closed kinetic chain exercises using the cuff link with one arm.

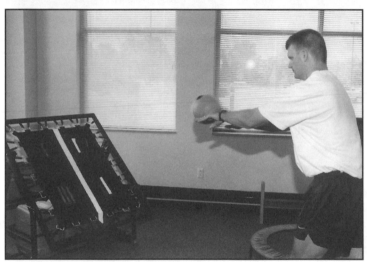

Figure 10-12. Plyometric training using a Plyoback system starting with two arms from the chest. Plyometrics are often progressed to replicate the throwing motion.

increased laxity in the anterior direction, our focus was on developing a posterior dominant shoulder.[11,12] Our goal was to change the normal unilateral ratio of the internal to external rotators from 3:2 to 4:3. Our operational definition of the posterior dominate shoulder is one in which the external rotators (ER) are strengthened an additional 10% and the unilateral ratio changes from approximately 66% of the internal rotators (IR) to 76% of the IR.[11,12] From the limited research and our empirically based clinical experiences, the following are examples of exercises that we used to address these deficits.

POSTERIOR DOMINANT SHOULDER TRAINING

- 90/90 surgical tubing training for external rotators
- Shoulder horn and Body Blade exercises
- Manual rhythmic stabilization perturbation training with emphasis on resisting the external rotators
- Plyometric training with retrothrowing

Specificity Training for Functional Rehabilitation for Return to Sport

Specificity training is the final stage of the rehabilitation program. These activities primarily replicate the demands of the sport and are imposed in a progressively challenging manner. If patients have difficulty performing these sport-specific activities in a controlled clinical setting, then most likely they will have problems when they try to return to practice or game/meet situations.

Patient one returned to competitive swimming 10 months postoperatively and has continued to swim for an additional 14 months without pain. She recently set her high school record in the 50 m and 100 m freestyle events. Patient two returned to baseball 8 months after surgery. He had no pain with throwing and remained asymptomatic for two more seasons of collegiate baseball.

DISCUSSION

Shoulder pain in the overhead athlete remains a challenging diagnostic problem. In the uninjured shoulder, static and dynamic stabilizers work in unison to maintain the relationship between mobility and stability. Excessive stress on these structures, due to repetitive overhead activities, may disrupt this equilibrium secondary to fatigue of the rotator cuff and scapular rotators. This leads to anterior glenohumeral translation and eventual attenuation of the capsulolabral complex with subsequent instability and secondary impingement, and possibly rotator cuff tearing.

The literature clearly supports the premise that a relationship exists between glenohumeral instability and pathologic changes in the rotator cuff.[4,6,71-74] In 1989, Jobe first reported a classification for overhead athletes with refractory pain. The athletes were placed in four groups based on a thorough history, physical examination, and diagnostic arthroscopy.[73]

- Group 1: Primary impingement without instability
- Group 2: Primary instability with subluxation with secondary impingement
- Group 3: Primary instability with secondary impingement associated with generalized hyperlaxity
- Group 4: Primary instability without impingement

The clinician must recognize that anterior shoulder pain in the overhead athlete involves failure of the static and dynamic stabilizers. The anterior capsulolabral reconstruction and its rehabilitation program were developed to address the underlying pathology. When the present surgical procedure was developed, it presented three major differences from prior surgical procedures aimed at decreasing anterior shoulder pain. First, the subscapularis is split and not detached, leading to less scarring. Second, the T-shaped capsulotomy addressees the redundancy by allowing a capsular shift; this is reinforced by overlapping the superior flap over the repair. Lastly, by splinting the arm in abduction, forward flexion, and external rotation, the capsule is allowed to heal with minimal contracture, thereby decreasing the amount of time it takes to regain full ROM.

In conclusion, the anterior capsulolabral reconstruction addressed fundamental pathology in the refractory overhead athlete who experienced shoulder pain due to instability. Since its initial description in 1991, the anterocapsulolabral reconstruction has been successful in returning overhead athletes to their prior competitive level. In a recent review, Montgomery and Jobe[6] reported 81% of overhead athletes returned to their prior competitive level, with an additional 13% returning to the same sport at a lower level of competition.

SUMMARY

The purpose of this case report was to provide current concepts and supportive research in surgical management using an anterocapsulolabral reconstruction and rehabilitation of patients with anterior instability. The examination findings, surgical procedure, rehabilitation techniques, follow-up and outcomes, and discussion of this case is included.

REFERENCES

1.   Tibone JE, Elrod B, Jobe FW, et al. Surgical treatment of rotator cuff tears in athletes. *J Bone Joint Surg Am.* 1986;68:887-891.

2.   Aamoth GM, O'Phelan EH. Recurrent anterior dislocation of the shoulder: a review of 40 athletes treated by subscapularis transfer. *Am J Sports Med.* 1977;5:188-190.

3.   Lombardo SJ, Kerlan RK, Jobe FW, et al. The modified Bristow procedure for recurrent dislocation of the shoulder. *J Bone Joint Surg Am.* 1976;58:256-261.

4. Rowe CR, Patel D, Southnagel WW. The Bankart procedure: a long-term end result study. *J Bone Joint Surg Am.* 1978;60:1-16.

5. Jobe FW, Giangarra CE, Kvitne RS, et al. Anterior capsule of the shoulder in athletes in overhead sports. *Am J Sports Med.* 1991;19:428-434.

6. Montgomery WH, Jobe FW. Functional outcome in athletes after modified anterior capsule-labral reconstruction. *Am J Sports Med.* 1994;22:352-358.

7. Kvitne RS, Jobe FW. Anterior capsulolabral reconstruction for instability in the throwing athlete. In; Craig EV, ed. *Master Techniques in Orthopaedic Surgery: The Shoulder.* New York, NY: Raven Press; 1995.

8. Kibler, WB. Biomechanical analysis of the shoulder during tennis activities. *Clin Sports Med.* 1995;14:79-85.

9. Pink MM, Screnar PM, Tollefson KD. Injury prevention and rehabilitation in the upper extremity. In: Jobe FW, ed. *Operative Techniques in Upper Extremity Sports Injuries.* St. Louis, MO: Mosby; 1996:3-15.

10. Kibler WB. Shoulder rehabilitation: principles and practice. *Med Sci Sports Exerc.* 1998;30:S40-S50.

11. Davies GJ. *A Compendium of Isokinetics in Clinical Usage.* 4th ed. Onalaska, Wis: S & S Publishers; 1992.

12. Davies GJ, Ellenbecker TS. Eccentric isokinetics. *Orthop Clinics North Am.* 1992;1:297-336.

13. Andrews JR, Wilk KE. *The Athlete's Shoulder.* New York, NY: Churchill Livingston; 1994.

14. Moseley JB, Jobe FW, Pink M, et al. EMG analysis of the scapular muscles during a shoulder rehabilitation program. *Am J Sports Med.* 1992;20:128-134.

15. Davies GJ, Ellenbecker TS. Total arm strength rehabilitation for shoulder and elbow overuse syndromes. *Orthopedic Physical Therapy Home Study Course.* LaCrosse Wis: Orthopedic Section, APTA;1993.

16. Schexneider MA, Catlin PA, Davies GJ, et al. An isokinetic estimation of total arm strength. *Isok Exerc Sci.* 1991;1:117-121.

17. Davies GJ, Fortun C, Romeyn R, et al. Computerized isokinetic testing of patients with rotator cuff (RTC) impingement syndromes demonstrates specific RTC external rotators power deficits. *Phys Ther.* 1997;77:S105.

18. Jobe FW, Moynes DR. Delineation of diagnostic criteria and a rehabilitation program for rotator cuff injuries. *Am J Sports Med.* 1982;10:336-339.

19. Townsend H, Jobe FW, Pink M, et al. Electromyographic analysis of the glenohumeral muscles during a baseball rehabilitation program. *Am J Sports Med.* 1991;19:264-272.

20. Davies GJ, Manske RC. The importance of evaluating muscular power (torque acceleration energy) in patients with shoulder dysfunctions. *Phys Ther.* 1999;79:S81.

21. Manske RC, Davies GJ. Rehabilitation outcomes assessing muscular power (torque acceleration energy) in patients with selected shoulder dysfunctions. *Phys Ther.* 1999;79:S81.

22. Manske RC, Davies GJ, Carney D. Correlation between isokinetic testing and a closed kinetic chain upper extremity stability test in patients with RTC impingement syndromes. *Clin J Sports Med.* In press.

23. Cain PR, Mutschler TA, Fu FH, et al. Anterior stability of the glenohumeral joint: a dynamic model. *Am J Sports Med.* 1983;2:247-270.

24. Perry J. Anatomy and biomechanics of the shoulder in throwing, swimming, gymnastics and tennis. *Clin Sports Med.* 1983;2:247-270.

25. Allegrucci M, Whitney SL, Irrgang JJ. Clinical implications of secondary impingement of the shoulder in freestyle swimmers. *J Orthop Sports Phys Ther.* 1994;20:307-318.

26. Brewster C, Moynes-Schwab DR. Rehabilitation of the shoulder following rotator cuff injury or surgery. *J Orthop Sports Phys Ther.* 1993;18:422-426.

27. Cordasco FA, Wolfe IN, Wooten, et al. An electromyographic analysis of the shoulder during a medicine ball rehabilitation program. *Am J Sports Med.* 1996;24:386-392.

28. Ginn KA, Herbert RD, Khouw W, et al. A randomized, controlled clinical trial of a treatment for shoulder pain. *Phys Ther.* 1997;77:802-811.

29. Janda DH, Loubert P. A preventive program focusing on the glenohumeral joint. *Clin Sports Med.* 1991;10:955-971.

30. Jobe FW, Bradley JP. Delineation of diagnostic criteria and a rehabilitation program for rotator cuff injuries. *Am J Sports Med.* 1982;10:336-339.

31. Jobe FW, Pink M. Classification and treatment of shoulder dysfunction in the overhead athlete. *J Orthop Sports Phys Ther.* 1993;17:427-432.

32. Kamkar A, Irrgang JJ, Whitney SL. Nonoperative management of secondary shoulder impingement syndrome. *J Orthop Sports Phys Ther.* 1993;17:212-224.

33. Kenal BT, Knapp LD. Rehabilitation of injuries in competitive swimmers. *Sports Med.* 1996;22:337-347.

34. Meister K, Andrews JR. Classification and treatment of rotator cuff injuries in the overhead athlete. *J Orthop Sports Phys Ther.* 1993;18:413-421.

35. Morrison DS, Frogameni AD, Woodworth P. Nonoperative treatment of subacromial impingment syndrome. *J Bone Joint Surgery Am.* 1997;79:732-737.

36. Wilk KE, Arrigo C. Current concepts in rehabilitation of the athletic shoulder. *J Orthop Sports Phys Ther.* 1993;18:365-378.

37. Wilk KE, Voight MIL, Keirns MA, et al. Stretch-shortening drills for the upper extremities: theory and clinical application. *J Orthop Sports Phys Ther.* 1993;17:225-239.

38. Bak K, Magnusson SID. Shoulder strength and range of motion in symptomatic and pain-free elite swimmers. *Am J Sports Med.* 1997;25:454-458.

39. Ballantyne BT, O'Hare SJ, Paschall JL, et al. Electromyographic activity of selected shoulder muscles in commonly used therapeutic exercises. *Phys Ther.* 1993;73:668-677.

40. Codine P, Bernard PL, Pocholle M, et al. Influence of sports discipline on shoulder rotator cuff balance. *Med Sci Sports Exerc.* 1997;29:1400-1405.

41. Cohen DB, Mont MA, Campbell KR, et al. Upper extremity physical factors affecting tennis serve velocity. *Am J Sports Med.* 1994;22:746-750.

42. Glousman R, Jobe F, Tibone J, et al. Dynamic electromyographic analysis of the throwing shoulder with glenohumeral instability. *J Bone Joint Surg.* 1988;70:220-226.

43. Leroux JL, Codine P, Thomas E, et al. Isokinetic evaluation of rotational strength in normal shoulders and shoulders with impingement syndromes. *Clin Orthop.* 1994;304:108-115.

44. Scovazzo ML, Browne A, Pink M, et al. The painful shoulder during freestyle swimming: an electromyographic cinematographic analysis of twelve muscles. *Am J Sports Med.* 1991;19:557-582.

45. Warner JP, Micheli U, Arslanian LE, et al. Patterns of flexibility, laxity and strength in normal shoulders and shoulders with instability and impingement. *Am J Sports Med.* 1990;18:366-375.

46. Jenp YN, Malanga GA, Growney ES, et al. Activation of the rotator cuff in generating isometric shoulder rotation torque. *Am J Sports Med.* 1996;24:477-485.

47. Kelly BT, Kadrmas WR, Kirkendall DT, et al. Optimal normalization tests for shoulder muscle activation: an electromyographic study. *J Orthop Res.* 1996;14:647-653.

48. Kronberg M, Brostrom LA. Electromyographic recordings in shoulder muscles during eccentric movements. *Clin Orthop.* 1995;314:143-150.

49. McCann PD, Wooten ME, Kadaba MP, et al. A kinematic and electromyographic study of shoulder rehabilitation exercises. *Clin Orthop.* 1993;288:179-188.

50. Keating JF, Waterworth P, Shaw-Dunn J, et al. The relative strengths of rotator cuff muscles: a cadaver study. *J Bone Joint Surg.* 1993;7513:137-140.

51. Ellenbecker TS, Davies GJ, Rowinski M. Concentric versus eccentric isokinetic strengthening of the rotator cuff: objective data vs functional test. *Am J Sports Med.* 1988;16:64-69.

52. Greenfield BH, Donatelli R, Wooden MJ, et al. Isokinetic evaluation of shoulder rotational strength between the plane of the scapula and the frontal plane. *Am J Sports Med.* 1990;18:124-128.

53. Hageman PA, Mason DK, Rydlund KW, et al. Effects of position and speed on eccentric and concentric isokinetic testing of shoulder rotators. *J Orthop Sports Phys Ther.* 1989;11:64-69.

54. Heiderscheit B, Palmer-McLean K, Davies GJ. The effects of isokinetic versus plyometric training on the shoulder internal rotators. *J Orthop Sports Phys Ther.* 1996;25:133-136.

55. Hughes RE, An KN. Force analysis of rotator cuff muscles. *Clin Orthop.* 1996;330:75-83.

56. Mont MA, Cohen DB, Campbell KR. Isokinetic concentric versus eccentric training of shoulder rotators with functional evaluation of performance enhancement in elite tennis players. *Am J Sports Med.* 1994;22:513-517.

57. Soderberg GJ, Blaschak MJ. Shoulder internal and external rotation peak torque production through a velocity spectrum in differing positions. *J Orthop Sports Phys Ther.* 1987;8:518-524.

58. Fortun C, Davies GJ, Kernozek TK. The effects of plyometric training on the shoulder internal rotators. *Phys Ther.* 1997;73(6):S88.

59. Litchfield R, Hawkins R, Dillman CJ, et al. Rehabilitation of the overhead athlete. *J Orthop Sports Phys Ther.* 1993;18:433-441.

60. McGee C, Kersting E, Palmer-McLean K, et al. Standard rehabilitation vs standard plus closed kinetic chain rehabilitation for patients with shoulder impingement: A rehabilitation outcomes study. *Phys Ther.* 1999;79:S65.

60. Wooden MJ, Greenfield B, Johanson M, et al. Effects of strength training on throwing velocity and shoulder muscle performance in teenage baseball players. *J Orthop Sports Phys Ther.* 1992;15:223-228.

61. Itoi E, Kido T, Sano A, et al. Which is more useful, the "full can test" or the "empty can test" in detecting the torn supraspinatus tendon? *Am J Sports Med.* 1999;27:65-68.

62. Borsa PA, Lephart SM, Kocher IVIS, et al. Functional assessment and rehabilitation of shoulder proprioception for glenohumeral instability. *J Sport Rehab.* 1994;3:84-104.

63. Davies GJ, Lawson K, Jones B. The acute effects of fatigue on shoulder rotator cuff internal/external rotation kinesthesia. *Phys Ther.* 1993;78(5):S87.

64. Guanche C, Knatt T, Solomonow M, et al. The synergistic action of the capsule and the shoulder muscles. *Am J sports Med.* 1995;23:301-306.

65. Jerosch J, Thorwesten L, Steinbeck J, et al. Proprioceptive function of the shoulder girdle in healthy volunteers. *Knee Surgery, Sports Traumatology, Arthroscopy.* 1996;3:219-225.

66. Lephart SM, Warner JP, Borsa PA, et al. Proprioception of the shoulder in normal, unstable and post-surgical individuals. *J Shoulder Elbow Surg.* 1994;3:371-380.

67. Lephart SM, Henry TJ. The physiological basis for open and closed kinetic chain rehabilitation for the upper extremity. *J Sports Rehab.* 1996;5:71-87.

68. Lephart SM, Pincivero DM, Giraldo JL, et al. The role of proprioception in the management and rehabilitation of athletic injuries. *Am J Sports Med.* 1997;25:130-137.

69. Davies GJ. The need for critical thinking in rehabilitation. *J Sport Rehab.* 1995;4:1-22.

70. Gainor BJ, Piotrowski G, Puhl J, et al. The throw: biomechanics and acute injury. *Am J Sports Med.* 1980;8:114-118.

71. Garth WP, Allman FL, Armstrong WS. Occult anterior subluxation of the shoulder. *Am J Sports Med.* 1988;15:579-585.

72. Hawkins RJ, Kennedy JC. Impingement syndrome in athletes. *Am J Sports Med.* 1980;8:151-158.

73. Jobe FW, Kvitne RS, Giangarra CE. Shoulder pain in the overhand or throwing athlete: the relationship of anterior instability and rotator cuff impingement. *Ortho Rev.* 1989;18:963-975.

74. Rowe CR, Zarins B. Recurrent transient subluxation of the shoulder. *J Bone Joint Surg Am.* 1981;63:863-872.

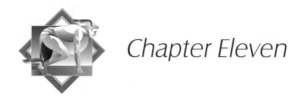

Chapter Eleven

Subscapularis Rupture Following an Anterior Capsular Reconstruction Surgery in a Competitive Wrestler

Martin J. Kelley, MS, PT, OCS

INTRODUCTION

Anterior glenohumeral instability of the shoulder is commonly encountered in the athletic population.[1] High velocity, end range activities can overload the static and dynamic glenohumeral restraints. Traumatic dislocations often result in Bankart lesions, and if the patient is to return to competitive activities, an anterior capsular reconstruction may be required. Complications can occur following anterior capsular reconstruction, including loss of motion, subscapularis failure, capsulorrhaphy arthroplasty, hardware migration, and neurovascular injury. An immediate postoperative examination of the patient is essential to establish baseline status, and re-examination during rehabilitation is required to assure proper progression. Numerous authors have proposed specific tests or signs to clinically assess shoulder joint stability,[2] tendon integrity,[3-6] and strength.[7-9]

Rehabilitation after anterior capsular reconstruction is essential for recovery, particularly in the athlete.[10-12] Indepth knowledge of glenohumeral joint instability, the associated surgical procedure, examination techniques, and the rehabilitation process allows the clinician to effectively treat the athlete, recognize complications, and facilitate appropriate intervention.

This case presentation describes a competitive wrestler who experienced a traumatic dislocation and underwent anterior capsular reconstruction. During the postoperative period he ruptured his subscapularis tendon but eventually returned to his sport, despite being unable to repair the rupture.

SUBJECT

The athlete is a left-hand dominant wrestler (150 lb weight class) in a National Collegiate Athletic Association (NCAA) Division 1 university. He was a 19-year-old sophomore when he suffered an anterior-inferior traumatic dislocation on November 13, 1994 during a wrestling match. The injury occurred with the right arm fixed on the mat in elevation and external rotation while his body was turned to the left. He was taken to the emergency room, and the shoulder was reduced without incident. He was seen by the team physician 3 days later and was neurovascularly intact but demonstrated limited active and passive motion. He was immobilized for 3 weeks and placed on a progressive range of motion (ROM) and strengthening program with the team athletic trainer. He went on to dislocate his shoulder three subsequent times; the first two events were classified as traumatic (wrestling) and the third event (August 25, 1995) occurred atraumatically when he was carrying luggage with his arm abducted and externally rotated over his head.[13] Each episode was reduced with the help of the athletic trainer or a friend. Three weeks after the last dislocation, he was again evaluated by the team physician and roentgenograms revealed a small Hills-Sachs lesion on the stryker notch view.

The physician's clinical examination revealed a positive anterior apprehension sign and relocation test. He was felt to anteriorly sublux while performing the apprehension sign. The sulcus sign was positive bilaterally but could be subluxed more on his right shoulder, and there was no posterior instability. Rotator cuff/deltoid strength was good. The athlete wanted to continue to wrestle but was made aware that future instability events were likely and surgery would be required. He chose conservative management and continued to work with the athletic trainers. He returned to the team physician 1 month later with complaints of daily instability episodes of an atraumatic nature and reported a sense of "looseness" in his left shoulder. He was no longer able to wrestle and decided to have surgery.

A common sequence of events in patients sustaining glenohumeral dislocations is movement from the classification of traumatic dislocations to atraumatic dislocations.[14] Most likely this athlete suffered a Bankart lesion during the first event, then further stretched the capsuloligamentous complex (CLC) with each subsequent episode, resulting in atraumatic dislocations and inability to participate in wrestling.

Surgical Procedure

On November 24, 1995 the patient underwent an open Bankart repair, anterior capsular shift, and rotator cuff interval closure. Using the grading system advocated by Silliman and Hawkins,[2] examination under anesthesia (EUA) revealed 3+ anterior instability with the right shoulder easily dislocatable. Inferior and posterior stability was graded as 1+ bilaterally. Anterior stability of the left shoulder was graded as 2+.

An incision was made at the axillary crease and the deltopectoral interval was found. The interval was entered and the deltoid and cephalic vein were retracted laterally. The subscapularis was located and a vertical incision made 1 cm from its musculotendinous junction beginning at the tendon's superior margin to the anterior humeral circumflex arteries. The tendon was freed from the anterior capsule and tagged. The anterior capsule was incised 0.5 cm lateral to the glenoid rim and a "T" incision continued right above the inferior glenohumeral ligament to the humeral insertion. The Bankart lesion was noted and the anterior glenoid rim was roughened using an osteome. Three large suture anchors were placed in the anterior-inferior glenoid, and the Bankart lesion was repaired. Next the capsular shift was performed with the inferior capsule shifted superiorly. A medium-size lesion of the rotator cuff interval was closed. The arm was able to be externally rotated to 30 degrees after the procedure. The subscapularis was repaired in vertical mattress fashion. The subcutaneous and skin incisions were closed in typical fashion.

Postoperative Physical Therapy Examination

The patient presented to physical therapy on December 4, 1995, 10 days after surgery. He was using a sling up to the point of seeing the physician 2 days previously. At that time, the surgeon said he could begin to wean off the sling, but should use it when in crowds or when the shoulder became painful. The patient did not wear the sling after this discussion with the surgeon.

The incision was healing with no drainage. Moderate edema surrounding the anterior shoulder was noted with mild global atrophy present. ROM findings are in Table 11-1. Cervical spine motion was assessed and an upper quarter neurologic examination was performed, excluding the internal rotators. Specific attention was paid to the deltoid. The middle deltoid was examined by supporting the arm in approximately 30 degrees of abduction and asking the patient to hold the arm as the examiner released it. The middle deltoid head was palpated during this unweighting procedure to assess tone and activity. The anterior head was evaluated in the same manner, but the arm was supported in approximately 30 degrees of flexion and slight external rotation. The posterior head was evaluated by supporting the arm in approximately 30 degrees of abduction and asking the patient to push gently backward (horizontal abduction). Palpation for intactness was noted for each deltoid head. Checking for deltoid intactness after any type of capsular reconstruction procedure (or glenohumeral dislocation) is important due to possible axillary nerve damage.[15] Occasionally, just the anterior branch to the anterior deltoid suffers a neurapraxia due to retraction in an effort to gain joint exposure.

Table 11-1			
RANGE OF MOTION			
Left	**12/4/95**	**12/19/95**	**1/23/96**
Active ROM			
Elevation 180 degrees	Not tested	135 degrees**	165 degrees
Functional internal rotation T5	Not tested	Not tested	L2
Passive ROM			
Elevation 180 degrees	90 degrees	140	165 degrees
Glenohumeral abduction (coronal) 115 degrees	50 degrees		90 degrees
External rotation (adduction) 75 degrees	-10 degrees	15	55 degrees
External rotation 90 degrees (coronal) 100 degrees	Not tested	Not tested	80 degrees
External rotation (plane of scapula) 105 degrees	35 degrees	60	90 degrees
Internal rotation (glenohumeral abduction) 50 degrees	30 degrees (50 degrees)*		40 degrees (90 degrees)*

ROM: range of motion

*Available coronal plane abduction

**Slight subscapularis substitution noted

This is particularly true in individuals who are well muscled, such as athletes. The risk to the axillary nerve has dramatically reduced since surgeons began using currently available fixation devices.

We examined the stability of the left shoulder (uninvolved) using load and shift testing, which revealed grade 2 anterior translation (the humeral head glides over the glenoid rim but spontaneously reduces).[2] Although the patient had significant translation of the uninvolved shoulder, he did not demonstrate generalized hyperelasticity (laxity). This is found when the patient can approximate the thumb to the volar aspect of the wrist, has metacarpophalangeal hyperextension, or elbow and knee recurvatum. The assessment of generalized laxity is an important guide to rehabilitation regarding ROM progression. Typically, ROM is progressed slower in patients who demonstrate generalized hypermobility. If return of motion appears too slow, the therapist then "dials in" motion by progressing the stretching program. Patients with generalized hypoelasticity are treated with more aggressive stretching.

TREATMENT AND REHABILITATION

The athlete was instructed to position his arm in sitting with the arm supported in slight plane of scapula (POS) abduction (20 to 30 degrees) and neutral rotation. This position reduces tension on the glenohumeral soft tissues and discourages formation of an internal rotation contracture. He was cautioned against actively lifting the arm, opening doors, or pushing inward (internal rotation such as lifting a box), as these motions could overload the subscapularis tendon repair site. Exercises included pendulum, passive supine forward elevation to 90 degrees, and external rotation to 0 degrees with the arm at 45 degrees of elevation in the POS. The reason for stretching into external rotation in the POS is based upon several studies. Turkel et al,[16] found that incising the subscapularis produced an 18-degree increase in external rotation when the arm was placed in adduction. Therefore, external rotation stretches with the arm at the side should be restricted to avoid excessive tension on the subscapularis repair site. Additionally, stretching the arm into external rotation in adduction could over tension the rotator cuff interval repair since the interval restricts external rotation with the arm in adduction.[17] He was encouraged to ice as frequently as possible through the day.

There was slight concern about his 10 degrees internal rotation contracture and his upcoming leave for holiday break. The patient was treated until December 19. The rationale for treatment was to reduce soft tissue edema and pain, improve ROM, promote dynamic stabilization, and begin active-assisted motion to facilitate collagen healing. He was treated with soft tissue mobilization over two sessions to reduce soft tissue edema and pain. Grade I and II joint mobilizations were performed to reduce pain and improve motion related to pain/muscle guarding.[18] Mobilization treatments were performed during his first three sessions of physical therapy. He was treated using submaximal manual isometric abduction/external rotation activity (to improve dynamic stabilization) on sessions three through five, and with active-assisted ROM (to facilitate collagen healing) to full available elevation motion and external rotation to 30 degrees from sessions three through five.[20]

ROM was assessed on December 19, 1995 and is presented in Table 11-1. The patient presented with 140 degrees of passive elevation and 135 degrees of active elevation with slight scapular substitution noted. Passively, external rotation at neutral was to 15 degrees, external rotation at 90 degrees, and the plane of the scapula was to 60 degrees. It is quite common to find external rotation (measured in adduction) lagging behind elevation 3 to 4 weeks after surgery. Assessing the arm at 90 degrees in the POS provides reliable insight as to the return of external rotation, without jeopardizing the surgical reconstruction or subscapularis.

Treatment on December 19 included review of phase I elastic band strengthening exercises for external rotation and extension. Internal rotation strengthening could begin 1 week later. He began biceps strengthening using three 16 lb weights with the arm supported. All exercises were performed with scapular muscle integration, meaning that the scapula is first retracted slightly using the medial scapular muscles and then the exercise is performed. This encourages scapular muscle activity while the glenohumeral dynamic stabilizers are activated.[12,20] The patient left for the holiday and was to continue exercises on his own. If he had any difficulties there was a therapist in his hometown to contact.

The patient returned to physical therapy on January 23, 1996, approximately 8 weeks after surgery. Examination revealed 165 degrees of active elevation, with active internal rotation to L2. Complete ROM assessment is listed in Table 11-1. He reported a sense of "insecurity" at the ends of motion, which is common in patients who have had multiple dislocations and are post-capsular reconstruction, but this does not truly reflect instability. Muscle strength testing with the arm at the side revealed 4-/5 strength for the abductors and internal rotators, and 4+/5 strength of the external rotators. He admitted that he did not consistently perform strengthening exercises over the break.

To assess subscapularis strength more closely, we used the lift-off test and belly press test, which were both positive for this athlete. The lift-off test was performed by placing the patient's hand on the lumbar spine (dorsum of hand) and having him attempt to lift the hand away. This requires the subscapularis to maximally activate and fully internally rotate the arm.[3,4,21] The athlete was unable to lift the hand off his back, yet did have the available passive ROM. For the test to be valid, the patient must have the available passive motion and/or it must not be limited by pain. For the belly press test[4] (abdominal compression test), the athlete placed his hand on his stomach with his elbow out to the side and slightly forward. He was asked to push his hand into his stomach and maintain the elbow out to the side. Unable to keep his elbow out to the side (maintaining internal rotation/abduction), he substituted with the adductors/internal rotators by pulling the arm into adduction/extension. To gain full appreciation of the subscapularis weakness, the examiner attempt-

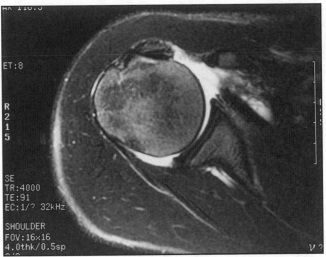

Figure 11-1. MRI demonstrating complete rupture of the subscapularis tendon.

ed to pull the hand off the stomach, even allowing the adduction substitution. The patient had dramatic weakness compared to the other side when pulling the hand off the stomach.

Considering the positive signs and tests specific to subscapularis insufficiency, the athlete was specifically questioned about any event that may have jeopardized the integrity of the subscapularis. He denied any incident and we concluded that the weakness was a result of the athlete not consistently performing his exercises. These findings were discussed with the surgeon and we decided to monitor his progress over the next 2 weeks. He was seen five times per week between January 23 and February 9, 1996. Treatment consisted of manual dynamic stabilization exercises using multiangle isometrics at 45, 90, 120, and 150 degrees. D1 and D2 proprioceptive neuromuscular facilitation (PNF) patterns were also used. The Body Blade was utilized at 30 and 60 degrees in the plane of the scapula with scapular muscle integration. He performed these exercises with one- and two-hand sagittal plane positioning at 90 degrees. These exercises were performed five times at 15-second intervals. This exercise is thought to encourage coactivation of all the glenohumeral and scapulothoracic dynamic stabilizers with bias toward certain groups depending upon the activity and position chosen. The patient's home strengthening program was progressed to include forward flexion and plane of the scapula abduction with a 3 lb weight to 90 degrees. The rationale for treatment was to improve dynamic stabilization and scapular muscle integration while working from nonprovocative to provocative positions.

On January 29, 1996, the third visit from his re-examination, the athlete disclosed that he did have an episode during the holiday break while wrestling with a friend at home. Apparently, his right arm was forced into external rotation with the arm toward the side. He reported feeling a sense of soreness over the next 2 days and then began to feel weakness when pressing into his body, such as washing his chest, legs, or opposite shoulder.

Over the next two sessions, his internal rotation strength had only improved slightly, but his abduction strength improved to 4+/5. He reported no sense of instability with activities of daily living (ADLs). Because he continued to demonstrate a positive lift-off and belly press test, an appointment was scheduled with his physician and an MRI was ordered. The MRI on February 13, 1996 revealed a complete subscapularis tear with discontinuity of 1.5 to 2 cm. The muscle was retracted but did not appear atrophied (Figure 11-1).

Isokinetic and isometric tests were performed on February 16, 1999 to objectively document his strength (Table 11-2). Testing was performed supine using the Lido dynamometer (Loredan, Davis, Calif) isokinetic unit. The arm was placed in 45 degrees of abduction and 30 degrees anterior to the coronal plane (the plane of the scapula). We use this position with all of our shoulder strength testing, as it has been found to be valid and reliable.[8,22,23] This test position offers several advantages when testing a patient who has glenohumeral joint instability. First, the provocative position of 90 degrees of abduction and 90 degrees of external rotation is avoided, thus, testing can be performed without promoting an unstable event and jeopardizing the recent

Table 11-2

ISOKINETIC AND ISOMETRIC STRENGTH VALUES 2 1/2 MONTHS AFTER SURGERY

| | External Rotation | | | Internal Rotation | | | |
	Right	Left	Right/left (%)	Right	Left	Right/left (%)	Deficit (%)
Isokinetic (90 degrees/second)							
Peak torque	23	27	85	37	39	95	5
Total work	156	190	82	233	256	91	9
Isometric							
0 degrees	-	-	-	32	48	66	34
-60 degrees	-	-	-	7	22	32	68

surgical intervention. Second, the POS may provide mechanical advantages related to the length-tension relationship of the rotator cuff.[23,24] Third, this position results in strength measurements that are similar to other functional test positions.[9,25]

The isokinetic testing was only performed at one speed to avoid overburdening the shoulder. We chose the slower speed to better represent strength deficits and limited ROM to 40 degrees of external rotation (instead of 60 degrees) and 60 degrees of internal rotation. The isokinetic results were very surprising since both peak torque and total work did not show significant deficits of the internal rotators. We suspected that it was possible for internal rotation peak torque to be symmetrical since peak torque occurs while the arm is in the externally rotated position (lengthened) and the pectoralis major, latissimus dorsi, and teres major may be lengthened enough to compensate. This is similar to what occurs when isokinetically testing the hamstrings in patients after ACL reconstruction using an autogenous /gracilis graft. One rarely finds peak torque deficits at the angle of peak torque (25 to 30 degrees of knee flexion) since strength deficits are seen at greater than 60 degrees of knee flexion where the semitendinosis/gracilis gain greater leverage and improved angle of application.[26] We were very surprised to find that total work did not show deficits since we expected to see strength loss as the arm moved into internal rotation and the larger internal rotators became too short to compensate. We assumed that he was over compensating with excessive scapular protraction as he moved into full internal rotation, thereby keeping the arm in relative external rotation. When testing was performed isometrically at neutral rotation and 60 degrees of internal rotation (similar to the belly test position), significant deficits of 34% and 68%, were noted respectively. Clinically, we have found isometric testing of the shoulder to be more accurate in detecting weakness in patients who have some degree of pain or apprehension, or who have a tendon rupture or peripheral nerve lesion. Continued mild weakness of the external rotators, noted during testing, has been found following anterior capsular reconstruction.[27]

Secondary to the clinical examination and positive MRI findings, the surgeon recommended re-operating as soon as possible, as studies show best results if subscapularis ruptures are operated on within 6 weeks of the injury.[3,4,28,29] Therapy was deferred until the patient saw the surgeon again. The athlete's father was contacted and informed of the need for surgery because his son had not returned to the physician. The athlete missed his surgery scheduled for February 26, 1996. He returned to the surgeon the next day and informed the surgeon that he wanted to go skiing the next week. Several conversations between the athletic trainers and the family occurred regarding the need for surgery as soon as possible. Finally, the patient underwent exploratory surgery again on March 18, 1999, approximately 3 1/2 months after the initial surgery and approximately 9 weeks after the subscapularis rupture. The surgeon was unable to identify and repair the subscapularis tendon secondary to retraction and scarring. He inspected the Bankart reconstruction and capsular shift and found both intact. Examination under anesthesia revealed a stable joint.

The patient returned for his postoperative visit to the surgeon on 3/26/96 and was referred back to physical therapy. He returned to therapy on April 1, 1996 and presented with 150 degrees of active elevation and 75 degrees of external rotation at 90 degrees. External rotation in adduction was 65 degrees. He was placed on active ROM exercises and was to return in 1 week to be reassessed and begin strengthening exercises. He returned in 1 week with full motion and 5/5 strength of the abductors and external rotators. He continued to demonstrate positive lift off and belly press tests. He denied any sense of instability. He was progressed in his elastic band strengthening program to 45 degrees of elevation for rotator strengthening. We discussed seeing the athlete one more time to progress his program, however, he canceled his next appointment. We called the athletic trainers regarding the progression of his program. He was able to return to free-weight strengthening, but bench pressing and behind-the-head lifting (latissimus dorsi pull down or military press) was to be modified to the front. The patient was discharged from therapy.

FUNCTIONAL OUTCOME

The patient continued with rehabilitation under the direction of the team athletic trainers. He was able to return to competitive wrestling the following season until suffering a traumatic dislocation of the left shoulder (other side). He went on to have a Bankart procedure on the left shoulder but did not return to competitive wrestling after that procedure. The patient actually had a fairly successful season up to his left shoulder dislocation, with a nine wins and six losses. He reported feeling the need to "protect his right shoulder from elevated positions" when wrestling but denied significant weakness.

The patient completed the Penn shoulder score on July 22, 1999 (approximately 4 1/2 years after the initial surgery). The survey is a subjective 100-point questionnaire assessing pain (30 points), satisfaction (10 points), and function (60 points). There is also a 100-point score evaluating sports participation related to pain, stability, strength, level of participation, and performance (20 points for each category). The sports participation questions related to his current involvement in tennis and basketball. He scored 94/100 on the Penn shoulder score and 68/100 in the sports participation score. He reported that he occasionally feels movement in his right shoulder but has not had any dislocations or painful subluxations. In addition, he feels limited in his ability to grab a rebound from another player with his arm elevated.

DISCUSSION

Complications following glenohumeral anterior joint reconstruction include recurrence of instability, loss of motion, subscapularis failure, capsulorrhaphy arthroplasty, hardware migration, and neurovascular injury. In this case the patient experienced subscapularis tendon failure. Greis[29] reported on four cases (4.5% incidence) of subscapularis failure after an open Bankart procedure. In three of the four cases, an excessive external rotation or abduction/external rotation event occurred within 5 weeks of surgery. The fourth case occurred 4 months after surgery due to a fall. A feeling of weakness and instability was reported in the three cases, and just weakness in the fourth. Two patients demonstrated increased external rotation with the arm at the side and two had disrupted the Bankart repair. All demonstrated a positive lift-off test (one patient had the reoccurrence on the same day as surgery so the lift-off test was not performed). All patients underwent exploration between 1 week and 16 months post initial surgery, and all had the subscapularis reattached. The patient who only experienced weakness without instability did not disrupt the initial Bankart repair. The wrestler presented in this case eventually reported an event that forced his arm into excessive external rotation at approximately 6 weeks postoperative. He also described a sense of weakness, however, like the one case in Greis' report but did not have a sense of instability. At the time of exploration, the Bankart repair and capsular shift were found to be intact, resulting in a stable shoulder. It appears that if the capsular reconstruction remains intact, some patients may remain stable and function well.[30]

Ziegler, et al[31] reported on 30 patients who disrupted the subscapularis after multiple instability procedures. They found the average delay in diagnosing the subscapularis rupture was 12 1/2 months. All of the patients had internal rotation weakness and a positive abdominal pull-off test. Sixty-six percent complained of instability, 56% complained of anterior tenderness, 46% had a palpable defect adjacent to the lesser tuberosity, and 80% demonstrated increased external rotation. Wirth[32] reported on 12 patients of 182 (6.5%) who had irreparable subscapularis ruptures after anterior reconstruction. Gerber, et al[3,4] reported on individuals who experienced traumatic isolated ruptures of the subscapularis without previous instability surgery. They found that the most important clinical findings were a positive lift-off test and increased external rotation when measured with the arm at the side. Although the wrestler in this case study demonstrated internal rotation weakness, a positive lift-off test, and a positive belly press test, he never demonstrated excessive external rotation motion with the arm at the side. Most likely this was due to the capsular reconstruction remaining intact and limiting motion. It is not known whether he went on to develop increased external rotation motion over time.

Impressive in this case was the patient's ability to return to a sport that demanded significant internal rotation strength and challenged both the static and dynamic stabilizers. For him to return to competitive wrestling is a feat, but for him to win 9 of 15 matches is phenomenal. Possibly, he was able to substitute during competition using the other internal rotators as he had during the isokinetic testing. A recent preliminary investigation by our group may shed some light on internal rotation strength related to function after surgery. We tested nine patients who were 11 months to 2 years post total shoulder arthroplasty. All had a positive belly press test and a positive lift-off test, but none had enough passive internal rotation to allow a valid lift-off test. What was very surprising was that objective strength measurements using an Isobex tensiometer, performed in the belly press test position, revealed dramatic deficits. In fact, only two of the nine patients could generate enough torque to register. However, eight of the nine patients scored greater than 80 on the Penn shoulder score, and none reported a sense of instability or significant weakness. Did all these patients disrupt their subscapularis? Was the subscapularis intact (along with the anterior capsule) but insufficient? It is difficult to imagine that all tore their subscapularis, particularly when correlating this finding to their outcome scores. Possibly the belly press test is not sensitive or specific enough.

The rehabilitation course in this case was thought to be a standard progression from ROM exercises to dynamic stabilization activities. The patient really never progressed to end-stage activities, such as plyometrics, due to the subscapularis findings. What this case elucidates is that subscapularis ruptures do occur after glenohumeral joint anterior capsular reconstruction procedures. The reported incidence is between 4.5%[29] and 6.5%.[32] The clinician must be aware of the associated signs and symptoms of a subscapularis tear; if disruption is suspected, prompt re-exploration is recommended. Additionally, specific patient education related to ROM, overuse of the internal rotators, and inappropriate activities is essential, particularly in the first 6 weeks after open repair. Specific instruction in ROM exercises are required with precautions of avoiding excessive external rotation (particularly with the arm at the side), and avoiding aggressive internal rotation strengthening exercise before 4 to 6 weeks. The clinician must also assess the "personality" of the patient. Although this patient was felt to be extremely stoic and was given specific precautions of the "do's and don'ts" he pushed the boundaries too far. I have become much more firm in my educational approach when working with an aggressive personality. The clinician must also consider the clinical examination findings and correlate them to objective strength measurements. If isometric testing had not been performed in this case, the clinical exam findings may have been ignored based upon isokinetic data.

SUMMARY

This case presentation focused on a wrestler who experienced a subscapularis rupture following a shoulder anterior capsular reconstruction procedure. Through specific examination procedures, the problem was identified and the patient was moved to the appropriate level of care. Even with a deficient subscapularis the patient was able to return to competitive wrestling until dislocating the opposite shoulder. The patient remains stable and able to participate in recreational activities 4 1/2 years after the surgical procedure and irreparable subscapularis rupture. As always, the concept of team management of the patient must be emphasized. The surgeon, physical therapist, and athletic trainer must work together and communicate in an effort to bring about optimal care to the patient, particularly when complications arise.

REFERENCES

1. Simonet WT, Cofield RH. Prognosis in anterior shoulder dislocation. *Am J Sports Med.* 1984;12(1):19-24.

2. Silliman JF, Hawkins RJ. Classification and physical diagnosis of instability of the shoulder. *Clin Orthop.* 1993; 291:7-19.

3. Gerber C, Krushnell, RJ. Isolated rupture of the tendon of the subscapularis muscle. *J Bone Joint Sur Br.* 1991;73:389-94.

4. Gerber C, Hersche O, Farron A. Isolated rupture of the subscapularis tendon. *J Bone Joint Surg Am.* 1996;78:1015-1023.

5. Hertel R, Ballmer FT, Lombert SM, et al. Lag signs in the diagnosis of rotator cuff rupture. *J Should Elbow Surg.* 1996;5(4):307-313.

6. Jobe FW, Moynes DR. Delineation of diagnostic criteria and a rehabilitation program for rotator cuff injuries. *Am J Sports Med.* 1982;10(6):336-339.

7. Wilk K, Andrews J, Arrigo C. The internal and external rotator strength characteristics of professional baseball pitchers. *Am J Sports Med.* 1993;21:61-66.

8. Kuhlman J, et al. Isokinetic and isometric measurement of strength of external rotation and abduction of the shoulder. *J Bone Joint Surg Am.* 1992;74:1320-1333.

9. Greenfield BH, Donatelli R, Wooden MJ, et al. Isokinetic evaluation of shoulder rotational strength between the plane of scapula and the frontal plane. *Am J Sports Med.* 1990;18(2):124-128.

10. Lephart SM, Pincivero DM, Giraldo JL, et al. The role of proprioception in the management and rehabilitation of athletic injuries. *Am J Sports Med.* 1997;25:130-137.

11. Lephart S, et al. Proprioception of the shoulder in healthy, unstable and surgically repaired shoulders. *J Should Elbow Surg.* 1994;3:371-380.

12. Kelley M. Anatomic and biomechanical rationale for rehabilitation of the overhead athlete. *J Sport Rehab.* 1995;4:122-154.

13. Thomas SC, Matsen FA. An approach to the repair of avulsion of the glenohumeral ligaments in the management of traumatic anterior glenohumeral instability. *J Bone Joint Surg Am.* 1989;71:505-513.

14. Matsen FA, Thomas SC, Rockwood CA. Glenohumeral instability. In: Rockwood CA, Matsen FA, eds. Philadelphia, Pa: WB Saunders Company;1990:1-33.

15. Ho E, Dofield R. Neurologic complications after shoulder stabilization procedures. Paper presented at AAOS annual meeting. San Francisco, Calif; February 14, 1997.

16. Turkel SJ, Panio MW, Marshall JL, et al. Stabilizing mechanisms preventing anterior dislocation of the glenohumeral joint. *J Bone Joint Surg Am.* 1981;63(8):12208-1217.

17. Harryman DT, Sidles JA, Harris SL, et al. The role of the rotator interval capsule in passive motion and stability of the shoulder. *J Bone Joint Surg Am.* 1992;74(1):53-66.

18. Maitland G. *Peripheral Manipulation.* London: Butterworth; 1977.

19. Kisner C, Colby L. *Therapeutic exercise: foundations and techniques.* Philadelphia, Pa: FA Davis; 1985.

20. Kelley M, Leggin B. Shoulder rehabilitation. In: Iannotti, ed. *Disorders of the Shoulder: Diagnosis and Management.* Philadelphia, Pa: Lippincott Williams & Wilkins; 1999.

21. Hawkins RJ. Electromyographic validation of the subscapularis during the lift off test. Paper presented at AAOS annual meeting. Atlanta, Ga; 1996.

22. Iannotti JP, Bernot MP, Kuhlman JR, et al. Postoperative assessment of the shoulder function: a prospective study of full-thickness rotator cuff tears. *J Should Elbow Surg.* 1996;5(6):449-457.

23. Sapega AA, Kelley MJ. Review: strength testing about the shoulder. *J Should Elbow Surg.* 1994;3(5):327-345.

24. Greenfield BH, et al. Isokinetic evaluation of shoulder rotational strength between the plane of scapula and the frontal plane. *Am J Sports Med.* 1990;18(2):124-127.

25. Whitcomb L, Kelley M, Leiper C. A comparison of torque production during isokinetic testing of shoulder abduction in the coronal plane and the plane of the scapula. *J Orthop Sports Phys Ther.* 1995;21:227-232.

26. Rogers K, et al. Concentric and eccentric isokinetic evaluation using two positions in patients two years post ACL reconstruction using the autogenous semitendinosis/gracilis graft. Paper presented at Pennsylvania Athletic Trainer's Association annual meeting. State College, Pa; 1996.

27. Sempo K, et al. Evaluation of isokinetic strength of recurrent dislocation and subluxation of the shoulder. *J Should Elbow Surg.* 1993;2:S41.

28. Warner J, Answorth A, Gerber C. Diagnosis and management of subscapularis tendon tears. *Techniques in Orthopaedics.* 1994;9(2):116-125.

29. Greis PE, Dean M, Hawkins RJ. Subscapularis tendon disruption after Bankart reconstruction for anterior instability. *J Should Elbow Surg.* 1996;5(3):219-222.

30. Williams GR. Personal communication. 1999.

31. Ziegler DW, Harryman DT, Matsen FA. Subscapularis insufficiency in the previously operated shoulder. Paper presented at AAOS annual meeting. Atlanta, Ga; 1996.

32. Wirth MA, Seltzer DA, Rockwood CA. Replacement of the subscapularis with the pectoralis muscles in anterior shoulder instability. Paper presented at AAOS annual meeting. Orlando, Fla; 1995.

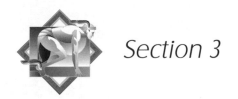

Section 3

Elbow, Wrist, and Hand

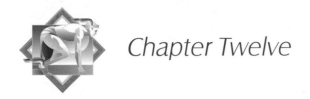

Chapter Twelve

Rehabilitation after Surgical Reconstruction of the Ulnar Collateral Ligament of the Elbow in a Baseball Player

Paul Mieling, MS, OTR, ATC

INTRODUCTION

Injuries to the elbow in the throwing athlete are common, complicated, and at times elusive. A thorough history and physical evaluation is necessary to determine the extent of the athlete's symptoms and disability. Care must be taken to conduct a systematic and exhaustive evaluation that delves into the athlete's subjective history, as well as the physical findings. In the case of injuries to the medial elbow in throwers, the subjective history will provide necessary clues that can lead to the correct diagnosis. Overhead throwing creates repetitive valgus stress that can result in medial elbow symptoms arising from four pathologic conditions:
1. Medial epicondylitis, also known as flexor pronator tendonitis
2. Ulnar collateral ligament (UCL) injury or insufficiency
3. Ulnar nerve tension neurapraxia
4. Medial elbow intra-articular pathology[1]

In the thrower, it is vital to determine if the signs and symptoms are acute or chronic in nature.[2] According to Andrews, et al,[2] chronic injuries include UCL strain or rupture, valgus extension overload, musculotendinous strains, and osteochondral defects that progress to degenerative changes.

Significant injury requiring intervention follows one of three scenarios: the experience of an acute "pop" or sharp pain on the medial aspect of the elbow leading to the inability to throw, the gradual onset of medial elbow pain over time with throwing, or pain following an episode of heavy throwing with the inability to throw above 50% to 75% of full function on successful attempts.[3] The patient may report associated recurrent pain or paresthesia radiating onto the ulnar aspect of the forearm, hand, and fourth and fifth fingers, especially with throwing.[3] In a study performed on 71 throwing athletes with valgus instability of the elbow, 40% had symptoms of impairment in the ulnar nerve as a result of valgus stress loading due to an incompetent ulnar collateral ligament.[4]

The ulnar collateral ligament or medial ligament complex consists of three distinct parts: the anterior, posterior, and transverse bundles (Figure 12-1).[5-7] The primary constraint resisting a valgus force on the elbow is the anterior band.[4,8] The act of throwing a baseball or javelin, or a similar activity, causes enormous valgus stresses on the elbow during the late cocking and acceleration phases of throwing that may exceed the tensile strength of the ligament.[4,9] According to Fleisig and Escamilla,[10] a large valgus torque is produced at the elbow during the arm cocking phase, caused in part by pelvis and upper torso rotation and rapid shoul-

Figure 12-1. Ulnar collateral ligament of the elbow showing anterior bundle, posterior bundle, and transverse bundle.

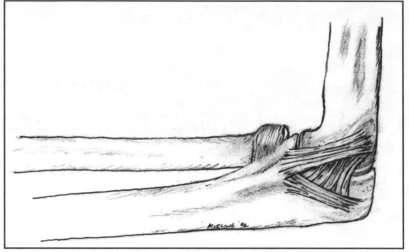

der external rotation. A maximum varus torque of 52 to 76 nm is generated shortly before maximum external rotation to resist valgus torque at the elbow.[10,11] Morrey and An,[12] studied the UCL and showed that the contributions of the ligament contributed approximately 54% of the resistance to valgus forces. Assuming that the UCL produces 54% of the 52 to 76 nm varus torque generated by an elite pitcher, the UCL would then provide approximately 30 to 40 nm of varus torque.[10] A failure load of 32 nm was reported by Dillman, et al,[13] which makes it apparent that the UCL is loaded to its maximum capacity. Other structures providing valgus resistance and minimizing stress on the UCL include the wrist flexor and pronator mass, as they originate on the medial epicondyle, as well as the anconeous and triceps.[14]

This case is presented to demonstrate one example of a National Collegiate Athletic Association (NCAA) Division 1 pitcher who was able to return to a high level of competition after reconstruction of the ulnar collateral ligament.

SUBJECT

The patient was a 22-year-old NCAA Division 1 baseball player who sustained an injury to his right ulnar collateral ligament of the elbow during the summer of 1995. He noted paresthesia in the ulnar nerve distribution at the same time he felt the pop. He was unable to continue throwing that game and took the rest of the summer off. He started throwing in the fall after 2 to 3 months of rest and had no problems until he experienced some aching in the winter. He was doing fairly well until March 3, 1996 when he was pitching in the third or fourth inning. He threw a curve ball and noted significant pain over the medial aspect of his elbow similar to what he had experienced the previous summer. After a few more pitches he was unable to continue. The patient rested for 1 1/2 weeks and attempted to throw lightly on March 14 but still experienced medial elbow pain. He rested for 2 more weeks and, on March 28, began a soft toss program in an attempt to return to throwing. He was not able to return to prior level of function. Each time, he complained of significant medial elbow pain. He also complained of a click and pain with the follow-through phase of pitching, although most of his pain was during the acceleration phase.

Examination was performed on April 25, 1996 by an orthopedic surgeon with experience diagnosing and treating ulnar collateral ligament injuries. The exam revealed full range of motion (ROM) and no gross instability to valgus stress. The patient did have some tenderness over the sublime tubercle with a positive milking sign (Figure 12-2) at 70 degrees of flexion and valgus stress that reproduced symptoms and resulted in soreness over the proximal ulna. He also had a positive Tinel's sign over the cubital tunnel and a positive ulnar flexion stress test (Figure 12-3). Plain radiographs were negative. Stress radiographs were obtained and were negative as well. Magnetic resonance imaging (MRI) showed mild medial epicondylitis with no significant

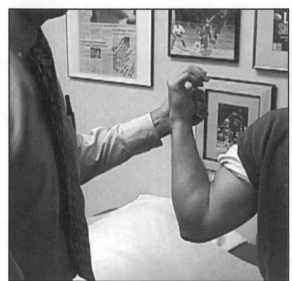

Figure 12-2. Milking sign. With the humerus at 80 to 90 degrees of abduction and the elbow flexed to 70 degrees, the examiner grabs the thumb (like milking a cow) and pulls the arm into external rotation. This gives a valgus force that replicates throwing or the force applied at the beginning of the acceleration phase.

Figure 12-3. Ulnar flexion stress test.

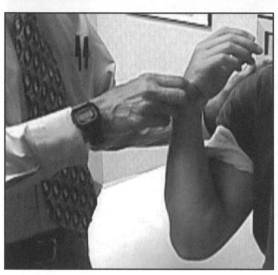

changes in the ulnar collateral ligament. Upon review of the MRI, there were some questionable areas in the distal aspect of the ulnar collateral ligament.

The physician diagnosed UCL insufficiency and recommended 3 to 4 weeks of rest, followed by a return-to-throwing program. If the athlete was unable to throw at that time, the surgeon was willing to perform an exam under anesthesia, arthroscopy and exploration, and possible reconstruction of the UCL using a palmaris longus graft. The alternative was for the athlete to stop throwing at a high level. The patient discussed these options with his parents, coach, and athletic trainers. The patient opted for the surgical intervention, as it was his junior year and the timetable for this treatment option would give him an opportunity to compete during his senior year.

Table 12-1

CONSERVATIVE PROTOCOL FOR ULNAR COLLATERAL LIGAMENT INSUFFICIENCY

Phase (Time from Injury)	Activity
Phase I (1 to 3 months)	Rest from throwing for 2 to 3 months. Take anti-inflammatory medication as needed. DonJoy IROM brace locked at 0 degrees extension and 120 degrees flexion during the day and 90 degrees extension and 90 degrees flexion at night. Active and passive ROM exercises three to four times per day for the elbow and forearm. Strengthening program for wrist flexors and pronators and the rotator cuff. Ice two to three times per day
Phase II (3 to 6 months)	If pain-free, patient can discontinue brace (elbow hyperextension brace with lateral support may be used for throwing and lifting). Progress upper extremity strengthening program to include all muscles. Impulse machine may be used for throwing exercises. Begin throwing progression.

PERIOPERATIVE REHABILITATION

Treatment Plan

PHASE I: PREOPERATIVE REHABILITATION

The patient was sent to our occupational therapy department and issued a conservative protocol for ulnar collateral ligament insufficiency that included ROM exercises and a strengthening program for the wrist flexors and pronators and the rotator cuff (Table 12-1). A DonJoy IROM brace (Smith & Nephew DonJoy, Inc, Carlsbad, Calif) was issued and set at 0 degrees extension and 120 degrees flexion during the day and 90 degrees extension and 90 degrees flexion at night. The patient performed active and passive ROM exercises three to four times per day for the elbow and forearm.

This throwing progression was designed to stress the elbow gradually and not disrupt the healing that had taken place. We found this to be an ideal time for the athlete to focus on throwing mechanics and make any adjustments necessary to avoid reinjury.

Surgical Procedure

On May 10, 1996 the patient underwent right UCL reconstruction ulnar nerve transfer. The palmaris longus was used as the graft. Under anesthesia, both elbows were stressed with the right elbow opening to valgus stress at 30 degrees, approximately 2 mm more than the left. The articular surfaces of the coronoid process and the trochlea were entirely intact. There was synovitis medially and 5 degrees of opening with valgus stress at 70 degrees of flexion. The radial head and capitellum were entirely intact. Some irregularity of the medial aspect of the tip of the olecranon was noted, and there were some changes in the olecranon fossa, consistent with posterior medial impingement or valgus extension overload syndrome. This was addressed by removing a posteromedial osteophyte. The ulnar nerve was identified and noted to be quite hyperemic and swollen, indicating the necessity of an anterior transfer of the nerve.

A significant amount of hemorrhage and degeneration of the distal portion of the ligament was noted. A longitudinal incision was made in the ligament and verified that the ligament had been torn from its distal attachment. Some fibers were moderately functioning, but they were quite attenuated. Valgus stress was applied and the joint opened approximately 3 to 4 mm, confirming the diagnosis of ulnar collateral ligament insufficiency. Two drill holes were made approximately 5 mm distal to the joint surface on the proximal ulna. The medial epicondyle was exposed further and drill holes were made beginning at the attachment of the ulnar collateral ligament to the medial epicondyle, one entering posterior to superior and one posterior to inferior along the superior aspect of the medial epicondyle. A posteromedial arthrotomy was performed, and the posterior olecranon osteophyte was identified and removed by means of an osteome.

An 18-cm palmaris longus tendon graft was harvested. Using a suture passer, the graft was passed through the tunnel in the ulna and through two tunnels in the medial condyle. With the elbow in the 30 to 40 degrees of flexion and varus configuration the three stands of palmaris longus were sutured to themselves. The graft was tested and felt to be satisfactorily isometric; good stability was noted with less than 1 mm opening at the joint line.

The ulnar nerve was then gently transferred anteriorly, and a superficial fascia subcutaneous flap was made and sutured to the anterior aspect of the flexor pronator mass. Compression dressings, burn dressing, Kerlix dressing (Kendall Company, Mansfield, Mass), elastic wrap, a long arm splint at 90 degrees of flexion and neutral forearm rotation were applied.

POSTOPERATIVE CLINICAL COURSE

The rehabilitation program involved a progressive approach to controlling patient ROM to promote tissue healing and graft site protection (Table 12-2). Gripping exercises were initiated on the day of the operation to minimize flexor muscle atrophy and scarring. Active and passive ROM of the wrist, forearm, and elbow were initiated 6 days postoperatively within a DonJoy IROM brace with adjustable locking for extension and flexion. Strengthening exercises that were specific to the throwing athlete, and a slow progression for return to throwing, were given to the patient.

PHASE II: 0 TO 6 DAYS

The patient was immobilized with a posterior elbow splint and bulky dressing with the elbow at 90 degrees of flexion and a neutral forearm. Active gripping with a sponge ball was initiated three to four times a day for 5 minutes each. The patient was also instructed to ice the elbow as much as possible. Six days postoperatively the staples and sutures were removed and Steri-strips (3M Corporation, St. Paul, Minn) were applied. Two-point discrimination was normal and motor function was intact. Elbow flexion was 110 degrees and extension was 30 degrees short of 0 degrees. Pronation was 85 degrees and supination was 70 degrees. The patient also had 55 degrees of wrist extension and 50 degrees of wrist flexion. Edema was minimal.

PHASE III: 7 TO 21 DAYS

The patient followed the perioperative rehabilitation program, which emphasized increasing ROM and minimizing pain and inflammation. The brace used preoperatively was applied with Tensogrip (Smith & Nephew, Germantown, Wis) and locked at 90 degrees of extension and 90 degrees of flexion at all times, with the exception of six sessions daily. During these sessions, the brace was moved to 30 degrees of extension and 110 degrees of flexion to perform active ROM and light passive ROM exercises for the elbow, forearm, and wrist. The exercises were performed 10 times and held for 10 seconds each. Ice was applied four to five times per day. The brace was adjusted 14 days after surgery by 10 degrees of extension and flexion so that exercises were being performed at 20 degrees extension and 120 degrees of flexion. The brace was then locked at 90 degrees extension and flexion with the forearm straps loosened so the patient could perform active and light

Table 12-2

POSTOPERATIVE REHABILITATION FOR ULNAR COLLATERAL LIGAMENT OF THE ELBOW

Phase (Time After Surgery)	Objective	Activity
Phase I (1 to 3 weeks)	Clinical goals	Maintain shoulder ROM. Elbow ROM of 30 degrees extension to 120 degrees flexion.
	Testing	Elbow and forearm ROM.
	Exercises	DonJoy IROM brace at 90 degrees between exercises and at night. Active ROM and light passive ROM exercises for the elbow within the brace (brace should be set at 30 degrees extension and 120 degrees flexion and the exercises should be performed six times per day). Active and light passive pronation/supination exercises within the brace with forearm straps loosened. Ice three to four times per day. Strengthening using putty three times per day for 5 to 10 minutes. Shoulder ROM exercises to maintain motion.
Phase II (3 to 6 weeks)	Clinical goals	Achieve full elbow and forearm ROM by 6 weeks.
	Testing	Elbow and forearm range of motion. Grip strength test at 6 weeks using a hand-held dynamometer.
	Exercises	Set brace at 20 degrees of extension and 120 degrees of flexion for exercises at 3 weeks. Initiate wrist flexor and pronator strengthening exercises at 3 weeks. The patient may remove the brace one to two times per day to fully flex elbow 10 times at 3 weeks. Continue to increase extension in brace 10 degrees each week to achieve full extension by 6 weeks.
Phase III (6 weeks to 6 months)	Clinical goals	Discontinue brace at 6 weeks. Increases shoulder and elbow strength.
	Testing	Elbow and forearm ROM. Grip strength.
	Exercises	Elbow strengthening; the patient should avoid valgus stress for 4 months. Shoulder strengthening can begin 1 week after elbow strengthening is initiated. HXT brace (United States Manufacturing Company, LLC, Pasadena, Calif) may be used if needed when gradually returning to a sport other than baseball.

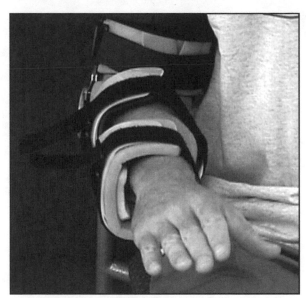

Figure 12-4. Active ROM exercise for pronation.

passive pronation and supination exercises (Figure 12-4). Putty exercises for grip strengthening were performed three times per day for 10 minutes each session.

PHASE IV: 3 TO 6 WEEKS

The goal of this phase was to achieve full elbow and forearm ROM by 6 weeks. At week 3, active ROM was 0-17-105 and passive ROM was 0-15-115; forearm and wrist active ROM was within normal limits compared to the left. Edema was minimal. Grip strength was 115 lbs on the right and 125 lbs on the left. Two-point discrimination was normal. The brace was set to 10 degrees of extension and 120 degrees of flexion. The patient was allowed to remove the brace one to two times per day to fully flex the elbow 10 times. At this time, the patient was to continue to increase extension by 10 degrees in the brace each week in order to achieve full extension by week 5 or 6. Wrist flexor and pronator strengthening was initiated at 3 weeks with TheraBand performing three sets of 12 repetitions two to three times per day. Ice was used two to three times per day, and the patient was weaned out of the Tensogrip (Rehabilitation Group, Smith & Nephew, Germantown, Wis) around week 3.

PHASE V: 6 WEEKS

This phase emphasized a balanced and progressive upper extremity strengthening and flexibility program and began the return-to-throwing progression (Table 12-3). At 6 weeks, the patient's elbow motion was 0-5-145 and forearm and wrist motion were normal compared to the left. Grip strength was 125 lbs bilaterally. If elbow and forearm ROM had not been within normal limits, dynamic splinting would have been considered. Elbow and rotator cuff strengthening were initiated at 6 weeks and the patient was allowed to return to the weight room, avoiding valgus stress for 6 more weeks. At 10 weeks, the patient's elbow ROM was 0-5-145 and had no evidence of instability or symptoms. At 3 months postoperatively the patient's elbow ROM remained 0-5-145 and grip strength was 125 lbs bilaterally. He was allowed to throw a sponge ball 15 to 20 feet for 2 weeks, then a tennis ball 20 to 30 feet for 2 weeks. At 4 months, he was throwing a baseball 30 feet at 50% velocity. At 5 months, the patient was throwing 60 feet at 50% velocity without problems. Six months after surgery he was throwing 90 feet at 75% velocity and was allowed to progress as tolerated. The patient reported throwing 100% off of the mound at 7 months and had no return of symptoms. At the 8-month period, the team began its spring workouts and the patient was unrestricted with all drills and workouts.

On February 28, 1997, 9½ months after surgery, the patient was able to throw one inning and reported no recurrence of symptoms. On March 3, 1997, 1 year from his initial injury, he threw 7 innings against the

Table 12-3

INTERVAL THROWING PROGRAM

Phase I: 30 Ft	Phase II: 45 Ft	Phase III: 60 Ft	Phase IV: 90 Ft
Warm-up throwing 30 ft	Warm-up throwing 45 ft	Warm-up throwing 60 ft	Warm-up throwing 90 ft
Rest 5 minutes	Rest 5 minutes	Rest 5 minutes	Rest 5 minutes
Warm-up throwing 30 ft	Warm-up throwing 45 ft	Warm-up throwing 60 ft	Warm-up throwing 90 ft
Warm-up throwing 30 ft	Warm-up throwing 45 ft	Warm-up throwing 60 ft	Warm-up throwing 90 ft
Warm-up throwing 30 ft	Rest 5 minutes	Rest 5 minutes	Rest 5 minutes
Rest 5 minutes	Warm-up throwing 45 ft	Warm-up throwing 60 ft	Warm-up throwing 90 ft
Warm-up throwing 30 ft	Warm-up throwing 45 ft	Warm-up throwing 60 ft	Warm-up throwing 90 ft
Rest 5 minutes	Rest 5 minutes	Rest 5 minutes	Rest 5 minutes
Warm-up throwing 30 ft	Warm-up throwing 45 ft	Warm-up throwing 60 ft	Warm-up throwing 90 ft
	Rest 5 minutes	Rest 5 minutes	
	Warm-up throwing 45 ft	Warm-up throwing 60 ft	
Warm-up throwing 30 ft	Warm-up throwing 45 ft	Warm-up throwing 60 ft	Warm-up throwing 90 ft
Rest 5 minutes	Rest 5 minutes	Rest 5 minutes	Rest 5 minutes
Warm-up throwing 30 ft	Warm-up throwing 45 ft	Warm-up throwing 60 ft	Warm-up throwing 90 ft
Rest 5 minutes	Rest 5 minutes	Rest 5 minutes	Rest 5 minutes
Warm-up throwing 30 ft	Warm-up throwing 45 ft	Warm-up throwing 60 ft	Warm-up throwing 90 ft
			Warm-up throwing 90 ft
			Rest 5 minutes
Warm-up throwing 30 ft			Warm-up throwing 90 ft
Rest 5 minutes			Rest 5 minutes
Warm-up throwing 30 ft			Warm-up throwing 90 ft
Rest 5 minutes			Assessment by orthopedic surgeon and athletic trainer
Warm-up throwing 30 ft			

Table 12-3 continued

Individual variability: The interval throwing program is designed so that each level is achieved without pain or complication, and the athlete progresses based on achieving goals rather than completing a certain time frame. Because of the length of the program, success will vary from athlete to athlete. Although the program recommends throwing every other day, some days may be worse than others and the athlete may have to throw every third or fourth day due to pain or swelling. Progression should be based on how the arm responds to the increased stress and should be judged by the orthopedic surgeon and athletic trainer.

Warm-up: Jogging increases blood flow to the muscles and joints and thus increases their flexibility and decreases the chance for injury. Since the amount of warm-up time will vary from athlete to athlete, he should jog until developing a light sweat and then progress to the stretching phase.

Stretching: Because throwing involves all of the muscles in the body, all muscle groups should be stretched before throwing. This should be carried out in a systematic manner beginning with the legs and including the trunk, back, neck, and arms.

Throwing: The warm-up throws should be performed at a comfortable distance (approximately 30 to 45 ft) and progress to the distance for that phase. The object of each phase is for the athlete to be able to throw the ball without pain to the specified number of feet. The amount of velocity should be controlled as well. The athlete should begin throwing at only 25% of his full velocity and progress only to 75%. Pitchers are not to "experiment" with breaking pitches, change-ups, split finger pitches, etc.

Interval throwing program: Each phase of the throwing program contains steps that must be performed pain-free before advancement is recommended. Each phase is designed to be performed for approximately 3 weeks for a total of 3 months, although this will vary from athlete to athlete. After the final phase, the orthopedic surgeon will assess the need for further advancement.

same team that his injury occurred. During the course of the spring season he accumulated a record of six wins and two losses with a 5.6 earned run average. He threw a total of 68 innings in 15 games. He reported his most significant victory as a win against a conference rival that clinched a spot for his team in the post-season tournament, giving him four wins and two losses against conference teams.

At the 4-year follow-up, the patient was still pitching. He was playing in a local traveling league and reported no complaints. When asked if his arm was able to respond to the demands he placed on it he said, "After the surgery and rehabilitation on my elbow I was able to throw harder and never experienced any more pain." Objectively he was symptom-free.

REFERENCES

1. Field LD, Altchek DW. Elbow injuries. *Clin Sports Med.* 1995;14(1):59-78.

2. Andrews JR, Whiteside JA, Buettner CM. Clinical evaluation of the elbow in throwers. *Op Tech Sports Med.* 1996;4(2):77-83.

3. Jobe FW, El Attrache NS. Treatment of ulnar collateral ligament injuries in athletes. In: Morrey BF, ed. *Master Techniques in Orthopedic Surgery.* New york, NY: Raven Press, Ltd; 1994:149-168.

4. Conway JE, Jobe FW, Glousman RE, Pink M. Medial instability of the elbow in throwing athletes. Treatment by repair or reconstruction of the ulnar collateral ligament. *J Bone Joint Surg Am.* 1992;74(1):67-83.

5. Guerra JJ, Timmerman LA. Clinical anatomy, histology, and pathomechanics of the elbow in sports. *Op Tech Sports Med.* 1996;4(2):69-76.

6. Morrey BF. Anatomy of the elbow joint. In: Morrey BF, ed. *The Elbow and its Disorders.* Philadelphia, Pa; 1993:16-52.

7. Timmerman LA, Andrews JR. Histology and arthroscopic anatomy of the ulnar collateral ligament of the elbow. *Am J Sports Med.* 1994;22(5):667-673.

8. Hotchkiss RN, Weiland AJ. Valgus stability of the elbow. *J Orthop Res.* 1987;5:372-377.

9. Hang YS, Lippert FG, Spolek GA, et al. Biomechanical study of the pitching elbow. *Int Orthop.* 1979;3:217-223.

10. Fleisig GS, Escamilla RF. Biomechanics of the elbow in the throwing athlete. *Op Tech Sports Med.* 1996;4(2):62-68.

11. Pappas AM, Vitolo J. Elbow anatomy and function. In: Pappas AM, ed. *Upper Extremity Injuries in the Athlete.* New York, NY: Churchill Livingstone; 1994:303-321.

12. Morrey BF, An KN. Articular and ligamentous contributions to the stability of the elbow joint. *Am J Sports Med.* 1983;11:315-319.

13. Dillman C, Smutz P, Werner S, et al. Valgus extension overload in baseball pitching. *Med Sci Sports Exer.* 1991;23:S135.

14. Werner SL, Fleisig GS, Dillman CJ, et al. Biomechanics of the elbow during baseball pitching. *J Orthop Sports Phys Ther.* 1993;17(6):274-278.

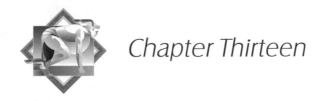

Chapter Thirteen

Adolescent Baseball Pitcher with Medial Elbow Pain and Diagnosis of Medial Epicondylitis

Todd S. Ellenbecker, MS, PT, SCS, CSCS, David G. Carfagno, DO

SUBJECTIVE HISTORY

The patient is a 15-year-old, right-handed baseball pitcher who weighs 140 lbs and is 71 inches tall. He presented with a primary complaint of right medial elbow pain that had been present for approximately 1 week. He played high school baseball and was involved in fall and summer ball in addition to his spring season of high school baseball.

INJURY MECHANISM

During the third inning of a high school baseball game the athlete described having focal elbow pain. He reported having tightness in the medial elbow for approximately 2 weeks before the onset of this pain. The patient continued to pitch for three more innings with discomfort, and after the game he reported a continued dull ache in the medial aspect of the elbow. The pain persisted despite rest for several days, and use of ice as recommended by his high school athletic trainer. The patient reported a pain level of 2/10 with rest and 7/10 with activities such as throwing or swinging. The patient denied any neural radiation of symptoms distally to the hand and forearm and did not feel or hear a pop in the elbow during one pitch. He had a history of medial elbow pain and upper right arm problems. He is generally in good health with the exception of exercise-induced asthma, for which he uses an inhaler as needed. The athletic trainer, coach, and parents reported that the athlete has been very fatigued in the last few weeks and that he was trying to do some light strengthening exercises in the gym for the past month. They also noted a change in his pitching mechanics, with an appearance of a "lagging arm" and dropped elbow, especially when he was throwing while fatigued.

COMPARISON OF INJURY TO THE ESTABLISHED NORM

According to Nirschl,[1,2] injuries to the medial elbow are typically caused by repetitive overuse and lead to breakdown or degeneration of the tendon, which he terms "tendonosis." Repetitive exertional activity, possibly a change of mechanics, or frequency of the exertional event often lead to the development of "tendonosis." This recent finding and change in nomenclature represents greater knowledge in the degenerative process within the tendon and the relative absence of inflammatory process during the histological examination and study of injured tendons.[2] The relatively avascular status of many humans' tendons couples with the large and repetitive eccentric overloads applied to them. This often leads to classic presentation of medial elbow pain, as described in this case study.[3]

CLINICAL EXAMINATION

The initial evaluation of this patient was performed by the athletic trainer and physical therapist following the game. The onsite, onfield evaluation was not conducted since the athlete did not tell the coach or sports medicine team that he was in pain until he was taken out of the game.

Observation of the patient showed a well-developed, lean, muscular, 140-lb high school sophomore. Muscular hypertrophy of the forearm muscles on the right elbow was immediately evident. No swelling or ecchymosis was present. The patient was evaluated without his shirt on and viewed from the posterior aspect. The right shoulder was lower than the left by approximately 1 inch and there was significant scapular winging. Pressing the hands against the wall exaggerated the prominence of the medial and inferior borders of the scapula. Active range of motion (ROM) of the right elbow was -12 degrees of extension and 138 degrees of flexion. Seventy-five degrees of wrist flexion and 55 degrees of wrist extension were measured on the right extremity. Full extension (0 degrees) and 138 degrees of flexion were present in the left elbow. Seventy-five degrees of flexion and extension of the wrist were measured on the left, nondominant arm. Gross manual muscle testing revealed 4/5 strength with provocation of medial elbow pain with testing of right wrist and finger flexion and forearm pronation. All measures were 5/5 and graded as normal with the exception of right shoulder external rotation which was 4/5. Gross grip strength was 60 kg on the dominant extremity and 58 kg on the nondominant extremity measured with a dynamometer. The patient was fully intact to light touch sensations in dermatomes C5 to T1 and showed full cervical spine rang of motion (ROM). Palpation revealed a region of tenderness about the size of a quarter over the medial epicondyle, just distal and medial to the medial epicondyle over the common flexor tendon. There was also mild tenderness in the flexor pronator muscle mass.

Special tests performed on the elbow included the valgus, which was bilaterally symmetrical with respect to laxity, but did provoke mild tenderness in the medial epicondyler region on the right elbow. The valgus extension overpressure test, varus stress test, radiocapitellar compression test, and Tinel's test were negative. The good hands test was positive. The patient's right shoulder showed increased anterior humeral head translation compared with the left (grade II+ compared to grade I+), with negative impingement signs.

CLINICAL EXAM BY A PHYSICIAN

The physician evaluated the patient in the office the following day and observed a slightly depressed right shoulder and increased carrying angle on the right elbow compared to the left. No ecchymosis or swelling was noted. Palpatory tenderness was present over the medial epicondyle on about a 2.5 cm diameter just medial and distal to the epicondyle. Mild tenderness was present over the flexor/pronator belly. ROM was approximately 10 degrees extension and full flexion. Manual muscle testing revealed 4+/5 right finger/wrist flexion and wrist pronation with provocation of pain. External rotation of the right shoulder was 4+/5. The remainder of the muscle groups in elbow, shoulder, hand, and wrist tested 5+/5. Cervical spine ROM was full with negative compression testing. A neurovascular exam was intact, including a negative Tinel's test. Special testing included a valgus stress test, which showed no laxity but did provoke pain in the medial epicondylar area. Good hands test was positive. Valgus extension overload, radiocapitellar compression, and varus stress tests were all negative. The athlete's right shoulder displayed 2+ anterior laxity compared with the left which was 1+ with negative apprehension/relocation. Impingement testing was negative.

DIFFERENTIAL DIAGNOSIS

Medial epicondyle is the primary change considered when a patient presents these signs and symptoms. The history of playing baseball year long without a break sets up the athlete for an overuse tendinous injury. Reproducibility of pain with palpatory/manual muscle test, and the lack of ligamentous laxity both help guide the clinician in the diagnosis. Diagnoses to consider include growth plate fracture, medial collateral ligament MCL sprain, and apophysitis. Type 1 avulsion is the most common growth plate fracture, and can be discovered on radiographs. Mild cases of MCL sprains may be difficult to differentiate from pure epicondylitis due to the absence of gross laxity with mild ligamentous injury. The provocative test in which the patient's wrist is taken into full flexion/pronation with application of a valgus stress test should not reproduce pain if true epicondylitis is present. True apophysitis also needs to be considered 9- to 13-year-old athletes.

Nerve entrapment syndromes of the ulnar nerve can be present concurrrently with medial epicondylitis. It has been reported that 40% to 60% of patients undergoing surgery for medial epicondylitis exhibited some signs/symptoms of ulnar nerve involvement.[4-6] Anterior interosseous nerve entrapment causes weakness with resisted pronation and the inability to sustain thumb and index apposition ("OK" sign). Radicular pain from the first thoracic T1 nerve root distal parenthesis may also be present. Our athlete had no such complaint, and neck and neurovascular exams were within normal limits.

DIAGNOSTIC IMAGING

Radiographs of the elbow showed no evidence of any ulnar tractions spurs, calcifications, loose bodies, or fractures/widening of growth plates. A magnetic resonance imaging (MRI) arthrogram was performed 4 weeks after the initial exam and showed edema within a pronator teres muscle test at the level of medial humeral epicondyle compatible with minor strain of the common flexor region. No abnormalities of the common flexor tendon of the medial epicondyle were identified. The ulnar collateral ligament was intact. Ellenbecker et al,[7] used stress radiography to study the medial ulnar collateral ligament in healthy, uninjured baseball pitchers. Their findings showed statistically significant increases in medial elbow laxity in the dominant elbow as compared with the nondominant, non-throwing elbow. This diagnostic test offers a cost-effective and noninvasive alternative to an MRI to rule out ligamentous injury. Research shows that only minor differences in medial elbow laxity exist, and cannot be reliably identified using manual clinical tests in a professional baseball pitcher.[9]

DIAGNOSIS: RIGHT ELBOW MEDIAL EPICONDYLITIS

Preoperative Rehabilitation for Medial Epicondylitis

IMMEDIATE MANAGEMENT

The initial treatment following physician evaluation was to decrease the patient's sign and promote healing. Providing an optimal environment in the region of the tendon, by reducing the stresses applied to the tendon, and increasing bloodflow helped accomplish this. The use of ultrasound, electrical stimulation, acupuncture, transverse friction massage, and anti-inflammatory medications have all been reported as effective methods to decrease pain.[9-13] The authors preferred the use of stimulation and iontophoresis with dexamethasone applied directly to the affected area. This combination has worked clinically and assists with the initial goal of decreasing pain and improving local bloodflow.[14]

Scientific research comparing therapeutic modalities allows clinicians to make educated decisions regarding the optimal modalities or combination of modalities for any given treatment. Dijs, et al[15] reviewed 70 patients with lateral epicondylitis and compared the effectiveness of a cortisone injection versus physical therapy. Ninety-one percent of the patients had initial short-term relief following a cortisone injection, compared to 47% who experienced initial short-term relief from physical therapy. Striking results from this study are the long-term recurrence rates using the two methods of treatment. When patients were treated with a cortisone injection, a 51% recurrence rate was reported, while only a 5% recurrence rate was reported in the patients who underwent physical therapy.[16]

Research by Kivi[16] reported no difference in pain or symptom reduction after two types of injection with an immobilizer and nonsteroidal anti-inflammatory medication in patients with humeral epicondylitis. Stratford, et al[17] studied the effects of ultrasound with a placebo, phonophoresis, and friction massage and found no significant differences for treatment of humeral epicondylitis. This review of literature clearly demonstrates that there is no superior method for decreasing initial pain levels. In a meta-analysis, Labelle, et al,[18] reviewed 185 articles that examined the treatment of humeral epicondylitis and found a glaring deficiency with no clearcut evidence on the proper modalities to apply in this stage of treatment based on prospective, randomized studies.

In addition to modality application, protection of the limb is emphasized, but complete immobilization of the extremity with a wrist splint is not recommended.[1,9] Use of the immobilizer may lead to further atrophy of the musculature and exaggerate the deficiency in strength and endurance of the involved musculature. This patient discontinued throwing and hitting activities to protect the elbow from stress. Cardiovascular exercises and fielding activities were continued to maintain baseball-specific conditioning levels.

Measures to promote full ROM and strengthening were initiated in this early post-injury phase. Nirschl[1,9] used the patient's tolerance to a firm handshake to determine when light, submaximal exercise could be initiated. Even when resistance application to the involved muscle tendon unit produces pain (in this case flexion and pronation), resistance exercise can submaximally be introduced to the wrist extensors and forearm supinators, often in a pain-free manner. Care was taken with all resistive exercises to ensure that the exercises were performed in a pain-free ROM and at a resistance level that did not provoke pain. Gradual initiation of exercises for the patterns of wrist flexion and extension, forearm pronation and supination, and radial and ulnar deviation of the wrist is recommended with a low resistance, high repetition format.[1,3,9] This not only serves to increase blood flow but also improves local muscular endurance.[19]

During the early phase of rehabilitation, mobilization of the elbow and gentle passive stretching were indicated to normalize joint arthrokinematics. Care was taken not to overly stretch the muscle tendon unit, which could replicate the stresses incurred during injury and provoke and prolong symptoms.[3,9] The anatomical presence of actual mid-muscle belly portions of the brachioradialis in the anterior aspect of the ulnohumeral joint can produce bleeding from aggressive stretching and can lead to myositis ossificans.[3] Active assistive and passive stretching using two to three repetitions for 30 seconds has been recommended to produce a plastic deformation in the soft tissue.[20] Mobilization techniques such as joint distraction were applied. In addition, specific movements of the ulnohumeral joint were utilized, including posterior glide of the ulna on the distal humerus to increase flexion.

One particularly important consideration for this patient, and in many baseball and tennis players, is the flexion contracture (lack of complete elbow extension).[3] Prolonged stretching of the elbow using the concept of "low intensity, long duration" was indicated to attempt to restore greater elbow extension.[3] The technique we prefer is to place the patient supine with the arm abducted 90 to 120 degrees and stretch the elbow. Additionally, combining elbow extension with wrist extension and forearm supination increased the stretch to the structures in the anteromedial aspect of the elbow, which is beneficial for throwing athletes.

As the patient's pain and local tenderness decreased, focus of the rehabilitation shifted to a phase termed, "total arm strength."[3] During this phase, the entire upper extremity is strengthened using a low resistance, high repetition format. Patterns emphasizing strengthening of the rotator cuff were shoulder internal and external rotation, prone horizontal abduction, prone external rotation, and prone extension. Seated rowing and scapular protraction punches were also included to strengthen the scapular stabilizers, which provide proximal stability and establish a strong base for the elbow to function. Additional recommended exercises were ball dribbling (using a basketball or Swiss ball), Body Blade, and medicine ball plyometric chest passes and side throws.

As the patient progressed to the point of tolerating the resistive exercise progression with the use of 3- to 5-lb resistance levels, isokinetic exercise was introduced to provide objective quantification of strength as well as controlled accommodative resistance at faster, more functional speeds.[22] The pattern of wrist extension/flexion was initiated first using speeds from 180 to 300 degrees per second. Three to five sets of 15 to 20 repetitions were used to improve local muscular endurance with a progression from submaximal to maximal training. The patterns of forearm pronation/supination and shoulder internal/external rotation were added to provide an isokinetic total arm strength training stimulus.

Re-Evaluation 14 Days after Medial Elbow Injury

The patient had minimal tenderness to direct palpation of the medial elbow and no pain with ligamentous testing or the good hands maneuver.[3] Active ROM showed 5 degrees of elbow extension, and the patient had 5/5 manual muscle test of the elbow, forearm, and wrist musculature. Gross grip strength using a hand grip dynamometer was 65 kg on the dominant injured extremity and 58 kg on the nondominant extremity.

An isokinetic evaluation was performed for shoulder internal/external rotation, wrist flexion/extension, and forearm pronation/supination. Results of the testing showed the patient had equal wrist flexion/extension between extremities, 15% greater pronation strength on the injured extremity, but 5% weaker supination strength. This information was particularly important because normative data on health elite tennis players and baseball pitchers have shown wrist flexors and extensors and forearm pronators to be 10% to 30% greater on the dominant arm. Forearm supination did not typically demonstrate a dominance effect in these studies. The isokinetic shoulder test showed 10% deficits in the injured shoulder for external rotation, but 30% to 40% greater internal rotation. External/internal rotation ratios ranged between 50% to 55% and were below the standard 66% to 70% ratio previously reported in healthy overhead athletes.[3,21-24]

A summary of re-evaluation findings highlights improved elbow extension, improved strength in the flexor and pronator muscle groups, and a moderate strength imbalance in the rotator cuff, as evidenced by the lower external/internal rotation ratios.

Functional Progression

The beginning of the functional progression started early in the rehabilitation process with the use of low resistance, high repetition exercises that mimicked the nature of the sport in which this patient played. Use of medicine ball plyometrics, ball dribbling, and patterns of exercise including shoulder internal/external rotation at 90 degrees of abduction all set the platform for the final functional progression and return to functional activity. Strict adherence to an interval sport-return program is of paramount importance. The use of an interval throwing program for this patient was indicated based on his current clinical results. The patient started throwing on level ground at 45 feet with two sets of 25 tosses. Two trials of successful, pain-free functional activity were required for progression to the next step. Throwing occurred on alternate days, allowing valuable rest and recovery between sessions. Progression to 60, 90, and 120 feet were followed using these guidelines.

During this critical time the patient's throwing mechanics were evaluated by the sports medicine team as well as the coaching staff. Small changes in torso segmental rotation, shoulder position, and elbow flexion angles can greatly affect the loads placed upon the medial aspect of the elbow.[25] The patient began throwing off the mound after successful completion of the 120-foot phase. Interval hitting programs were also followed with initial batting taking place off a tee, then using a "soft-toss" feeding type skill, and finally progressing to "live" batting practice.

Careful monitoring of this patient by all members of the sports medicine team produced a successful return to both throwing and hitting activities. Continued resistive exercises were recommended, particularly for the shoulder external rotators, scapular stabilizers, and the distal forearm musculature since this patient's isokinetic shoulder and grip strengths were near normal. Additional monitoring of this patient's elbow extension was recommended since a flexion contracture would increase demands on the ligamentous and muscle-tendon structures when compared to an elbow with complete extension.[26]

Surgical Indications

According to Nirschl and Sobel,[9] in 3000 cases of epicondylitis, 92% responded favorably to nonoperative management. Characteristics of patients who did not respond favorably were chronic symptoms of pain, pain in the contralateral elbow and shoulder, intense pain in the involved elbow even at rest, exacerbation of symptoms following cortisone injection, and nonoperative treatment interventions.

The athlete in this case study would have had to fail conservative management, including physical therapy modalities as described; and a local steroid injection, before being considered a candidate for surgical intervention.

The surgical procedure indicated for this type of patient would be an amendment of recalcitrant medial epicondylitis. Histological evaluation of the diseased tendon usually shows the absence of acute inflammatory cells. This consistent finding, which has been stated in other studies, is angiofibroblastic hyperplasia tendinosis and fibrillary degeneration of collagen. The lack of inflammatory cells and, presence of degenerative tissue is more accurately termed tendinosis.

SUMMARY

The importance of an accurate initial diagnosis and comprehensive evaluation is clearly highlighted in this case study. The use of a multidisciplinary approach encompassing the athletic trainer, physician, physical therapist, and coach allowed for early initiation of treatment and a return to full activity. Careful monitoring of throwing mechanics and strict, individualized adherence to an interval throwing program, as well as use of functionally specific rehabilitative exercises, are all integral parts of complete rehabilitation of this adolescent baseball pitcher with medial epicondylitis.

REFERENCES

1. Nirschl RP. Tennis elbow. *Primary Care.* 1997;4:367-382.

2. Kraushaar BS, Nirschl RP. Tendonosis of the elbow: current concepts review. *J Bone Joint Surg Am.* 1999;81(2):259-278.

3. Ellenbecker TS, Mattalino AJ. *The Elbow in Sport.* Champaign, Ill: Human Kinetics; 1996.

4. Kibler WB. The role of the scapula in athletic shoulder function. *Am J Sports Med.* 1998;26(2):325-337.

5. Nirschl RP. Lateral and medial epicondylitis. In: Morrey BF, ed. *Master Techniques in Orthopaedic Surgery: The Elbow.* New York, NY: Raven Press; 1994.

6. Nirschl RP. Sports and overuse injuries to the elbow. In: Morrey BF, ed. *The Elbow and its Disorders.* 2nd ed. Philadelphia, Pa: WB Saunders; 1993.

7. Vangsness CTJ, Jobe FW. Surgical treatment of medial epicondylitis. *J Bone Joint Surg Br.* 1991;73:409.

8. Ellenbecker TS, Mattalino AJ, Elam EA, et al. Medial elbow joint laxity in professional baseball pitchers: a bilateral comparison using stress radiography. *Am J Sports Med.* 1998;26(3):420-424.

9. Ellenbecker TS, Boeckmann RB. Interrater reliability of manual valgus stress testing of the elbow joint and its relation to an objective stress radiography technique in professional baseball pitchers. *J Orthop Sports Phys Ther.* 1998;27(1):95.

10. Nirschl RP, Sobel J. Conservative treatment of tennis elbow. *The Physician and Sports Medicine.* 1981;9(6):43-54.

11. Bernhang AM, Dehner W, Fogerty C. Tennis elbow: a biomechanical approach. *Am J Sports Med.* 1974;2:235-260.

12. Kamien M: A rational management of tennis elbow. *Sports Med.* 1990;9:173-191.

13. Ingham B. Transverse friction massage. *The Physician and Sports Medicine.* 1981;9(10):116.

14. Rosenthal M. The efficacy of flurbiprofen versus piroxicam in the treatment of acute soft tissue rheumatism. *Curr Med Res Opin.* 1984;9:304-309.

15. Griffin JE, Karselis TC. *Physical Agents for Physical Therapists.* Springfield, Ill: Charles C. Thomas Publishers; 1982.

16. Dijs H, Mortier G, Driessens M, et al. A retrospective study of the conservative treatment of tennis elbow. *Medica Physica.* 1990;13:73-77.

17. Kivi P. The etiology and conservative treatment of tennis elbow. *Scan J Rehabil Med.* 1982;15:37-42.

18. Stratford PW, Levy DR, Gauldie S, et al. The evaluation of phonophoresis and friction massage as treatments for extensor carpi radialis tendonitis: a randomized controlled trial. *Physiotherapy Canada.* 1989;41:93-99.

19. Labelle H, Guibert R, Joncas J. Lack of scientific evidence for the treatment of lateral epicondylitis of the elbow. *J Bone and Joint Surg Br.* 1992;74:646-651.

20. Fleck SJ, Kramer WJ: *Designing Resistance Training Programs.* Champaign, Ill: Human Kinetics; 1987.

21. Zachezewski JE, Reischl S. Flexibility for the runner: specific program considerations. *Topics in Acute Care and Trauma Rehabilitation.* 1986;1:9-27.

22. Davies GJ. *A Compendium of Isokinetics in Clinical Usage*, 2nd ed. LaCrosse, Wis: S&S Publishers; 1992.

23. Ellenbecker TS, Mattalino AJ. Concentric isokinetic shoulder internal and external rotation strength in professional baseball pitchers. *J Orthop Sports Phys Ther.* 1997;25(5):323-328

24. Ellenbecker TS. Rehabilitation of shoulder and elbow injuries in tennis players. *Clin Sports Med.* 1995;14(1):87-109.

25. Warner JJP, Micheli LJ, Arslanian LE, et al. Patterns of flexibility, laxity, and strength in normal shoulders and shoulders with instability and impingement. *Am J Sports Med.* 1990;18:366-375.

26. Marshall RN, Noffal GJ, Legnani G. *Stimulation of the Tennis Serve: Factors Affecting Elbow Torques Related to Medial Epicondylitis.* Paris: Biomechanics ISB; 1993.

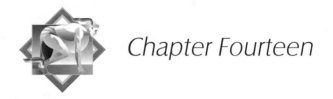

Chapter Fourteen

Rehabilitation After Open Reduction and Internal Fixation of a Displaced Intra-articular Metacarpal Head Fracture

Cheri Alexy, OTR, CHT

INTRODUCTION

Sports-related metacarpal fractures are usually stable due to the supportive soft tissues around the metacarpals, including the interosseous muscles and the distal intermetacarpal ligaments. These fractures typically heal well with treatment of continuous splinting for 1 to 2 weeks, followed by active ROM exercises. The splint is continued at night and between exercises for approximately 2 more weeks, then splint wear is gradually decreased, worn only as needed for protection. Athletes are often able to return to play during the first or second week after the injury with a padded splint, or playing cast, and buddy taping, depending on the sport and position they play.[1,2]

Displaced intra-articular and comminuted fractures of the head and neck metacarpal are usually caused by high energy trauma. The patient is most likely to achieve full joint mobility and hand function after open reduction and internal fixation (ORIF) to anatomically reduce the fracture and apply rigid fixation.[2-8] Following internal fixation, the patient is allowed to begin early ROM exercises, often during the first few days postoperatively.[5,8] Early motion helps to ensure minimal joint and ligament contracture and tendon adherence to the fracture site, the most common problems following metacarpal fracture.

The return of function and fine motor coordination in the hand after a fracture is dependent upon free muscle and tendon gliding and the restoration of full joint mobility.[8,9] The success of the rehabilitation program depends upon the patient being educated and involved in the process. It is the responsibility of the therapist or athletic trainer to ensure patient understanding of the importance of edema control, brief but regular exercise sessions, and appropriate splint wear.

Controlling edema is one of the most important components of the postoperative therapy program. Untreated edema in the hand can lead to extensive scarring, tissue inelasticity, and limited ROM. While arterial blood flow into the hand occurs on the volar aspect, the return flow of blood occurs primarily on the dorsum of the hand. The return of venous and lymphatic fluid requires a pumping action of the fingers, which is usually diminished after injury secondary to limited ROM.[10] Failing to keep the hand elevated will increase fluid as it pools in the hand.

As the swelling continues, fluids rich in protein surround the joints, tendons, and ligaments. The soft tissues gradually become shortened and tight due to their distension with fluid. As the proteins in the fluid consolidate, the fluid becomes rigid.[10] This can be described to the patient as pouring glue along the joints and tendons, making it difficult to move the fingers.

Figure 14-1. Hand based ulnar gutter splint with MCP joints in flexion for mid-shaft, head, and neck metacarpal fractures.

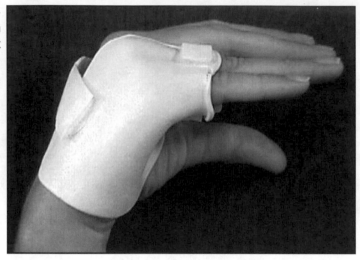

Keeping the hand elevated above the heart creates a negative relative pressure around the injured area and encourages drainage of the fluid.[5] After surgery patients are often issued large foam pillows to elevate the hand while sitting or lying. The patient can also rest the arm on a stack of pillows. A light compressive dressing consisting of an elastic bandage wrapped over gauze or an elastic sleeve applied over the hand and forearm helps to decrease swelling in the hand. If the fingers are swollen, Coban (3M, St. Paul, Minn) may be wrapped lightly around the finger, beginning at the tip and wrapping proximally to the base of the finger. The patient is instructed in the use of ice packs or a Cryo/Cuff, which can be beneficial for both edema control and pain management.[11] The patient needs to understand that by decreasing edema, the amount of pain experienced during the rehabilitation process will also be decreased, and lessening the degree of edema and pain will greatly enhance the return of motion and function in the hand.[5,10,11]

Scar adhesions around the fracture site may limit the glide of the extensor tendons on the dorsum of the hand, resulting in limited active extension of the metacarpophalangeal (MCP) joints as well as limited active and passive flexion. It is important for the patient to understand that frequent but brief exercise sessions, as many as eight to 10 times a day, are needed to achieve and maintain tendon gliding. The exercise sessions should not cause a significant amount of pain, however, some discomfort is normal, and the patient is encouraged to take the prescribed pain medications as needed to achieve the best results from therapy.[5]

Fractures at the base and proximal portion of the metacarpal are splinted in a forearm based wrist immobilization splint, well molded around the metacarpals. When the fracture is in the head, neck, or mid-shaft of the metacarpal, the hand is splinted in a hand based safe-position splint (Figure 14-1). The interphalangeal joints are usually left free, and the involved finger is buddy taped to an adjacent finger if there is a need to control rotation. The safe-position splint holds the MCP joints in 60 to 80 degrees of flexion, maintaining the length of the collateral ligaments and preventing significant MCP joint extension contractures.[4,8,11,12]

SUBJECT

The patient was a 21-year-old NCAA Division I softball player who injured her right ring finger while catching a ball during a game on October 10, 1998, one of the last games of the fall season. She was a senior and was planning on playing in the spring, as well as the following year as a second year senior. The patient stated that while attempting to catch the ball with her left hand, the ball glanced off of her glove and hit the base of the ring finger of her throwing hand. She stated that the finger felt dislocated, and was reduced by the athletic trainer in the dugout. The patient and the athletic trainer reported that secondary to minimal pain or swelling the finger was taped to an adjacent finger and she returned to the game, playing first base with little discomfort. By the end of the game, there was significant swelling in her hand and pain was increasing. The athletic trainer wrapped the hand, applied ice, and referred the patient to a physician at the university. Radiographs revealed a displaced, intra-articular fracture of the ring metacarpal head. The athlete was referred to an orthopedic hand surgeon, where she was seen 2 days after the injury.

PHYSICAL EXAMINATION

When performing an initial examination of a possible metacarpal fracture, the athletic trainer or physician has to decide if the injury requires immediate medical attention or if the athlete can continue playing, possibly with some type of protection. The goal is to determine the stability of the fracture. The evaluation should determine the presence of bony tenderness, crepitus, obvious shortening of the metacarpal, angulation, and rotation. Mild rotational deformities of the metacarpals are often difficult to see when the fingers are extended. With full active flexion, fingertips should point to the scaphoid tubercle, without crowding or overlapping of the fingers. Fractures are typically stable if the athlete can fully extend and flex the fingers with no malrotation.[3,10]

Physician's Evaluation

The orthopedic hand surgeon evaluated the patient on October 12, 2 days after the injury. She brought x-rays from the university, which revealed an intra-articular fracture of the fourth metacarpal head, with disruption of the articular surface. The physician's exam revealed significant tenderness and swelling over the fourth MCP joint. Two point discrimination was normal, but there was significant limitation of motion. The physician discussed the nature of the injury with the patient and her family and recommended ORIF of the fracture to reconstitute the articular surface of the metacarpal head. They discussed the procedure in detail and decided to schedule surgery for the following day.

Without ORIF, intra-articular fractures, especially those with displacement and comminution, often result in articular incongruity. This can cause rotational and angular deformities, pain, decreased ROM, tendon and joint contractures, and functional impairment.[4,8]

PREOPERATIVE CARE

The patient was first seen in therapy on October 12, 1998, the day before surgery. Moderate to severe edema was present in the hand, and she was in a significant amount of pain. On a subjective pain rating scale of one to 10, with 10 being severe pain, the patient rated her pain as nine. ROM was minimal. All clinical findings are presented in Table 14-1.

Surgery was scheduled for the next day, so the only goals were to protect the hand and decrease the edema and pain as much as possible. A light compressive dressing and a hand based safe-position splint were applied, and the ring and small fingers were buddy taped. The patient was instructed to keep the hand elevated above the heart, and to use ice packs four to six times a day for 20 minutes. Light motion to the uninvolved digits was encouraged to help pump the edema from the hand.

SURGICAL PROCEDURE

On October 13, 1998, the patient underwent ORIF of an intra-articular, comminuted fracture of the fourth metacarpal head. The extensor digitorum communis tendon of the ring finger and the joint capsule beneath it were incised longitudinally to expose the MCP joint. There was an impacted volar fracture involving approximately one third of the metacarpal head, with a small comminuted fragment ulnarly. The surgeon was able to obtain anatomic reduction of the fracture, and then achieve internal fixation by means of two small Herbert screws, using one 12 mm and one 10 mm screw. The joint was stable as it was moved through full ROM. After irrigation of the joint with normal saline solution, the dorsal capsule and extensor tendon were closed. The wound was injected with 0.25% Marcaine (Winthrop, New York, NY) with epinephrine solution, and the skin was closed. A postoperative compressive dressing was applied, and a forearm based dorsal splint was secured with an elastic bandage and tape, holding the wrist in a neutral position and the MCP joints in flexion. The patient was issued commercial ice wraps that she kept wrapped around the hand and

Table 14-1

CLINICAL FINDINGS

	1 Day Preoperatively	2 Days Postoperatively	9 Days Postoperatively	15 Days Postoperatively	3 Weeks Postoperatively	7 Weeks Postoperatively
Edema	Moderate/severe	Moderate (+)	Moderate	Minimal (+)	Minimal (+)	Minimal
Active Range of Motion	MCP ext: 30 degrees MCP flex: 45 degrees PIP ext: 25 degrees PIP flex: 45 degrees DIP ext: 0 degrees DIP flex: 20 degrees	MCP ext: 20 degrees MCP flex: 40 degrees PIP ext: 10 degrees PIP flex: 60 degrees DIP ext: 5 degrees DIP flex: 35 degrees	MCP ext: 25 degrees MCP flex: 50 degrees PIP ext: 0 degrees PIP flex: 90 degrees DIP ext: 0 degrees DIP flex: 70 degrees	MCP ext: 23 degrees MCP flex: 65 degrees PIP ext: 0 degrees PIP flex: 100 degrees DIP ext: 5 degrees DIP flex: 75 degrees	MCP ext: 0 degrees MCP flex: 80 degrees PIP ext: 0 degrees PIP flex: 105 degrees DIP ext: 0 degrees DIP flex: 80 degrees	MCP ext: 0 degrees MCP flex: 90 degrees PIP ext: 0 degrees PIP flex: 105 degrees DIP ext: 0 degrees DIP flex: 85 degrees
Passive Range of Motion	Not tested	MCP ext: 5 degrees MCP flex: 50 degrees PIP ext: 5 degrees PIP flex: 75 degrees DIP ext: 0 degrees DIP flex: 50 degrees	MCP ext: 0 degrees MCP flex: 60 degrees PIP ext: 0 degrees PIP flex: 100 degrees DIP ext: 0 degrees DIP flex: 80 degrees	MCP ext: 5 degrees MCP flex: 70 degrees PIP ext: 0 degrees PIP flex: 105 degrees DIP ext: 0 degrees DIP flex: 80 degrees	MCP ext: 0 degrees MCP flex: 90 degrees PIP ext: 0 degrees PIP flex: 105 degrees DIP ext: 0 degrees DIP flex: 85 degrees	Not tested
Pain	9/10	9/10	4/10	2/10	2/10	0/10
Grip Strength	Not tested	Not tested	Not tested	Not tested	Right 40 lbs, Left 70 lbs	Right 65 lbs Left 70 lbs

MCP = metacarpalphalangeal; PIP = proximal interphalangeal joint; DIP = distal interphalangeal joint; Ext = extension; Flex = flexion

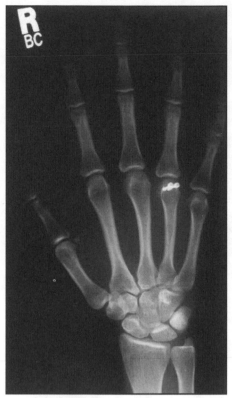

Figure 14-2. Fixation of intra-articular, comminuted fracture of the fourth metacarpal head using two small Herbert screws.

forearm until her first postoperative visit 2 days later. She was also issued a large foam pillow to keep her hand elevated at night and while sitting.

POSTOPERATIVE REHABILITATION

2 Days Postoperatively

The first postoperative therapy visit was on October 15, 1998, 2 days after surgery. X-rays showed good anatomic position with the two small Herbert screws in place (Figure 14-2). The wound was clean and dry and edema was minimal to moderate. Because she had to drive herself from school, which was over an hour away, she had not taken any pain medications that morning and was in a significant amount of pain. Clinical findings are in Table 14-1.

Because the fracture was now stable, the patient was instructed in active and gentle passive ROM exercises to be performed eight to 10 times a day for 5 to 10 minute sessions. Each exercise was to be performed ten times, holding each passive stretch for 10 seconds and each active stretch for 5 seconds. The exercises included gentle passive composite flexion and extension of the digits, active composite flexion and extension, isolated MCP joint extension, isolated MCP joint flexion, blocking exercises to the proximal interphalangeal (PIP) and distal interphalangeal (DIP) joints, isolated PIP joint extension, and composite wrist and finger flexion stretches (Figures 14-3 to 14-6).

An elastic compression sleeve was applied over light gauze, and the ring finger was wrapped in Coban to control the swelling. After taking a mild pain medication, the patient was able to perform the exercises. Ice was then applied as her hand was elevated on pillows. We recommended that she use cold packs for 20 minutes after exercise sessions and at least three to four times a day. She was encouraged to take prescribed pain medication as needed in order to perform her exercises correctly. The safe-position splint was refitted to accommodate the decrease in swelling. The patient was instructed to wear the splint at all times except when

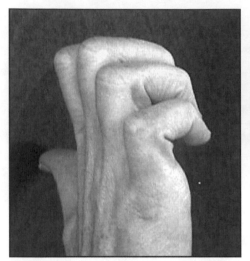

Figure 14-3. Isolated MCP joint extension exercise.

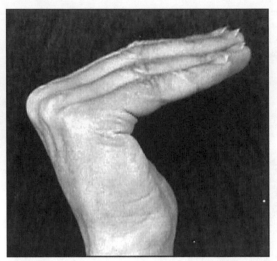

Figure 14-4. Isolated MCP joint flexion exercise.

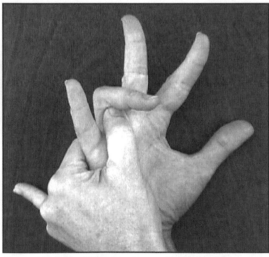

Figure 14-5. Blocking exercise for the proximal interphalangeal joint.

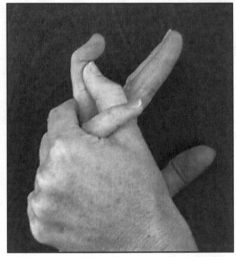

Figure 14-6. Blocking exercise for the distal interphalangeal joint.

doing exercises. Table 14-2 summarizes the postoperative rehabilitation after ORIF of the fourth metacarpal head fracture.

Nine Days Postoperatively

The hand surgeon saw the patient on October 22, 1998, 9 days after surgery, for removal of stitches. The x-ray showed no change in the position of the fracture, and the wounds were healing well. There was a small area of drainage noted around the stitches, proximally. The patient was then seen in therapy, where she stated that her pain had decreased to three or four out of 10. The wound was slightly open and red, possibly from an infected stitch. Other clinical findings are in Table 14-1. The exercises were reviewed emphasizing MCP flexion and extension and adding an extension exercise for the ring finger.

Table 14-2

SUMMARY OF EXERCISES AFTER ORIF OF FOURTH METACARPAL HEAD FRACTURE

Date (Time After Surgery)	Goal	Activity
10-12-98 (1 day preoperatively)	Edema control	Light compressive dressing with Coban to ring finger. Immobilization and elevation. Ice pack 4 x to 6 x a day for 20 minutes
	Splinting	Hand-based safe-position splint to the ring and small fingers, with buddy tape, to be worn at all times until surgery the next day
	Exercises	Light active motion to uninvolved digits, with the splint on
10-15-98 (2 days postoperatively)	Edema control	Elastic sleeve over light gauze with Coban to ring finger. Elevation. Ice 4 x to 6 x a day for 20 minutes, after exercise sessions.
	Splinting	Hand based safe-position splint to the ring and small fingers, with the PIP and DIP joints left free, to be worn between exercises and at night
	Exercises	Active and gentle passive ROM exercises, to be performed 8 x to 10 x a day for 5 to 10 minute sessions: passive composite flexion and extension, active composite flexion and extension, isolated MCP joint flexion, isolated MCP joint extension, blocking exercises to the PIP and DIP joints, interphalangeal joint extension exercise, and composite wrist and finger flexion and extension.
10-22-98 (9 days postoperatively)	Edema control	Elastic sleeve, with Coban to the ring finger. Elevation. Ice 3 x to 4 x a day for 20 minutes, after exercise sessions.
	Splinting	Safe-position splint is continued between exercises and at night
	Exercises	Exercises initiated last visit are continued, with emphasis on isolated MCP joint flexion and extension
10-28-98 (15 days postoperatively)	Edema control/scar management	Elastic sleeve. Ice 3 x a day for 20 minutes after exercise sessions. Scar massage 4 x to 5 x a day. Elastomer pad over scar at night.

Table 14-2 continued		
Date (Time after Surgery	**Goal**	**Activity**
	Splinting	A hand-based extension gutter splint was fabricated to be worn 4 x a day for 30 minutes. Hand based safe-position splint is continued at all other times between exercises.
	Exercises	Same exercises are continued 8 x a day. Finger flexion taping is initiated, to be performed 3 x a day for 20 minute sessions before exercises.
11-5-98 (3 weeks postoperatively)	Edema control/scar management	Elastic sleeve over elastomer pad at night. Retrograde/scar massage 4 x a day. Ice 2 x to 3 x a day for 20 minutes.
	Splinting	Safe position splint at night for 2 more weeks as needed during day. Extension gutter splint 2 x to 3 x a day, PRN, to maintain extension.
	Exercises	Continue hand exercises 5 x a day for 5 minutes. Finger flexion taping 2 x a day for 20 minutes before exercises. Strengthening exercises added: exercise putty 3 x a day for 10 minutes to increase thenar and grip strength, wrist flexion and extension and forearm rotation strengthening exercises once a day (two sets of 10 repetitions each, with 3 lbs), elbow flexion and extension strengthening exercises once a day (two sets of 10 repetitions, with 5 lbs), patient was instructed to begin shoulder strengthening exercises the following week with her trainer at school, and 4 to 5 weeks postoperative the patient started swinging a bat and tossing a softball with no pain.
11-30-98 (7 weeks postoperatively)	Edema control	Ice after strengthening exercises, softball practice as needed.
	Splinting	The patient had not worn any splints for 2 to 3 weeks.
	Exercises	The patient was progressing to full batting, throwing, and weight lifting with her athletic trainer at school, with no limitations. She did begin spring practice in February and finished the season with no pain or problems with her hand.

The patient was instructed to clean the suture site with hydrogen peroxide three times a day and to apply a sterile dry dressing before reapplying the splint. She was to continue performing the exercises eight to 10 times a day, and icing three to four times a day for 20 minutes. Because her pain was improving, she had been using her hand more, possibly causing the increase in edema. Elevation and rest were encouraged as much as possible between exercise sessions.

15 Days Postoperatively

ROM, edema, and pain had all continued to improve when the patient was seen again in therapy 6 days later, on October 28, 1998 (see Table 14-1). The wound was closed, but the scar on the dorsum of the hand and MCP joint was raised and becoming hardened. Because scar formation was restricting the gliding action of the extensor tendon over the fracture site, and limiting MCP joint mobility, scar massage was initiated. The patient was taught scar retraction, massaging in the opposite direction of tendon excursion. With digital flexion, massage was performed in a proximal direction, and with digital extension, massage was performed in a distal direction, to help loosen and stretch scar adhesions. An elastomer insert was fabricated to wear over the scar at night and part of the day. The firm, positive pressure helped soften and decrease the size of the scar, and realign the collagen fibers, facilitating tendon excursion.[1,4]

Because we knew the fracture was stable, finger flexion taping was performed to increase passive flexion of the MCP joint. Flexion taping is similar to dynamic or static progressive splinting in that it provides a gentle, passive stretch for a prolonged period of time, to gradually increase passive motion of a joint. Fractures without rigid fixation must be determined by the physician to have healed sufficiently before taping can be initiated. A thin cotton glove may be worn to prevent the hairs from being pulled off of the hand. The MCP joint is taped into flexion with paper tape, beginning at the wrist, just proximal to the involved metacarpal. The tape is brought over the dorsum of the MCP joint, gently pulling the joint into flexion. The tape is secured near the center of the wrist, following the natural alignment of the finger. The finger is retaped every 5 minutes for a total of 15 to 20 minutes, gradually increasing the passive flexion of the digit. It is important to monitor the extension of the joint as well as the flexion, to assure that a lag in extension does not increase as flexion improves. Because an extension lag of 23 degrees was present in this athlete, a hand based extension gutter splint was made to hold the MCP joint in full extension. The patient was instructed to wear the splint four to five times a day for 30 minutes.

3 Weeks Postoperatively

X-rays showed excellent position of the fracture on November 5, 1998. The physician ordered a strengthening program and planned to see the patient in 3 weeks, at which time he probably would release her to practice softball.

During therapy the patient reported a feeling of tightness, but minimal pain (see Table 14-1).

Recommendations were to wear the safe-position splint at night, with the elastomer pad for 2 to 3 more weeks and as needed during the day for protection; and to wear the extension gutter splint two to three times a day as needed to maintain MCP joint extension. Finger flexion taping was continued once or twice each day as long as the finger felt tight in flexion. Exercise sessions were decreased to five or six times a day, and the patient removed the splint part of the day. Exercises using putty were prescribed to increase grip strength, extensor tendon strength, and to gradually apply pressure to the fracture site. She began using the putty three times a day for 5 minutes, and gradually increased to four times a day for 10 minutes. Wrist and forearm strengthening exercises were begun using a two to three pound weight, while a five pound weight was used for the elbow. Two sets of 10 repetitions were performed for wrist flexion, extension, radial and ulnar deviation, forearm rotation, and elbow flexion and extension. Weight was gradually increased after the first week, when she began shoulder strengthening exercises with her athletic trainer at school. Icing was continued once or twice a day, after strengthening exercises.

7 Weeks Postoperatively

A final x-ray on November 30, 1998 showed excellent position of the fracture. She stated that she had already been swinging a bat and tossing a softball for a week or 2 with no pain in her hand. Mild swelling occurred only after strengthening sessions. Grip strength measured 65 lbs in the right hand and 70 lbs in the left hand (see Table 14-1). The physician released her to progress to full batting, throwing, and lifting, with the supervision of the athletic trainer at school.

During a follow-up telephone call in July of 1999, 8 months after the injury and surgery, the patient reported that she had gained full strength in her hand and arm, had no pain in her hand, and was back to full batting and throwing soon after her last doctor visit. She had not needed any type of protective padding when she returned to throwing and lifting, and played throughout the spring softball season with no pain or limitations.

DISCUSSION

Athletes with metacarpal fractures who are injured early in the season usually are able to return to play within a few weeks with some type of protective device, once the physician has determined that the fracture is stable. Rettig, et al studied 56 metacarpal fractures in athletes and found that 82% were either minimally displaced or nondisplaced and were treated with casting or splinting. The average time away from practice or competition for this group was 12.3 days. The athletes who had required ORIF with plate and screws lost an average of 13.6 days, with the overall range for the whole group being 0 to 56 days.[12] The majority of the athletes were football players and were able to return with a protective silicone-rubber playing cast and buddy taping.

Another option is to cover the cast or hard splint with 0.5 inch closed cell foam, secured with prewrap and tape for practice and competition.[1] While the playing cast may no longer be needed after 4 to 6 weeks, buddy taping is usually recommended for the remainder of the season. Foam pads may then be used on the back of the hand for protection, while a gel type pad such as Akton padding (Smith Nephew, German, Wis) has been found to be effective for diffusing pressure in the palm.

Most metacarpal fractures occurring in athletes are stable, and are treated with splint immobilization and an early return to sports with an appropriate protective device and buddy taping. Intra-articular fractures of the metacarpal head with comminution require ORIF to reestablish congruity of the joint surface. Incongruity of the joint surface can lead to rotational deformities, pain, limited ROM, and functional impairment.[4,8] In addition to reestablishing the joint surface, ORIF allows for the initiation of early motion, usually within the first few days following surgery, and the earliest possible return to sports.[12] Early motion minimizes problems caused by prolonged immobilization, such as scar adhesions and tendon and joint contracture.

The physician decides when the athlete can return to play based on the stability of the fracture and the sport and position being played. Once the athlete has returned to play, it is important to x-ray the fracture at regular intervals to assure that stability has been maintained.[12] A football lineman or linebacker with an injury and surgery similar to the one being discussed in this case study might be able to return to football with a playing cast and buddy tape within 2 weeks of the surgery. However, an athlete requiring more use of the hand, such as a quarterback, basketball player, tennis player, or a gymnast, would probably lose 4 weeks of play. These athletes would require close to full ROM and grip strength with no tenderness over the fracture site in order to fully participate in their sports.

SUMMARY

The patient in this case study had gained almost full range of motion and 60% of her grip strength 3 weeks after ORIF of a displaced fourth metacarpal head fracture in her throwing hand. Approximately 4 weeks after surgery she was beginning to bat and throw a softball. The fall season ended shortly after her injury, so she was able to make a gradual return to weight training and full play before spring training began. She reported no pain or limitations in her hand 6 1/2 weeks after surgery and completed a successful spring softball season.

REFERENCES

1. Rettig AC, Patel DV. *Wrist and Hand Injuries in Athletes: Physician's Handbook.* Indianapolis, Ind: American College of Sports Medicine; 1996.

2. Rettig AC, Ryan R, Shelbourne KD. Metacarpal fractures in the athlete. *Am J Sports Med.* 1989;17(4):567-572.

3. Hastings H, Capo JT. Metacarpal and phalangeal fractures in athletes. *Clin Sports Med.* 1998;17(3):493-511.

4. Light TR, Bednar MS. Management of intra-articular fractures of the metacarpalphalangeal joint. *Hand Clin.* 1994;10(2):303-314.

5. Margles SW. Early motion in the treatment of fractures and dislocations in the hand and wrist. *Hand Clin.* 1996;12(1):65-71.

6. McElfresh EC, Dobyns JH. Intra-articular metacarpal head fractures. *J Hand Surg.* 1983;81:383-388.

7. Ouellette EA, Freeland AE. Use of minicondylar plate in metacarpal and phalangeal fractures. *Clin Orthop.* 1996;327:38-46.

8. Diao E. Metacarpal fixation. *Hand Clin.* 1997;13(4):557-567.

9. Mannarino S. Skeletal injuries. In: Stanley B, Tribuze S, eds. *Concepts in Hand Rehabilitation.* Philadelphia, Pa: FA Davis; 1992:285.

10. Reynolds C. Causes of stiffness. In: Malick M, Kasch M, eds. *Manual on Management of Specific Hand Problems.* Pittsburgh, Pa: Aren Publications; 1984:89-95.

11. Alexy C, DeCarlo MS. Rehabilitation and use of protective devices in hand and wrist injuries. *Clin Sports Med.* 1998;17(3):635-655.

12. Sadler JA, Koepfer JM. Rehabilitation and splinting of the injured hand. In: Strickland J, Rettig AC, eds. *Hand Injuries in Athletes.* Philadelphia, Pa: WB Saunders; 1992:236-242.

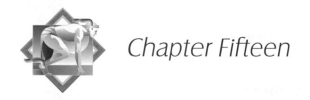

Chapter Fifteen

Management of a Scaphoid Fracture in a College Football Player

Tab Blackburn, PT, ATC

INTRODUCTION

Management of mid-shaft scaphoid fractures presents problems to the athlete and the sports medicine team. The primary goal of treatment is to insure a healed fracture site, return of full motion and strength, and return to all previous activity. The sports medicine philosophy supports this and one other tenet—return to all previous activities as soon as possible.

There are a number of ways to return an athlete with a mid-shaft scaphoid fracture to play quickly, some of which present risk. According to Langhoff and Anderson,[1] 95% of patients with minimally or nondisplaced fractures heal within 9 to 12 weeks when immobilized in a long- or short-arm thumb spica splint. A 4-week delay in treatment caused the healing rate to drop to 60%. Taking 3 months or longer to return to play puts most athletes out of their sports season.

Sports physicians have utilized playing casts or splints for athletes in sports such as football, hockey, or soccer because most athletes in these sports don't need quite as much dexterity as athletes in basketball and baseball. Reister et al[2] and Rettig et al[3] report a 90% and 92% healing rate, respectively, in athletes who continue to play sports with their fractures immobilized in playing casts. This clearly is a minimal risk to the athlete, yet allows early if not immediate return to play. The drawback is reduced dexterity.

What about the athlete who demands more use of his or her hand while competing? The alternative for athletes who require fine motor function from their hands is open reduction and internal fixation (ORIF). Rettig et al, Schroeter et al, and Rettig and Kollias have reported successful use of internal fixation and early, safe return during the same sports season.[3-5] Rettig, et al reported athletes returning to activity between 7 and 8 weeks after surgery. In 1996, Rettig and Kollias reported athletes returning to activity at an average of 5.8 weeks after surgery with no failure or reinjury.

This case study describes a unique scenario in which a starting athlete injures his wrist midway through an undefeated season presenting the medical team with difficult choices to make regarding treatment. This was a different situation from those presented in the literature, and ultimately a different fixation device was utilized than has previously been described.

SUBJECT

The athlete was a 21-year-old, right-hand throwing senior quarterback for a Division I college football team. He was 6 feet tall and weighed 216 lbs. His team was 6 weeks into what would become an undefeated season including a bowl victory. One week before the most important game of the season against the team's biggest rival the athlete sustained an injury to his wrist.

Figure 15-1. Axial compression of the scaphoid.

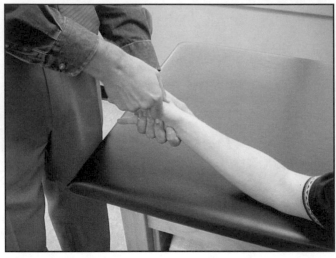

MECHANISM OF INJURY

On September 26, 1998, during the third play of the third quarter, the athlete was tackled while running with the ball. He fell to his left, landing on an outstretched left hand. His wrist dorsiflexed and radially deviated severely. There was some discomfort that he disregarded since he made a first down and the team was driving for a touchdown. He completed the entire game.

INITIAL EVALUATION

In the locker room after the game the athlete brought his sore left wrist to the attention of the athletic trainer and team orthopedist. He described the injury mechanism, pointed to his dorsal medial wrist as an area with increased tenderness, and demonstrated that there was an increase in pain with wrist extension.

The athletic trainer palpated tenderness over the anatomical snuff box that increased with wrist dorsiflexion. The team orthopedist then supported the athlete's wrist in neutral, extended his thumb, and squeezed the anatomical snuffbox, eliciting increased pain. Axial loading of the thumb also increased pain (Figure 15-1). Palpation over the snuffbox at the distal end of the scaphoid over the tubercle elicited no pain (Figure 15-2). Resisted pronation in the handshake position also increased pain. Mild swelling was apparent at the anatomical snuffbox. There was a slight reduction in range of motion (ROM) and strength secondary to pain.

Both the athletic trainer and physician suspected a scaphoid fracture to the left, nonthrowing wrist of their team's quarterback. Ice was applied and the athlete's wrist was elevated and immobilized in a compression dressing. Radiographs were taken the next day. Only nonsteroidal anti-inflammatory medication was administered, and instructions were given on caring for the wrist overnight.

The left wrist was x-rayed in the usual fashion with anterior-posterior, lateral, and oblique pictures taken at 45 degrees from the horizontal. There was a horizontal oblique fracture at the waist of the scaphoid that demonstrated less than 1 mm of displacement. The athlete's wrist was placed in a thumb spica immobilization splint.

The physician, athletic trainer, and athlete discussed three options for treatment. The type of fracture, with its location and time of discovery, lent itself to healing in 9 to 12 weeks, although at this point the season was half over. The quarterback could play wearing a full thumb spica cast, but the athlete vetoed this idea. He felt that in order to play his aggressive running and passing style, he would need more use of his left hand.

Option two was surgery, which the quarterback was not willing to undergo because he would miss 5 to 7 weeks and the season would be over. The hope for an undefeated season rested on his shoulders and there was a chance he could be drafted by the National Football League (NFL) the following spring.

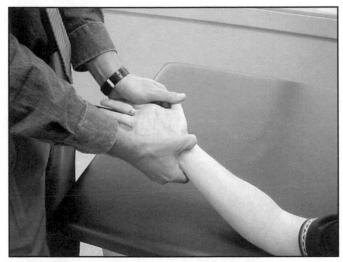

Figure 15-2. Wrist extension and scaphoid tubercle compression.

The remaining choice was to immobilize the wrist in a thumb spica cast and remove it weekly before each game. He would be taped in a molded thermal plastic splint that would allow enough mobility for him to perform and would be placed back in the cast after the game. This alternative was risky because the chance of delayed or nonunion fractures leading to bone grafting increases. Even more devastating would be avascular necrosis of the scaphoid.

The athlete felt he could not be effective as a quarterback with any treatment protocol other than the latter. His goals of an undefeated season and obtaining an NFL draft position hinged on his playing well. He was willing to take a chance even after being warned about the risks and possible complications.

Initially, the quarterback wore a compression glove for swelling. While in the cast, the athlete used hand putty to maintain strength in his left wrist and hand. He performed light, high repetition exercises daily to maintain biceps and triceps strength, rotator cuff and deltoid strength, and scapular stabilizing strength. He was unable to perform his usual upper body weight room program but carried out all lower body activities along with running and conditioning. The athlete had two removable casts, one for practice and one for the rest of the day. The daily cast was a typical thumb spica and restricted the thumb's movement in all directions. The playing cast restricted extension of the thumb but allowed gripping of the ball.

The quarterback stated he had very little discomfort while wearing his playing orthosis. He started the game after the injury and the rest of the season, including a late December bowl game. His team went undefeated, ending up seventh in the national polls and he received a number of personal awards and honors. He even played in the senior bowl in front of a number of NFL scouts.

Radiographs taken several times during the remaining portion of the season continued to show the fracture with less than 1 mm displacement. On October 21, there was some callous bridging (Figure 15-3). The athlete denied much discomfort and took no medication. At each evaluation he was reminded that he may need surgery for complete healing of his fracture.

After the Senior Bowl, the quarterback decided to have the injury surgically repaired. A magnetic resonance image (MRI) on January 14 clearly revealed a delayed union. With the upcoming NFL draft and rookie tryout later in the spring, time became very important.

The team orthopedic surgeon performed ORIF on January 26, 1999. The patient was placed in a supine position under general anesthesia. His left wrist was prepped and draped, and the tourniquet was applied at 200 mmHg. The first incision was 3 cm in length placed over the volar aspect of the wrist from the distal wrist crease to the flexor carpi radialis. The soft tissue was mobilized through the capsule and the fracture was seen in the scaphoid waist. The fracture was nondisplaced, but there was movement along the fracture line. A threaded guide wire was placed distally and proximally to the fracture under fluoroscopy radiographs. The surgeon over-drilled the distal cortex with a 2-0 cannulated drill. The distal pole of the scaphoid was then

Figure 15-3. Scaphoid fracture AP view, October 21.

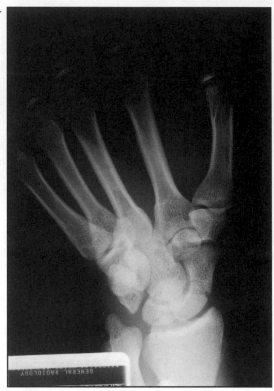

countersunk 7.5 mm with a 4.5 drill, and a washer was put into position. The screw length was measured at 28 mm. The surgeon threaded a 3-0 cannulated Synthes screw over the guide pin and screwed it into the washer. There was a very good purchase on the bone. Anterior-posterior and lateral fluoroscopy radiographs verified the placement of the screw as being appropriate, and direct vision of the fracture site revealed slight depression, but there was no displacement. The threaded guide was removed and the area was reimaged to find everything in place. The soft tissue was closed, the wound irrigated with antibiotic solution and saline, the tourniquet let down, and the patient was put in a thumb spica splint.

On February 1, 6 days after surgery, the wound was healed, stitches were removed, and the quarterback was placed in a short-arm thumb spica cast. Radiographs demonstrated excellent position. The patient continued putty squeeze exercises for the hand, as well as the upper extremity program described previously.

Examination on February 22 showed the wound continuing to heal. Three x-ray views showed the screw in good position with only a small amount of gapping. The athlete was placed in a thumb spica splint, which he was only allowed to remove for bathing. The rehabilitation program was continued.

The athlete was invited to the NFL rookie tryout. The surgeons at the tryout evaluated his progress and took new radiographs. Since the injury was healing so well, he passed the tryout medical evaluation.

On the March 10 visit, there was minimal pain in the anatomical snuffbox. There was good evidence of healing on radiographs, especially the anterior-posterior view. Gentle active ROM progressed over the next month to active assistive exercises for all motions of the wrist. Light resistance at five sets of 10 repetitions was utilized with tubing or dumbbells for wrist extension, flexion, radial and ulnar deviation, pronation, supination, and biceps and triceps curls. The splint was worn when not bathing or exercising. Most exercises were done in a home program situation.

On April 5, the quarterback's scaphoid was 95% healed. He lacked only 20 degrees of dorsiflexion of his wrist. All other wrist motions were within normal limits. Manual muscle test showed 4/5 strength on wrist flexion, extension, pronation, and supination. The rest of the upper extremity manual muscle test was 5/5.

Grip strength was reduced by 25% comparing the involved and uninvolved sides. A computed tomography (CT) scan confirmed the healing level.

The surgeon decided at 10 weeks to let the patient progress to weight room activities as tolerated. The NFL draft occurred 2 weeks later. The quarterback was drafted in the second round.

DISCUSSION

The scaphoid is an intricate bone in the wrist. Mechanically, it bridges the proximal row of carpal bones to the distal row. Because of this linkage, high stresses are transmitted through it. It is the most frequently injured carpal and the management of its injury presents several problems including blood supply and instability issues. Healing time for some types of fractures does not lead to a quick return to activity. Since symptoms of a scaphoid fracture can mimic a simple wrist sprain, the injury may go undiagnosed for a length of time that can hinder healing.[6]

The anatomical configuration of the scaphoid demonstrates bone almost entirely covered with articular cartilage, making intra-articular fractures the rule rather than the exception. Incomplete or improper healing can lead to significant wrist dysfunction. Biomechanically, the scaphoid is subjected to compression, rotation, and shearing forces. Its relationship to the thumb makes it a direct extension of this all-important digit. Blood supply enters the scaphoid at its midportion (or waist) and a small amount at the distal pole. Fractures through the proximal portion of the scaphoid reduce blood supply to the proximal pole leading to avascular necrosis.[7] The more proximal the fracture, the more likely this is to occur.

Scaphoid fractures are classified as stable or unstable. Potentially unstable fractures occur when the fracture line is seen through both cortices.[8] Cooney, et al reported that unstable fractures demonstrated greater than 1 mm of displacement on anterior-posterior or oblique radiographs, or were angled on lateral x-rays.[9] Scaphoid fractures are also considered unstable if the lateral radiograph shows malalignment of the carpal bones suggestive of a fracture dislocation. Carpal widening on the anterior-posterior view suggests ligament disruption.

Fortunately, most scaphoid fractures are stable and occur at differing orientations. The horizontal oblique and the tubercle fractures are most stable. Fractures that have a vertical oblique orientation are the most unstable, whereas transverse fractures may or may not be unstable. Some authors suggest that long-arm casts allow nondisplaced stable fractures to heal more quickly than short-arm casts, but they recognize that immobilization hinders activities of daily living.[10] Tubercle and distal fractures do very well with a short-arm cast. Proximal fractures typically need ORIF, as do vertical oblique fractures.[11]

Every injury has a variety of factors that affect the way it is managed. In the case of this college quarterback, there were a number of issues that influenced the pathways chosen. His primary function on the team was to take a snap, run, and throw the football. The injury was to the nonthrowing hand, but being able to use both hands was critical to his style of play. Strict immobilization of the left arm in a long-arm thumb spica would not be conducive to play. Utilizing a short-arm cast for practice and a thumb and wrist splint during games gave maximum function but risked the healing of this stable fracture. The treatment protocol caused no discomfort to the player. Since there were over 3 more months of football, the fracture would fall into the 40% group that would have trouble healing and might require surgery. Acute surgical intervention would require anywhere from 5 to 8 weeks of noncontact activity, which was not suitable to this athlete.

The athlete decided that he had to play. There was a distinct possibility of an undefeated season and bowl game along with a professional football opportunity if he continued to play. Of course, there was also a distinct possibility of a nonunion of his wrist fracture, which could have lead to surgery and difficulty in gaining a position in the NFL draft. The team physician had experience with a new type of screw thought to be more effective than the commonly used Herbert screw. Both the physician and the athlete planned for a delayed union and surgical repair after the season that would allow the scaphoid to heal in time for the NFL draft. If the wrist proved too symptomatic, the quarterback would have accepted the surgery sooner.

In our opinion, the use of the Synthes screw provided better compression and, hence, better fixation. Enhanced fixation allowed for more rapid return of function. The two major advantages of this fixation over the Herbert screw are better compression and a simple and straightforward surgical technique.

The rehabilitation program during the season and after surgery was quite straightforward. High repetition, low weight activities maintained the athlete's strength around the injured joints. Because of the nature of the fracture, the quarterback could not perform his regular in-season upper body program. Putty and other hand exercises were encouraged. Once the wrist was healed, mobilization techniques of the wrist joint were employed.

REFERENCES

1. Langhoff O, Anderson JL. Consequences of late immobilization of scaphoid fractures. *J Hand Surg.* 1988;13:77-79.

2. Reister JN, Baker BE, Mosher JF, et al. A review of scaphoid fracture healing in competitive athletes. *Am J Sports Med.* 1985;13:159-161.

3. Rettig AC, Weidenbener EJ, Gloyeske R. Alternative management of midthird scaphoid fractures in the athlete. *Am J Sports Med.* 1994;22:711-714.

4. Schroeter TA, Bassett FH, Strickland JW, et al. *Orthop Trans.* 1993;17:439-440.

5. Rettig AC, Kollias SC. Internal fixation of acute stable scaphoid fractures in the athlete. *Am J Sports Med.* 1996;24:182-186.

6. Leslie IJ, Dickson RA. The fractured carpal scaphoid. *J Bone Joint Surgery Br.* 1981;63:225-230.

7. Gelberman RH, Wolock BS, Siegel DB. Fractures and non-unions of the carpal scaphoid. *J Bone Joint Surg Am.* 1989;71:1560-1565.

8. Herbert TJ, Fisher WE, Leicester AW. The Herbert bone screw: a ten-year perspective. *J Hand Surg Br.* 1992;17:415-419.

9. Cooney WP, Dobyns JH, Linscheid RL. Fractures of the scaphoid: a rational approach to management. *Clin Orthop.* 1980;149:90-97.

10. Gellman H, Caputo RJ, Carter V, et al. Comparison of short and long thumb-spica casts for non-displaced fractures of the carpal scaphoid. *J Bone Joint Surg Am.* 1989;71:354-357.

11. Cooney WP, Linscheid RL, Dobyns JH. *Fractures and Dislocations of the Wrist in Rockwood and Green's Fractures in Adults.* 3rd ed. Philadelphia, Pa: JB Lippincott Co; 1991.

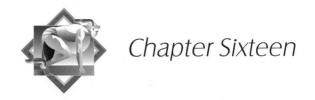

Chapter Sixteen

Radial and Ulnar Fracture in a College Football Player

Mike Matheny, PT, ATC

INTRODUCTION

The athlete was 30 years old, 66 inches tall, and weighed 125 lbs. He played wide receiver and kick return-er on a National Collegiate Athletic Association (NCAA) Division III football team and injured his non-dominant left forearm on November 15, 1997 during a game. He was at the end of his third year of eligibility.

INJURY MECHANISM

The athlete reported that while returning a kickoff, he attempted to jump over a tackler and was hit by an opposing player's helmet. The opponent's helmet made initial contact with the athlete's left forearm in which he was carrying the football. The force of the impact drove the patient's wrist and hand into his own chest, resulting in the patient having the wind knocked out of him.

CLINICAL EXAMINATION

Once the athlete was able to breathe normally, the athletic trainer performed an on-field examination, which revealed a lacerated thenar eminence, probably from contact with a shoulder pad buckle. The athletic trainer also suspected a closed radial and ulnar fracture that was tented dorsally. The orthopedic surgeon pres-ent at the game applied gentle traction to improve alignment. The laceration was covered with sterile gauze, the athlete's arm was immobilized in a vacuum splint, and he was transported to the emergency room.

DIAGNOSTIC IMAGING

At the emergency room, x-rays revealed that the athlete had a fracture at the junction of the middle and distal thirds of the left ulna and radius (Figure 16-1). Closed reduction was performed and the arm was placed in a posterior splint. The laceration of the thenar eminence was sutured and the athlete was instructed to fol-lowup with the orthopedic surgeon the next day.

DIAGNOSIS

The orthopedic surgeon examined the athlete the next morning in the training room. The splint was tem-porarily removed and the surgeon verified that there was no tenting of the skin by the fracture, nor were there any neurovascular impairments. The distal radial ulna joint and left elbow were within normal limits.

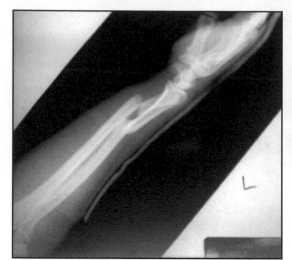

Figure 16-1. X-ray showing fracture at the junction of the middle and distal thirds of the ulna and radius.

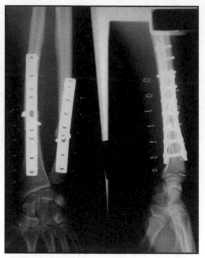

Figure 16-2. X-ray showing placement of plates and screws during open reduction and internal fixation of the fractures.

SURGICAL TREATMENT

Based on Schatzker and Tile's the rationale of operative fracture care (ORIF),[1] the standard of care for this injury is open reduction with internal fixation. Therefore, on November 17, 1997, 2 days after the injury, the patient underwent the procedure with plating of both his radius and ulna. After the initial incision was made, a significant hematoma was identified and aspirated. With the aid of bone reduction clamps, the radius fracture was reduced and an appropriately sized 35 DC plate was clamped in place. After a second incision, an appropriately sized 35 DC plate was clamped on the ulna. At this point, an intraoperative film was obtained. Based on the film, the location of both plates was adjusted and they were screwed in place. Eight cortices were placed above and below the fracture site on the radius. For the fracture of the ulna, eight cortices were placed proximal to the fracture site and four cortices and a lag screw were placed distal to the fracture on the ulna (Figures 16-2). The wound was closed in the standard fashion and standard dressings were applied. Neurovascular status was determined to be normal and the patient was transported to the recovery room, having tolerated the procedure extremely well.

POSTOPERATIVE REHABILITATION

Beginning on postoperative day 3, a progressive rehabilitation program was instituted (Table 16-1). Rehabilitation focused on allowing bony healing to occur and regaining normal motion, equal strength, and function. Progression of rehabilitation was based on the rate of bony healing, as determined by x-ray (Table 16-2) and consultation with the orthopedic surgeon. The first 10 days after surgery consisted of cryotherapy and gentle active range of motion (ROM) for the wrist and fingers only. At day 10 we began gentle active ROM for wrist pronation and supination, along with passive ROM for wrist and finger flexion and extension. The thenar eminence sutures were removed and warm whirlpool was begun as a precursor to therapeutic exercises. This regimen was followed on a daily basis until week 7, when strengthening exercises began and were performed every other day as outlined in Table 16-2. All resistive exercises progressed using the principles of progressive resistance exercises (PRE) established by DeLorme and Watkins.[2] At week 10, the athlete began elbow and shoulder strengthening exercises using TheraBand, cuff weights, and dumbbells less than 10 pounds. By week 15, full return to all upper and lower extremity weight training was allowed, in accordance

Table 16-1	
REHABILITATION PROTOCOL AFTER ORIF OF THE RADIUS AND ULNA	
Postoperative Time	**Activity**
3 to 10 days	Active range of motion: wrist flexion/extension, finger flexion/extension.
10 days	Active range of motion: begin pronation/supination. Passive range of motion: begin gentle wrist and finger flexion/extension. Begin warm whirlpool.
7 Weeks	Begin grip strengthening using therapy putty. Begin wrist flexion/extension strengthening using TheraBand, initially advancing to hand weights. Begin forearm pronation/supination strengthening using bar and cuff weights.
10 Weeks	Begin elbow and shoulder strengthening using TheraBand, cuff weights, and dumbbells.
15 Weeks	Full return to all upper and lower extremity weight training.

with Schatzker and Tile's recommendation that heavy lifting not be allowed "prior to evidence of bony union."[1] At week 15, the athlete began participating fully in the football team's off-season weight training program and continued to do so until the end of the academic year 4 weeks later. Before leaving campus for summer break, the athlete was instructed to continue active and assisted ROM exercises to regain the 10 degrees of supination he was still lacking.

FUNCTIONAL PROGRESSION

Beginning at week 2, the athlete was encouraged to perform light activities of daily living with the involved extremity. As strength and motion increased during the rehabilitation process, normal function returned. By week 10, the athlete was fully functional, performing all activities of daily living, but lacked 10 degrees of supination. At week 15, he was allowed to begin pass-catching drills with teammates, and these continued for 4 weeks, until the end of the academic year.

CLINICAL OUTCOMES

At the time of the athlete's final check before returning to football (38 weeks postoperatively), he demonstrated full active ROM in all hand, wrist, and elbow movements. All manual muscle tests of the hand, wrist, and elbow were scored 5/5. Upon his return to football the season following the injury, he experienced no limitations and completely resumed his previous role of receiver and kick returner.

Table 16-2	
PROGRESSION OF HEALING	
Postoperative Weeks	**Status**
0	X-rays showed metallic fixation plates holding the comminuted fractures in anatomic position.
1	X-rays showed normal alignment had been maintained.
2	Sutures removed from thenar eminence laceration. Staples removed from the radius and ulna incisions.
3	Incisions well healed. X-rays showed the fragments remained in excellent position with minimal callus formation.
9	X-rays showed that the fractures were healing. Obvious fracture line still visible on radius. No loosening of hardware.
12	X-rays showed ulna virtually healed, lucent line on radius.
18	X-rays showed abundant callus formation about the ulna, radius not completely healed at this point.
24	X-rays showed complete bridging callus on the ulna circumferentially and near complete bridging callus circumferentially on the radius.
38	X-rays showed radius and ulna completely healed; no evidence of nonunion.

REFERENCES

1. Schatzker J, Tile M. *The Rationale of Operative Fracture Care*. Philadelphia, Pa: Lippincott; 1984.
2. DeLorme TL, Watkins AL. *Progressive Resistance Exercise*. New York, NY: Appleton-Century-Crofts; 1951.

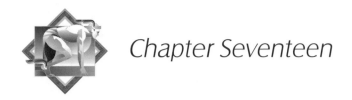

Chapter Seventeen

Recurrent Elbow Instability in a Professional Football Player

Arthur Rettig, MD, Christopher Price, MD, Hunter Smith, ATC

INTRODUCTION

The elbow is a highly constrained joint combining a hinge-like bony articulation, the dynamic tension of the opposing muscles, and medial and lateral stabilizing ligaments. However, elbow dislocations are relatively common, accounting for 10% to 25% of all injuries to the elbow.[1] Only the shoulder is dislocated more frequently than the elbow.[2] A fall onto an outstretched hand is the most common cause of elbow dislocation when all age groups are included.[3] Sports, motor vehicle accidents, and other high-energy mechanisms account for most of these injuries in young patients. Josefsson found the highest incidence of elbow dislocation associated with sports injuries in the second decade.[4,5]

The most common type of dislocation, making up approximately 90% of cases, is posterior or posterolateral displacement of the ulna on the humerus.[1,6] The standard treatment of elbow dislocation is closed reduction followed by assessment of stability. This is done by taking the elbow through a range of motion (ROM) and evaluating its propensity to subluxate. Instability, if present, usually occurs in extension; therefore, the elbow is generally splinted in flexion. The elbow is immobilized for 5 to 7 days and then ROM is initiated. Mehlhoff found that immobilization for periods greater than 13 days led to significant increase in long-term flexion contractures and pain.[1] Protzman found an average 3-degree loss of extension in patients immobilized less than 5 days, 11-degree loss when immobilized for 10 to 15 days, and a 21-degree loss when immobilized for greater than 21 days.[6]

In a prospective, randomized trial, Josefsson, et al compared open and closed treatment of simple elbow dislocations. There were no statistically significant differences in outcome with regard to extension, pronation, supination, or instability. In those surgically explored, the medial and lateral ligaments were found to be torn in all cases.[5] Even in the face of medial and lateral ligament tears, the bony architecture provides ample stability to allow gentle ROM after a dislocation while allowing the ligaments to heal in most cases. Recurrent instability is rare, occurring in less than 1% to 2% of simple elbow dislocations.[7] The instability can be characterized as a sense of instability or frank dislocation.

Posterolateral rotatory instability (PLRI) is a rare variant of instability that can occur after a dislocation or an elbow sprain.[8] Instability occurs when the ulna and radius subluxate off the humerus in a posterolateral fashion. This instability pattern is due to insufficiency of the ulnar part of the lateral collateral ligamentous complex.[8-10] O'Driscoll demonstrated that the elbow can subluxate or dislocate with an intact anterior band of the medial collateral ligament by sequentially sectioning the ligaments in cadavers. He proposed that elbow instability is a spectrum ranging from PLRI to dislocation (Figure 17-1).[9] In the acute setting, the lateral collateral ligament will heal with the elbow protected in flexion and pronation. Chronic insufficiency of the lateral collateral ligament can occur after dislocation with subsequent healing of the medial collateral ligament but not of the ulnar part of the lateral collateral ligament or after isolated injury to this ligament. Unlike acute

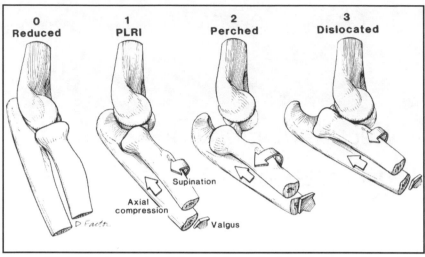

Figure 17-1. Spectrum of soft tissue injury. The lateral ulnar collateral ligament (LUCL) is disrupted in stage 1, the other lateral ligamentous structures along with the anterior and posterior capsule in stage 2, and in stage 3 the medial ulnar collateral ligament (MUCL) is disrupted partially or completely (reprinted with permission from O'Driscoll, Morrey BF, Korinek, et al. Elbow subluxation and dislocation: a spectrum of instability. *Clin Orthop Res.* 1992;280:186-197).

dislocations, PLRI presenting in the subacute or chronic setting does not typically resolve with conservative management. The following case study is an example of the clinical course of PRLI treated in a professional football player.

SUBJECT

The patient was a 24-year-old right hand dominant professional football player who played linebacker. He dislocated his dominant right elbow on November 23, 1993 when he fell on an outstretched arm during an intercollegiate football game. The team physician reduced the posterior dislocation on the field. Postreduction radiographs demonstrated a well-reduced elbow without fracture. He was immobilized in a cast for 2 weeks and was able to play in a bowl game on January 1, 1994 wearing a hinged brace with a terminal extension block. After the bowl game, the athlete continued to rehabilitate his elbow. He regained full ROM and felt that his elbow was stable.

The athlete participated in the National Football League (NFL) combine in the spring of 1994. Clinical exam demonstrated no instability of the right elbow. Radiographs showed no evidence of fracture, post-traumatic changes, or subluxation of the elbow. He was drafted into the NFL in the spring of 1994, participated in 2 weeks of training camp in July without taping or bracing, and reported no problems. During a preseason game on August 5, 1994, the athlete fell onto his right arm early in the game and felt discomfort. His elbow was taped and placed in a brace to limit extension to 30 degrees and he continued to play. Later in the game he fell onto his outstretched right hand and felt what he described as a similar sensation to when he originally dislocated his elbow in college. He was unable to return to the game.

CLINICAL EXAMINATION

On-field examination revealed significant edema and tenderness but no evidence of dislocation. The lateral elbow, especially the lateral humeral epicondyle, was more tender than the medial side, and ROM was painful. Twelve hours later, a significant joint effusion was present. ROM was now 40 degrees to 100 degrees.

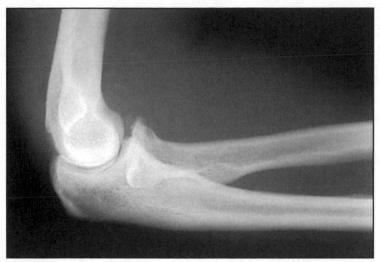

Figure 17-2. X-ray showing a type I avulsion fracture of the coracoid process.

No gross instability of the elbow was noted on clinical exam; however, the exam was limited by the athlete's pain and guarding.

DIAGNOSTIC IMAGING

Plain radiographs revealed satisfactory position of the elbow, but there was a small type I avulsion fracture of the coracoid process (Figure 17-2). Magnetic resonance imaging (MRI) revealed a large effusion, edema in the medial collateral ligament, lateral collateral ligament disruption, widening of the ulnohumeral joint, and posterior subluxation of the radial head.

DIAGNOSIS

Based on the clinical history of a sense of instability, tenderness over the lateral elbow and MRI results, the team orthopedic surgeon diagnosed PLRI of the elbow. Patients with PLRI typically present with chronic instability. They often complain of painful clicking, snapping, or locking, or of a generalized sense of elbow instability. In this case, the elbow was examined and the diagnosis made shortly after an acute injury limiting the history and clinical exam. It should be remembered, however, that the clinical exam is often nonspecific even in the chronic setting. O'Driscoll described the lateral pivot shift apprehension test used to aid in making the diagnosis (Figure 17-3). A positive response produces apprehension with reproduction of the patient's symptoms and a sense that the elbow is about to dislocate.[8] Often the patient will not allow an adequate exam and anesthesia is required to reliably perform the test. When performed under anesthesia, a prominence can be visualized posterolaterally over the radial head as it subluxates. A clunk can be heard when the reduction occurs.

SURGICAL TREATMENT

As the athlete demonstrated recurrent instability and desired to return to competition as rapidly as possible, he elected for operative management. The ulnar portion of the lateral collateral ligament was reconstructed using a plantaris graft harvested from the athlete's left leg. The plantaris graft was harvested through a small incision just proximal to the posteromedial aspect of the ankle. A tendon stripper was used to remove the graft. An ipsilateral palmaris longus allograft is usually used for this procedure; however, this athlete did not have one. Drill holes were made in the ulna and lateral epicondyle. The plantaris graft was weaved through the holes and sutured to itself. The elbow capsule was closed and plicated over the graft. The anterior band of the medial collateral ligament was also plicated as the athlete had some valgus instability and edema on the MRI.

Figure 17-3. Test for posterolateral instability of the elbow.

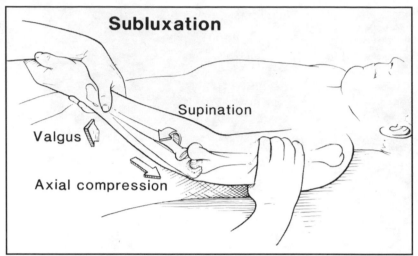

Postoperative Rehabilitation

The postoperative rehabilitation after lateral collateral ligament reconstruction varies widely. O'Driscoll reported rehabilitation ranging from immediate motion in a cast brace for 6 weeks to immobilization for 6 weeks followed by bracing for up to 3 months. He recommends 3 weeks of immobilization and at least 6 weeks of cast bracing. Normal activities are allowed at 6 months.[8,9]

The goals for this professional athlete were to regain ROM, strengthen surrounding muscle groups, and return to play as rapidly as possible.

Lower Extremity

The morbidity from a plantaris harvest is low, as this vestigial muscle does not significantly add to the strength of the leg. Lower extremity rehabilitation consisted of immediate ice and compression for local edema control. ROM exercises for ankle plantar flexion and dorsiflexion were started on the day after surgery. One week postoperatively, stationary bicycle and stretching of the posterior leg was initiated to maintain ankle ROM, as well as lower extremity and cardiovascular conditioning. Lower extremity strengthening included leg presses, toe raises, and stair climbing, and began at postoperative week 2. The athlete showed no residual lower extremity deficits by postoperative week 3. He resumed running 6 weeks after surgery when his elbow had progressed sufficiently to warrant increased cardiovascular conditioning.

Upper Extremity

Immediately after surgery, a hinged brace was placed on the elbow with the arm in pronation and the brace locked at 90 degrees of extension. The arm was placed in a pronated position, which allows the flexor pronator mass to act as a secondary stabilizer of the lateral elbow, thus protecting the repair.[8] Ice, compression sleeve, antiinflammatory, and elevation were used for pain and edema control. ROM was allowed from full flexion to 90 degrees, but no formal ROM exercises were started.

Postoperative Week 1

Ice and a compressive Ace wrap (Becton, Dickinson, and Company, Franklin Lakes, NJ) were continued. The extension block was decreased to 70 degrees and ROM exercises consisting of flexion and extension in the brace were performed three times per day.

Postoperative Week 2

The patient's wound was well-healed and the sutures were removed. Elbow ROM was 45 degrees extension to 125 degrees flexion. The extension block in the hinged brace was decreased to 45 degrees.

Postoperative Week 3

Elbow ROM was 15 degrees extension to 145 degrees flexion, and the extension block was set at 20 degrees. Water resistance with the Hydrobell (Hydro-tone, Freeport, NY) resistive device was used for shoulder strengthening.

Postoperative Weeks 4 and 5

ROM remained at 15 degrees extension to 145 degrees flexion. The hinged brace was now limited to use at night and when the patient was outside his house. He performed ROM exercises with the brace off three times a day. Water resistance exercises for the shoulder continued, as well as for the biceps and triceps while the elbow was maintained in a pronated position.

Postoperative Week 6

ROM of the elbow remained 15 degrees extension to 145 degrees flexion with full pronation and supination (pronation and supination were not measured earlier, as the elbow was being maintained in pronation). Water resistance exercises continued for elbow flexion/extension. The patient began bench press exercises in the weight room. Brace wear was continued at night and when in public.

Postoperative Week 7

Pronation and supination exercises were added to the water resistance exercises program. Weight room activities increased to include bench press, pull downs, and overhead press. Closed kinetic chain exercises were added, utilizing a therapy ball for catching and throwing. The elbow brace was worn while performing these exercises.

Postoperative Weeks 8 Through 11

Isokinetic resistance exercises were initiated daily for pronation/supination and elbow flexion/extension. Pronation was performed at 150 degrees/sec and supination was performed at 180 degrees/sec. Full weight training was resumed. At postoperative week 10 the athlete was allowed to participate in limited practice with elbow taping and bracing with a 20-degree extension block and the arm in pronation.

Postoperative Week 12

The athlete returned to full practice while wearing the brace.

Postoperative Week 13

The athlete was cleared to play while wearing the brace. He had normal pronation/supination, and extension remained at 15 degrees while flexion remained at 145 degrees. Grip strength assessment using a hand-held dynamometer revealed a measure of 195 foot pounds on the involved side compared to 165 foot pounds on the noninvolved side.

CLINICAL OUTCOME

At 6 months postoperatively, the athlete reported no incidence of further instability. He was cleared to play without his brace. Elbow ROM was 15 to 140 degrees with full pronation and supination. Loss of the terminal 10 to 20 degrees of the extension is common after elbow dislocation.[6] This loss of extension is generally well-tolerated and does not interfere with function. The patient felt that he returned to his previous level of activity and was pleased with the outcome.

Summary

This case presentation focused on the treatment of chronic elbow instability in a professional football player. After undergoing elbow ligament reconstruction and progressive rehabilitation, the patient was able to return to his previous level of activity without a sense of instability. Rehabilitation after lateral collateral ligament reconstruction of the elbow should focus on early protected ROM with care to limit extension and maintain the arm in pronation. By following these precautions, the repair can be protected while allowing the patient to regain ROM and strength in an expedient fashion.

References

1. Mehlhoff TL, Noble PC, Bennett JB, et al. Simple dislocation of the elbow in the adult: results after closed treatment. *J Bone Joint Surg Am*. 1988;70:244-249.

2. Josefsson PO, Johnell O, Gentz CF. Long-term sequelae of simple dislocation of the elbow. *J Bone Joint Surg Am*. 1984;66:927-930.

3. Morrey BF, ed. *The Elbow and Its Disorders*. 2nd ed. Philadelphia, Pa: WB Saunders; 1993.

4. Josefsson PO, Nilsson BE. Incidence of elbow dislocation. *Acta Orthop Scand*. 1986;105:313-315.

5. Josefsson PO, Gentz CF, Johnell O, et al. Surgical versus nonsurgical treatment of ligamentous injuries following dislocation of the elbow joint: a prospective randomized study. *J Bone Joint Surg Am*. 1987;69:605-608.

6. Protzman RR. Dislocation of the elbow joint. *J Bone Joint Surg*. 1978;60:539-541.

7. Linscheid RL, Wheeler DK. Elbow dislocations. *JAMA*. 1965;194:1171-1176.

8. O'Driscoll SW, Bell DF, Morrey BF. Posterolateral rotatory instability of the elbow. *J Bone Joint Surg*. 1991;73:440-446.

9. O'Driscoll SW, Morrey BF, Korinek S, et al. Elbow subluxation and dislocation: a spectrum of instability. *Clin Orthop*. 1992;280:186-197.

10. Morrey BF, An KN. Functional anatomy of the ligaments of the elbow. *Clin Orthop*. 1985;201:84-90.

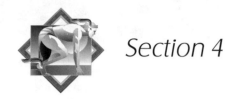

Section 4

Knee

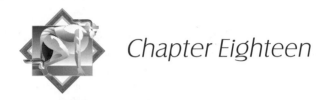

Chapter Eighteen

Rehabilitation Program for Arthroscopic Monopolar Radiofrequency Treatment of a Posterior Cruciate Ligament Insufficiency

Michael L. Voight, DPT, OCS, SCS, ATC, Geoff Kaplan, PT, ATC

INTRODUCTION

Posterior cruciate ligament (PCL) injuries are probably more common than once thought. Depending on the setting, PCL injuries are reported to account for 3% to 37% of knee ligament injuries.[1,2] To date, there is no data that accurately describe the incidence of PCL injuries in athletics. Given that the most common mechanism of injury is falling on a flexed knee, the incidence is expected to vary according to sport. Following injury to the PCL, patients have two treatment options; surgical and nonsurgical. Patients with posterior cruciate deficient knees tend to decrease their level of activity to accommodate the degree of instability. Nonsurgical treatment includes activity modification, therapeutic exercise to strengthen the dynamic restraints to abnormal posterior tibial translation, and external bracing. When patients are either unable to modify their activity or exceed the capacity of their body to stabilize the knee, functional instability occurs. The surgical goals of PCL reconstruction are threefold: prevent repetitive episodes of knee instability and subsequent secondary damage, normalize joint kinematics, and allow a return to normal activities of daily living, including high-demand sports.[3]

PCL insufficiency secondary to ligamentous disruption traditionally has been managed by reconstruction. Reconstructive methods vary from surgeon to surgeon because there are many technical details that require consideration, including graft choice, type of fixation, and number of bundles. Adequate graft choices include:

- Autograft bone patellar-tendon bone
- Quadrupled hamstring (gracilis and semitendonosis)
- Allograft bone patellar-tendon bone
- Allograft Achilles' tendon
- Autograft quadriceps tendon
- Contralateral bone patellar-tendon bone
- Contralateral hamstring
- Contralateral quadriceps tendon

Controversy regarding timing and type of reconstruction still exists because there are no long-term studies to determine which, if any, procedure is best. Surgery is technically demanding and associated with a variety of complications, including the recurrence of instability, stiffness, and neurovascular injury. Failures of PCL reconstruction include the loss of fixation, interstitial ligamentous creep, and gross disruption.

The use of thermal energy to modify collagenous soft tissues has been successfully applied to patients with glenohumeral instability.[4-9] Shrinkage of attenuated ligamentous and capsular soft tissue has restored functional stability in these patients. Based on multiple in vivo and in vitro studies that explored the interaction between therapeutic heat, collagen shrinkage, and healing, we hypothesized that the therapeutic application of nonablative thermal energy could shrink the attenuated PCL and thereby restore objective and subjective stability.[10-15] The primary contraindication for this radiofrequency mediated ligament repair is discontinuity of the ligament. Detachment proximally, distally, or in the midportion makes it impossible to retension the ligament and would, therefore, doom the electrotherapeutic repair to failure. Therefore, in order to retain attenuated ligamentous soft tissues, the PCL structure to be tightened must be attached on both the femur and the tibia.

We are presenting this case to demonstrate the use of a focused rehabilitation program following thermal shrinkage of the PCL. Initial alterations in the biomechanics of heat-treated ligaments highlight the need for specialized postoperative rehabilitation protocols. The patient presented in this case was a professional football player who wanted to return too full, unrestricted play as soon as possible. This is the first report, to our knowledge, of a patient who underwent monopolar radiofrequency treatment for the primary purpose of returning to full unrestricted sports participation.

Subjective History

The patient was a 29-year-old, 5'8", 188 lbs, professional football player who injured his left knee on September 6, 1998 while participating in a regular season football game.

Injury Mechanism

At the time of injury, the athlete was covering a punt. In the process of engaging a defender, he fell on the artificial surface with his knee bent approximately 90 degrees, landing on his anterior knee. While the athlete denied hearing an audible "pop," he did report immediate, severe pain and an inability to bear weight. Review of the injury on videotape revealed that in fact the athlete did land on his flexed knee.

Examination

An onfield examination was conducted by the team physician. The athlete's knee was tender to palpation posteromedially and while there was no medial instability, he experienced pain with a valgus stress test. Posterior drawer stress was positive (2 to 2+) and painful. In addition to the increased laxity with the posterior drawer test, a soft end point was noted. All other ligamentous stability testing was unremarkable.

Postgame examination was similar to the onfield examination and revealed joint line pain and grade 2 to 2+ post drawer test; all other ligament stability tests were normal. Patellofemoral crepitus was also noted. The athlete's knee was placed in a compression sleeve and long-leg brace. Clinical exam the following day revealed a grade 2 to 3 effusion, 0 to 120 degrees range of motion (ROM) secondary to the effusion, antalgic gait with decreased hip and knee flexion, good quadriceps tone, and a grade 2 posterior drawer test. Posterior drawer testing was difficult to perform due to swelling and muscle guarding.

Diagnostic Imaging

Radiographic examination was normal. Magnetic resonance imaging (MRI) revealed a partial tear of the PCL involving the posterior aspect of the ligament extending to the tibial attachment. In addition, a bone bruise on the anterior aspect of the lateral femoral condyle and chondral changes in the trochlear groove was noted.

Diagnosis

The athlete was diagnosed with a partial tear of the PCL with associated chondromalacia.

REHABILITATION

Preoperative Rehabilitation

Rehabilitation was initiated 1 day after the injury. Initial treatment goals centered on controlling inflammation. The athlete's treatment program consisted of ice, compression, and elevation. In addition, the athlete was instructed to continue wearing the long-leg brace. Eventually, the athlete was allowed to discontinue the brace as tolerated. As soon as the effusion was controlled, an aggressive quadriceps strengthening and proprioception rehabilitation program was implemented to maintain quadriceps strength and regain function. Hamstring exercises were avoided for 6 to 8 weeks to avoid stressing the healing PCL and associated structures

Days 1 to 7 Post-Injury

To reduce effusion and pain and to maintain quadriceps tone, treatment was performed twice a day (Table 18-1). Proprioception and balance training was also progressed. As soon as effusion subsided, ROM was restored and maintained through bicycling and wall slides.

Days 7 to 10

Quadriceps strength was increased with various exercises and balance training was progressed. Functional activities were initiated without complication.

Days 11 to 14

The athlete's functional activity program increased to include sport-specific and position-specific (defensive back) drills. All of these were initiated without complication.

The athlete was cleared for return to play 14 days after the injury and participated in full unrestricted activity. He completed the rest of the season and did not miss any remaining game action because of the PCL injury. Throughout the season, however, he did have recurrent episodes of effusion and anterior knee pain. Due the combination of PCL laxity and associated chondromalacia, the team physician felt that surgery was indeed indicated. This decision was based on the premise that PCL laxity increased the articular pressure in the trochlear groove and, thus, caused further damage with continued effusion and pain.

SURGICAL TREATMENT

As soon as the season was completed, the athlete had arthroscopic chondroplasty and radiofrequency probe tightening of the PCL. While thermal ligament shrinkage in the knee is not a common procedure, we felt that it was the most viable option for this athlete. Type I collagen is the main component of both ligaments and the joint capsule. These highly ordered dense collagen fibers serve to provide tissues with their mechanical stiffness and strength. It is a well-known phenomenon that collagenous tissue shrinks when it is heated. When threshold levels of temperature are reached, the heat labile bonds in the collagen molecule breakdown and the collagen molecule contracts into a less organized random coil configuration.[4] When enough collagen molecules are heated in this manner, a visible contraction of the treated tissue occurs.

In the early 1900s, the holmium laser was found to be a useful tool for thermally contracting the shoulder capsule and improving shoulder stability in a young active population. A pilot study by Thabit, et al[16] confirmed that laser-assisted capsulorrhaphy was an effective and less invasive method of clinically tightening the shoulder capsule that achieved success rates equal to or better than other arthroscopic techniques.

Because of its superficial thermal effects, the holmium:YAG laser is an inappropriate device for the treatment of this entity.[3] However, the deeper heating effects of the monopolar radiofrequency device makes it ideal for such a purpose. Studies have shown that thermal heating of joint capsules, ligaments, and tendons resulted in significant shrinkage that is both temperature and time dependent.[4,16-18] The degree of tissue modification (shrinkage) is influenced by the quality of the tissue (eg, collagen content crosslinks) and direc-

Table 18-1

REHABILITATION PROGRAM

Time after Injury/Surgery	Goals	Activity
Post-Injury		
1 to 7 days	Decrease pain and effusion	Ice, compression, elevation, wear long-leg immobilizer, and anti-inflammatory medication.
	Quadriceps tone	Isometric quadriceps sets, straight leg raising, bilateral mini-squats, and closed chain terminal knee extensions (TKE).
7 to 10 days	Proprioception	Bilateral to unilateral stance on uneven surfaces and foam matting.
	Quadriceps strength	Single-leg mini-squats with resistance tubing, unilateral leg press, wall squats, and side stepping against resistance tubing.
	Proprioception	Unilateral stance activities with the eyes open to single-leg training with the eyes closed. Stable base training progressed to unstable surfaces.
	Functional activities	Step-ups, stair machine, slide board, fitter, and straight ahead field jogging.
11 to 14 days	Functional activities	Jogging, side stepping, carioca, back pedaling, cutting drills, figure eights, change of direction drills, and covering receiver running routes.
Postoperative		
0 to 10 days	Promote healing and decrease pain and swelling	Knee placed in DonJoy IROM knee brace locked in full extension.
3 to 5 weeks	Maintain quadriceps tone	Straight leg raises, hip abduction, adduction, and extension, quadriceps sets, single-leg balance in immobilizer for proprioception training, ankle pumps, and patella mobilization.
	Rehabilitation exercises	Biking, active ROM exercises, passive ROM exercises (wall slides), patella mobilizations, unilateral leg press with elastic tubing, single-leg proprioception on uneven surfaces, closed chain TKE, standing calf raises, bilateral mini-squats progressing to unilateral

Table 18-1 continued		
Time after Injury/Surgery	**Goals**	**Activity**
		against elastic tubing, precor EFX elliptical trainer, stair machine climbing program.
5 to 8 weeks	Rehabilitation exercises	Progression with the unilateral leg press, step-up (both forward and lateral steps), single-leg squats, and forward and backward walking on a treadmill.
	Functional activities	Side-to-side stepping against elastic resistance, slide board, fitter, mini-stepper, elliptical trainer, stair machine, and spinner bike classes.

tion of the collagen fibers. Both animal and human tissue studies have confirmed that the temperature required for collagen contraction and stabilization of the human joint capsule is approximately 65°C.[4,14,17] Using a temperature of 67°C and 40 watts of power, significant shrinkage and heating effects, up to 5 mm of depth, can be achieved.[3]

Surgical rationale for this athlete was centered on the surgeon's vast experience with radiofrequency thermal capsular shrinkage. In addition, the thermal procedure offered a lower chance of post-surgical morbidity and a faster rehabilitation time than traditional PCL reconstruction, which influenced the decision-making process. On January 6, 1999, the patient underwent arthroscopic knee surgery, which included chondroplasty and radiofrequency probe thermal shrinkage tightening of the PCL.

POSTOPERATIVE REHABILITATION

0 to 10 Days

Immediately after surgery, a DonJoy IROM knee immobilizer was placed on the athlete's knee and locked in full extension. Full weightbearing as tolerated was allowed. The goal of early rehabilitation was to promote healing, decrease swelling and pain, and maintain quadriceps tone.

10 Days to 3 Weeks

The rehabilitation program continued as outlined above, adding prone passive knee flexion to 90 degrees. The rationale for prone knee flexion instead of supine is that in this position gravity against the PCL is eliminated. Rehabilitation goals were modified to include gradual increases in PROM, quadriceps tone, and promotion of an optimal healing environment for the PCL.

3 to 5 Weeks

At 3 weeks, the postoperative brace was discontinued and we initiated gait training. Lower extremity strengthening and proprioception training were progressed in intensity. Specific rehabilitation included bicycling, AROM, PROM (wall slides), patella mobilizations, single leg press with elastic tubing, single leg proprioception on uneven surfaces, closed chain TKE, standing calf raises, bilateral mini squats progressing to single leg mini squats against elastic tubing, Precor EFX elliptical trainer (Precor USA, Inc, Bothell, Wash.), and a stair machine climbing program.

5 to 8 weeks

During the second month postoperatively, both ROM and strengthening exercises were progressed in intensity and duration. Proprioception and balance training were progressed from eyes open to eyes closed and from stable to unstable surfaces. By the end of the second month, the athlete displayed full active pain-free ROM.

8 to 12 Weeks

During the third month postoperatively, the athlete's rehabilitation program continued to emphasize lower quarter strengthening and proprioception training.

12 to 16 Weeks

During the fourth month, strengthening exercises emphasized sport-specific drills for return to sport. It is important to note that hamstring exercises were not initiated until the athlete started working out with an isokinetic machine after 16 weeks. We restricted hamstring strengthening to avoid placing increased tension on the PCL, which can occur if there is strong and powerful hamstring contraction during the time of biological healing of the PCL.

FUNCTIONAL PROGRESSION

Since our athlete was a professional football player who played defensive back, the functional progression drills were designed to incorporate the necessary movement and skills needed to play that position. All field rehabilitation sessions started with the exercises presented in Table 18-2.

In the initial stages of the functional progression, these exercises were followed by straight line jogging and running. As soon as the athlete was able to perform these drills without any gait deviations, pain, or swelling, activities were progressed and are outlined in Table 18-2. The speed, duration and intensity of each drill were adjusted to challenge the player and test the knee. Position-specific drills were also incorporated into the functional progression. The criteria for full unrestricted return to activity was the performance of the full array of drills without pain, swelling, or dysfunction. Throughout the functional training period, the athlete did not utilize any supportive taping or bracing. The athlete did want to wear a Neoprene sleeve for comfort and warmth.

DISCUSSION/CONCLUSIONS

In vivo and in vitro animal studies have consistently documented a trade-off between soft tissue shrinkage and maintenance of soft tissue strength immediately after the deposition of thermal energy.[3,16,19] Thabit, et al showed a restoration of biomechanical tissue strength/stiffness by 8 weeks with the YAG laser and 12 weeks with the monopolar radiofrequency device in glenohumeral and patellofemoral joint capsules.[16] Near normal histology appeared by 3 months for both the Ho:YAG laser and radiofrequency devices for chronic ACL instability.[3] Jackson, et al suggested that devitalized ACL tissue treated by freezing thermal stress became "normal" compared with controls somewhere between 6 weeks and 6 months.[19] Our rehabilitation program is based on previous animal studies and our clinical experience with thermal radiofrequency shrinkage of the glenohumeral joint capsule. It is important to note that at this early developmental stage of our rehabilitation program we tend to err on the side of conservatism.

CLINICAL OBJECTIVE OUTCOME FINDINGS

The athlete has returned to full unrestricted participation in professional football without any recurrence of PCL problems. Objective clinical outcome data is presented in Table 18-3.

Table 18-2

FUNCTIONAL PROGRESSION

Stage	Repetitions	Activity
Initial stages		
Warm-up	2 repetitions of each exercise were performed at 25 yards before each field session	High knee jogging, buttock kicks, side steps, carioca, back pedaling, and skipping.
Functional progression		
Later stages		
Warm-up	Same as above	Straight line jogging and running, double leg hops, single-leg hops, bounding, and back pedal weave.
Change-of-direction drills		Forward weave the width of the field, zig-zag weave the length of the field, figure of eights starting larger and gradually making smaller and faster cuts.
Position-specific drills		Speed drills covering different passing routes: with receiver present and without receiver present.

CONCLUSIONS

Thermal repair of PCL insufficient knees represents an emerging treatment alternative to standard PCL reconstruction techniques. The minimal morbidity of PCL thermal repair, however, must be by the success rate of the well-documented PCL repair techniques. Patients must be observed closely in the first 3 months after surgery. A high degree of patient compliance is required to protect the healing ligament in the early stages. Ongoing basic science projects will help to further delineate the complex interaction between the therapeutic shrinking on the insufficient, unreconstructed PCL as well as failed reconstructions or repairs. The key question yet to be answered is not whether the PCL can be tightened, but when is the best time to release the athlete back to full, unrestricted sports? The animal data provided by Jackson, et al suggest that a minimum of 6 weeks and a maximum of 6 months may be required to restore tissue structure and function. Our clinical experience to date suggests that a 4-month period of activity modification and rehabilitation is both prudent and successful.

REFERENCES

1.   Fanelli G, Edson C. The posterior cruciate ligament injuries in trauma patients. Part II. *Arthroscopy.* 1995;11:526-529.
2.   Miyasaka K, Daniel D. The incidence of knee ligament injuries in the general population. *Am J Knee Surg.* 1991;4:3-8.

Table 18-3

CLINICAL OUTCOMES

	Preoperatively	20 Weeks Postoperatively
Range of motion	0-0-120 degrees	0-0-135 degrees
Strength (isokinetic testing)	Not tested	Quadriceps strength was within 10% of the non-involved knee at 90 degrees, 180 degrees, and 300 degrees per second
Ligament stability	Not tested	Normal compared to athlete's pre-injury scores
Subjective evaluation		
• Lysholm	Not tested	100/100
• Cincinnati knee	Not tested	94/100
• Score	Cincinnati knee score	Cincinnati knee score

3. Thabit G. The arthroscopic monopolar radiofrequency treatment of chronic anterior cruciate ligament instability. *Op Tech Sports Med.* 1998;6:157-160.

4. Fanton GS. Arthroscopic electrophysiologic surgery of the shoulder. *Op Tech Sports Med.* 1998;6:139-146.

5. Hayashi K, Markel MD. Thermal modification of joint capsule and ligamentous tissues. *Op Tech Sports Med.* 1998;6:120-125.

6. Hayashi K, Thabit G, Massa KL, et al. The effect of thermal heating on the length and histological properties of the glenohumeral joint capsule. *Am J Sports Med.* 1997;25:107-112.

7. Obrzut SL, Hecht P, Hayashi K, et al. The effect of radiofrequency energy on the length and histologic properties of the glenohumeral joint capsule. *Arthroscopy.* 1998;14:395-400.

8. Anderson K, McCarty EC, Warren RF. Thermal capsulorrhaphy: where are we today? *Sports Medicine and Arthroscopy Review.* 1999;7:117-127.

9. Ellenbecker TS, Mattalino AJ. Glenohumeral joint range of motion and rotator cuff strength following arthroscopic anterior stabilization with thermal capsulorrhaphy. *J Orthop Sports Phys Ther.* 1999;29:160-167.

10. Hayashi K, Markel MD, Thabit G. The effect of nonablative laser energy on joint capsular properties: an in vitro mechanical study using a rabbit model. *Am J Sports Med.* 1994;23:482-487.

11. Thabit G, Hayashi K, Markel MD. The effect of nonablative laser energy on joint capsular properties. *Jpn J Orthop Sports Med.* 1995;15:144-146.

12. Hayashi K, Markel MD, Bogdanske JJ. The effect of nonablative laser energy on ultrastructure of joint capsular collagen. *Arthroscopy.* 1996;12:474-481.

13. Hayashi K, Thabit G, Vailas AC. The effect of nonablative laser energy on joint capsular properties: an in vitro histological and biochemical study using a rabbit model. *Am J Sports Med.* 1996;24:640-646.

14. Hecht P, Hayashi K, Cooley AJ. The thermal effect of radiofrequency on joint capsular properties: an in vivo histological study using a sheep model. *Am J Sports Med.* 1998;26:808-814.

15. Lopez MJ, Hayashi K, Fanton GS. The effect of radiofrequency energy on the ultrastructure of joint capsular collagen. *Arthroscopy.* 1998;14:495-501.

16. Thabit G, Thorpe W, Horne R. Treatment of unidirectional and multidirectional glenohumeral instability by an arthroscopic holmium: YAG laser-assisted capsular shift procedure. Paper presented at: First Congress of International Musculoskeletal Laser Society; 1994; Neuchatel, Switzerland.

17. Naseef GS, Foster TE, Trauner K. The thermal properties of bovine joint capsule. *Am J Sports Med.* 1997;25(5), 670-674.

18. Vangsness CT, Mitchell W III, Nimni M. Collage shortening: an experimental approach with heat. *Clin Orthop.* 1997;337, 267-271.

19. Jackson DW, Grood ES, Cohn BT, et al. The effects of in situ freezing on the anterior cruciate ligament. An experimental study in goats. *J Bone Joint Surg Am.* 1991;73:201-213.

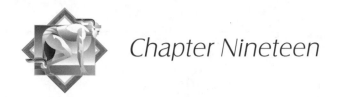

Chapter Nineteen

Knee Dislocation in a Collegiate Track Athlete

Joseph S. Lueken, MS, ATC, John R. McCarroll, MD

INTRODUCTION

Strong ligamentous and tendinous support provides stability of the knee. The incidence of knee dislocations is very low. However, the reported low incidence of dislocations is likely due to the idea that most dislocations reduce spontaneously before they are detected.[1-5]

Knee dislocations are classified in terms of the position of the tibia with respect to the femur and include anterior, posterior, medial, lateral, and rotary. Anterior dislocations, most often caused by a hyperextension force to the joint,[6-9] are the most common, and rotary dislocations are the most rare.[1,7,10] The etiology of dislocations ranges from high- to low-velocity injuries.

Dislocation of the knee invariably results in damage to several major structures. Soft tissue injuries occur to the ligaments, cartilage, muscles, and tendons. Fractures of the tibial plateau and avulsed fragments from the proximal tibia or distal femur have been reported.[1,3,11] Vascular and neurological injuries can have devastating complications resulting in long-term problems. The popliteal artery, which is tethered proximally at the adductor hiatus and the soleal arch distally, is especially vulnerable to injury due to its limited mobility. Popliteal artery injuries occur in approximately one-third of knee dislocations, ranging from intimal injury to complete disruption of the blood vessel.[1,12] Stretching of the artery is commonly seen in an anterior dislocation, whereas complete disruption is common in posterior dislocations.[1,3] An arteriogram should be performed to evaluate the integrity of the vascular supply following knee dislocations. Undiagnosed vascular injuries can lead to amputation.[1,3,6,7,12] The reported incidence of nerve injury is approximately 25% in most cases with common peroneal nerve involvement.[3]

SUBJECT

The patient was a 21-year-old National Collegiate Athletic Association (NCAA) Division I track athlete. She was 5'3", 106 lbs, with severe bilateral genu varum and knee hyperextension. She competed in several events including hurdles, middle distance, and relays. On April 27, 1995, during the second leg of the women's 4 x 400 meter relay, she suffered a hyperextension injury. The injury occurred after taking the baton and entering the first turn. Videotape of the injury, as well as subjective information from the athlete, revealed that while trying to jockey for position she was bumped by another competitor and thrown off balance. As she tried to regain her balance, she overstrided, hyperextended her knee, fell, and rolled onto the track (Figure 19-1). An orthopedic surgeon and certified athletic trainer examined her. There was an observable deformity and palpation of the femoral heads in the calf, which confirmed that she had sustained an anterior knee

Figure 19-1. Mechanism of injury. Athlete was running the 4 x 400 m relay. She hit the side rail of the track, hyperextended her knee, and her knees went into varus. She then had an anterior lateral dislocation of her knee.

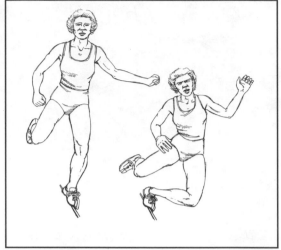

Figure 19-2. Lateral view showing dislocation.

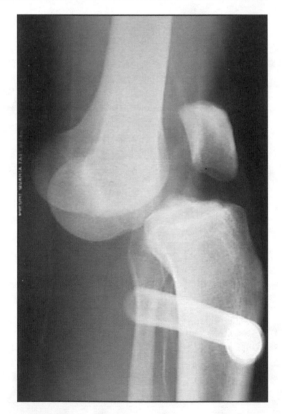

dislocation. The pedal pulse was normal, as were the sensory evaluations of the lower leg and foot. The athlete was placed in a vacuum splint, boarded, treated for possible shock, and taken to the hospital. At the emergency room, x-rays confirmed the anterior knee dislocation (Figures 19-2).

The athlete was placed under a general anesthetic and a closed reduction was performed. Post reduction, an arteriogram indicated no injury to the vascular supply. The following day, an MRI was obtained (Table 19-1 and Figures 19-3a and 19-3b).

Table 19-1

MRI RESULTS

- Moderate size joint effusion.
- Increased signal intensity in the inner aspect of the posterior horn of the lateral meniscus, but no definitive tear.
- Complete tear of the anterior cruciate ligament.
- Posterior cruciate ligament—partial tear.
- Lateral collateral ligament—complete tear.
- Popliteal tendon—partial tear.
- Medial and lateral gastrocnemius muscle—partial tear.
- Contusion to the outer aspect of the lateral femoral condyle.

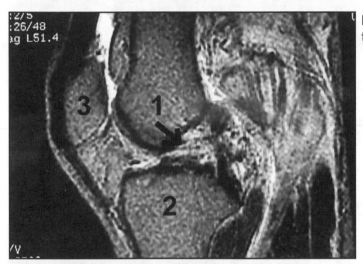

Figure 19-3a. MRI results showing the torn anterior cruciate ligament.

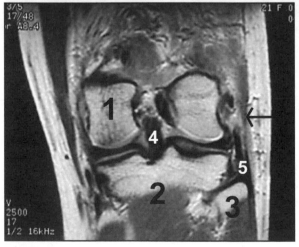

Figure 19-3b. MRI results showing the torn posterior cruciate ligament.

Figure 19-4. Anatomical drawing of the injured ligaments.

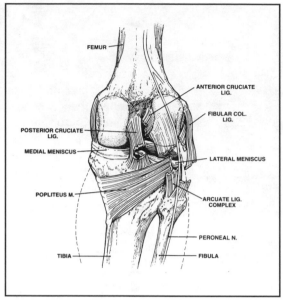

On April 29, 1995, 3 days after the injury, she was released from the hospital to return home. She was nonweightbearing and in an immobilizer. On May 1, 1995, she was evaluated by her team orthopedic surgeon and scheduled for surgery.

SURGICAL PROCEDURE

On May 8, 1995, the athlete underwent examination under anesthesia (EUA) and surgery to repair or reconstruct the damaged structures (Figure 19-4).

On EUA, the athlete had 3+ lateral instability at 30 degrees flexion and 0 degrees extension. The reason to examine instability at 0 degrees flexion is to also evaluate the posterior cruciate ligament (PCL). Patients with an absent PCL demonstrate joint opening in full extension, but not if the PCL is intact. She had a posterior draw sign of 1+ to 2+ with an end point. The Lachman's and anterior drawer signs were 3+ with no end point. We were unable to do a pivot shift due to the massive ligamentous injuries to the lateral side of her knee. Valgus instability was zero. There was severe posterolateral instability with positive external rotation and recurvatum tests.

An arthroscopy was not performed. The amount of intra-articular fluid required to inflate the knee joint during arthroscopy would not have been contained within the joint due to the lack of an intact lateral capsule. This would have compromised the leg due to increased swelling.

At the time of surgery, we found that there was about one-third of the PCL still attached to the medial femoral condyle, the anterior cruciate ligament (ACL) was completely torn, and the popliteal tendon was avulsed off the lateral femur. The lateral collateral ligament (LCL) was completely avulsed from the femur. The peroneal nerve and lateral meniscus were intact. The arcuate complex was completely disrupted off the femur with some damage to the lateral gastrocnemius muscle.

We repaired the PCL by placing sutures through it and attaching the sutures to the original PCL attachment on the medial femoral condyle using drill holes. We harvested a bone-patellar tendon-bone graft from the central one-third of the patellar tendon and performed a standard ACL reconstruction.

We then directed our attention to the lateral side. We reattached the popliteal tendon and LCL to their insertions on the femur, and then repaired and advanced the arcuate complex to the femur. The wounds were closed and the athlete's knee was placed in an Cryo/Cuff (AirCast, Summit, NJ) with an immobilizer set at 10 degrees flexion to relax the lateral repair.

We considered this a low-velocity knee dislocation.[13] The rationale for this surgery was:

1. To restore all the ligamentous stability to the knee via direct repair or reconstructive surgery.
2. To correct and keep the knee in the proper alignment in order for this knee to be functional for daily activities and sports.

In patients with lateral side instability it is very important to repair the structures as early as possible, otherwise they become shortened and retracted, thus, very difficult to repair if surgery is delayed for more than 2 weeks. It is also important to try to gain some early range of motion (ROM) in knee dislocations to prevent stiffness following the initial injury.

REHABILITATION

The primary goals of all rehabilitation programs are the same—to return the athlete to sport with full ability, as quickly and safely as possible.[14] Long-term goals were established with this athlete, considering the following:

1. The amount of trauma to her knee.
2. She would be entering her last year of NCAA eligibility.
3. She would not compete again for approximately 1 year due to the required rehabilitation.

Realizing that rehabilitation would be a long and, slow initially, the athlete set her long-term goals to first recondition her knee to perform activities of daily living, and second to possibly compete again for her university in middle distance running events.

Phase I: Preoperative Phase

The goals of the preoperative phase were to control pain and reduce swelling. Rehabilitation consisted of icing and elevation daily. A Cryo/Cuff was used throughout the course of the day and taken off at night. The athlete remained nonweightbearing using crutches during this period of time. A continuous passive motion (CPM) device was used from 0 degrees to 30 degrees to gain motion and prevent stiffness.

Phase II: 0 to 14 Days

Table 19-2 outlines the rehabilitation program. The athlete was restricted from activity the first week postoperatively to minimize the chance for injury to the repaired structures and to minimize swelling and pain. The athlete spent the week at home under her parents' supervision and was instructed to use the Cryo/Cuff, elevate the leg throughout the day and to stay in the immobilizer, nonweightbearing. During the second week postoperatively, the athlete was placed in a CPM device set at 10 degrees to 30 degrees of knee flexion. More ROM was not permitted because additional healing time was needed for the lateral structures. Active ROM exercises were initiated for the quadriceps in order to gain strength and control, while ankle pumping with the leg elevated was performed to help decrease swelling.

Phase III: 2 to 6 Weeks

The main goals of phase III included controlling pain and swelling, increasing ROM and strength, gait training with crutches, and returning to full weightbearing ambulation by week 6. To control pain and swelling, the athlete continued using the Cryo/Cuff and performing ankle pumps with the leg elevated. ROM exercises were performed including patellar mobilization, heel and wall slides, prone hangs, and passive knee flexion and extension. Stationary bike for gaining ROM was also initiated, with partial pedal turns until full pedal turns could be accomplished. Strengthening involved both the thigh and lower leg musculature. Ankle exercises included sport cord strengthening in inversion, eversion, dorsiflexion, and plantarflexion. The eccentric phase of heel raises progressed to unilateral heel raises. Exercises for the thigh included active straight leg raises in four directions and standing weight shifts. Bilateral squatting was initially done on the Shuttle 2000-1 (Contemporary Design Company, Glacier, Wash) with only one band so as to eliminate the effects of gravity and to provide a more controlled environment. After the athlete could perform squats against three bands of resistance, she progressed to one-quarter to one-half bilateral wall squats, and unilat-

Table 19-2

REHABILITATION PROTOCOL FOLLOWING SURGERY FOR ANTERIOR KNEE DISLOCATION

Phase	Activity
Phase I: Preoperative Phase	Nonweightbearing, crutches, and elevation.
Phase II: 0 to 14 days	
1 to 6 days	Cryo/Cuff, nonweightbearing, immobilizer, elevation, and active-assisted ROM and straight leg raises for the quadriceps.
7 to 14 days	Nonweightbearing, immobilizer, Cryo/Cuff, and CPM machine set from 10 to 30 degrees flexion when not in rehabilitation. Passive ROM: 10 to 30 degrees of flexion. Quadriceps steps and active ROM.
Phase III: 2 to 6 weeks	Partial weightbearing. Gait training with crutches to full weightbearing ambulation. Cryo/Cuff, CPM 5 to 100 degrees of flexion when not in rehabilitation, ankle pumps with the lower leg elevated, cross friction massage to the surgical scars, prone hangs to promote extension, heel/wall slides to promote flexion, patellar mobilization for ROM, stationary bike for ROM, passive ROM 0 to 100 degrees, sport cord lower leg strengthening (inversion, eversion, plantarflexion, and dorsiflexion), heel raises, straight leg raises in four directions, weight shifts, bilateral Shuttle 2000-1 squats to bilateral wall squats and unilateral Shuttle 2000 squats, and trampoline balancing, single leg.
Phase IV: 6 to 12 weeks	Full weightbearing ambulation, prone hangs to promote extension, heel/wall slides to promote flexion, patellar mobilization for range of motion, stationary bike for range of motion and strengthening, and unilateral 1/2 squats.
Phase V: 13 weeks and on	Unilateral Shuttle 2000-1 squats with basic plyometrics in later stages, walking lunges, stool walking for hamstrings, stationary bike for range of motion and strengthening, stair machine, weight room strengthening, unilateral plyometrics (Shuttle 2000-1 plyometrics, jumping rope, directional jumping on the floor and more advanced plyometrics in the later stages), weight room strengthening (leg press, squats, hamstring curls, over head lifts, step-ups and lunges), increased functional activities (cariocas, side stepping, backward running, sprinting, and cutting), increased distance runs to 3 to 5 miles, and increased speed training and conditioning under the supervision of the track coach.

eral squats on the Shuttle. A ball was placed between the thighs during bilateral squatting to involve the adductor muscle group. Bilateral trampoline balancing progressed to unilateral balancing. As strength and balance improved, the athlete was weaned off her crutches, and full weightbearing ambulation was achieved at the end of week 4. Electrical stimulation and ice was used after daily rehabilitation.

Phase IV: 7 to 12 Weeks

At the beginning of week 7, the athlete's ROM was 0-2-90 degrees, her stability was excellent, and her gait was good. The goals of phase IV included increasing knee flexion and strength, beginning basic functional activities, and returning to the weight room for upper body and limited lower body activities. Gaining original hyperextension was not a goal, as we felt that being 2 to 3 degrees short of 0 degrees of extension would further promote lateral stability. The exercises in phase IV were very similar to phase III with an increase in sets, repetitions, and resistance. Basic unilateral plyometrics on the Shuttle 2000-1 were added, as well as walking lunges, stool walking for the hamstrings, and the Stair machine. Weight room activities for the lower extremity included bilateral and unilateral leg press, step-ups with resistance, hamstring curls, and the thigh abductor/adductor machine. Walking functional activities were initiated, including walking backward, side steps, and cariocas. Jogging began at week 10 with a one-half mile run every other day. The distance was increased to 1 mile at the end of week 12.

Phase V: 13 Weeks

The goal of this phase emphasized a balanced program of strengthening, flexibility, functional activities, and return to competition. Most strengthening was performed in the weight room under the supervision of the certified athletic trainer and the strength and conditioning coach. Between weeks 16 and 20, the athlete was performing functional activities, including cariocas and side stepping at quicker speeds and one-half to three-quarter speed sprints. By the beginning of November, the athlete was working with the track coaches and training with the team. Her ROM at this time was 2-0-126 degrees.

Clinical Outcome

The patient's final ROM was 2-0-130 degrees, ACL Lachman negative, KT-1000 was 1 mm at 30 lbs of pull. She was able to return to track, although she lost some speed due to the injury.

SUMMARY

Considering the extent of injury this athlete sustained, she did an extraordinary job following through with rehabilitation. By February 1996, the athlete was competing in sprinting events for her university. In April 1996, she competed in hurdles. Her sprinting times were comparable to how she had previously performed. Her hurdle times were not as fast. She was unable to regain the form and confidence she needed to hurdle. Overall, she was excited to be competing and had accomplished the goals she set for herself.

REFERENCES

1. Cole BJ, Harner CD. The multiple ligament injured knee. *Clin Sports Med.* 1999;18:241-262.
2. Cooper DE, Speer KP, Wickiewicz TL, et al. Complete knee dislocation without posterior cruciate ligament disruption. *Clin Orthop Res.* 1992;284:228-233.
3. Good L, Johnson RJ. The dislocated knee. *Journal of the American Academy of Orthopedic Surgeons.* 1995;3:284-292.
4. Henshaw RM, Shapiro MS, Oppenheim WL. Delayed reduction of traumatic knee dislocation. *Clin Orthop.* 1996;330:152-156.
5. Wascher DC, Dvirnak PC, DeCoster TA. Knee dislocations: initial assessment and implications for treatment. *J Orthop Trauma.* 1997;11:525-529.
6. Holmes CH, Bach BR. Knee dislocations. *Phys Sports Medicine.* 1995;23:69-82.
7. Kremchek TE, Welling RE, Kremchek EJ. Traumatic dislocation of the knee. *Orthop Review.* 1989;18:1051-1057.

8.   Hill JA, Rana NA. Complications of posterolateral dislocation of the knee. *Clin Orthop Res.* 1981;154:212-215.

9.   Meyers MH, Harvey JP. Traumatic dislocation of the knee joint: a study of eighteen cases. *J Bone Joint Surg Am.* 1971;53:16-29.

10. Shapiro MS, Freedman EL. Allograft reconstruction of the anterior and posterior cruciate ligaments after traumatic knee dislocation. *Am J Sports Med.* 1995;23:580-587.

11. Noyes FR, Barber-Westin SD. Reconstruction of the anterior and posterior cruciate ligaments after knee dislocation. *Am J Sports Med.* 1997;25:769-777.

12. Frassica FJ, Sim FH, Staeheli JW, et al. Dislocation of the knee. *Clin Orthop.* 1991;263:200-205.

13. Shelbourne KD, Porter DA, McCarroll JR, et al. Low velocity knee dislocations. *Orthop Review.* 1991, XX:11; 995-1004.

14. Shelbourne KD, Nitz P. Accelerated rehabilitation after anterior cruciate ligament reconstruction. *Am J Sports Med.* 1990;18:292-299.

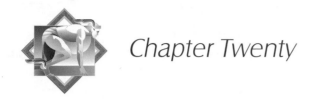

Chapter Twenty

Combined Ligament Injuries with Peroneal Nerve Injury in a College Football Player

Walter L. Jenkins, MS, PT, ATC, Mike J. Hanley, MS, ATC/L,

Tally Lassiter Jr, MD, James E. Tracy, MS, PT, ATC

INTRODUCTION

Rehabilitation following multiple knee ligament injuries can be among the most challenging of cases seen in athletic settings. When combined with nerve or vascular pathology, the clinician is presented with a unique challenge in which there is minimal literature to gain insight. Pertinent literature includes a review of existing case studies, biomechanical studies on ligaments, and the biomechanics involved in surgical techniques, including graft fixation. Problem solving in such cases is complex when one has so many variables from which to render an evaluation. A team approach with the team physician, orthopedist, athletic training staff, and other allied health professionals who may become involved is essential to the maximization of the athlete's recovery potential.

SUBJECT

The athlete was a 6-foot tall, 186 lb, freshman defensive back for an intercollegiate football team. He was injured near the conclusion of a fall football practice session while fighting with another player. A third player, who was trying to break up the fight, landed on the medial aspect of the athlete's right knee while his foot was planted, resulting in a varus opening. The athlete stated that he felt as if his knee "rolled outward." He denied hearing or feeling a pop.

An onfield evaluation was performed immediately by a certified athletic trainer. At the time of injury, the athlete did not have a knee effusion, but 5 to 10 minutes after the initial evaluation there was significant generalized swelling. The athlete was unable to actively move the injured knee secondary to pain. There was active plantarflexion and inversion of the ankle; however, the athlete was unable to perform active dorsiflexion or eversion at the time of injury. Active and resisted great toe flexion was within normal limits (WNL), while resisted ankle dorsiflexion and eversion, and great toe extension were absent (0/5). Full passive extension of the knee was observed. Palpation of the lateral aspect of the knee was acutely tender. Distal pulses in the foot were intact on initial evaluation. An orthopedic evaluation was performed the same day by one of the team physicians.

The athlete was placed in a compressive wrap and knee immobilizer. He was asked to use two axillary crutches with toe touch weightbearing. Standard ice, compression, and elevation were followed prior to the initial surgery.

Preoperatively, it was decided that the knee joint would be evaluated arthroscopically and a lateral repair would be performed approximately 1 month prior to an ACL/PCL reconstruction. The rationale for a two-stage operation in this case was the lack of immediate access to allograft tissue for the ACL/PCL reconstructions and the need for an acute repair of the posterolateral corner. The posterolateral corner needs to be repaired immediately in order to keep the tissue planes clear. After about 4 to 10 days, the scar tissue in the posterolateral corner makes anatomic repair difficult. Once the posterolateral repair was performed, an arthroscopic-assisted ACL/PCL reconstruction could be performed with minimal surgical morbidity.

SURGICAL PROCEDURE #1: LATERAL REPAIR (3 DAYS POST-INJURY)

The initial surgery consisted of arthroscopic evaluation under general anesthesia with debridement of the anterior and posterior cruciate stumps. Additionally, there was an open repair of the torn lateral collateral ligament, iliotibial (IT) band, biceps tendon, lateral meniscus, arcuate complex, and a decompression of the peroneal nerve. The lateral collateral ligament and the biceps tendon were avulsed from the fibula and reattached to their insertion by screw anchors and suture. The lateral meniscus was likewise reattached to the tibia via screws and sutures. The arcuate complex and the IT band had midsubstance tears and were primarily repaired with suture. The peroneal nerve was attenuated, but intact. There was evidence of hemorrhage within the peroneal nerve. The peroneal nerve was decompressed distally where it entered the lateral calf muscles by splitting the fascia and making a larger opening in the nerve canal with a hemostat.

The athlete was admitted to the hospital following the first procedure for observation and was discharged the next day. He was given heprin prophylactically for deep vein thrombosis and started on continuous passive motion (CPM) with the range of motion (ROM) set to his pain tolerance. Additionally the athlete was placed in a postoperative hinge brace and had a custom-made rigid ankle foot orthosis (AFO) ordered for his drop foot.

Rehabilitation was initiated 2 days postoperatively. The athlete was started on submaximal isometrics for the quadriceps/hamstrings in a cocontraction fashion so as to minimize the sagittal plane forces. ROM was limited to a pain-free arc of motion in flexion. Knee extension ROM was limited to approximately 10 degrees secondary to the posterior and lateral repairs performed during the initial surgery.[1] Care was taken to avoid positioning the knee in a varus alignment during this and subsequent postoperative periods. Swelling and pain control were performed with a combination of modalities and medication. The athlete was nonweightbearing on two axillary crutches until the second surgical procedure. Throughout the rehabilitation process, following all surgical procedures the lateral reconstruction was considered. A particular area of concern was varus loading in either an open or closed kinetic chain. Abduction straight leg raises or single limb strength training in a closed kinetic chain were prohibited due to the varus opening forces that occur with these activities.[2] A postoperative hinge brace was used early in rehabilitation and a functional knee brace was used later in the rehabilitation process so as to assist with decreasing the forces on this ligament complex.[3] Table 20-1 summarizes rehabilitation following the lateral repair.

The athlete tolerated the first surgery very well. He had consistent progress with his ROM and swelling throughout the first month postoperatively. There was a small fracture-type blister on the distal aspect of the lateral incision that healed well during the first week postoperatively. The staples that were used for the lateral incision were removed approximately 10 days post-surgery. The knee was stable with varus stress testing. ROM was 10 degrees from full extension to 120 degrees of flexion by the end of this period. There was no change in the peroneal nerve function prior to the second surgical procedure.

SURGICAL PROCEDURE #2: ACL/PCL RECONSTRUCTION (1 MONTH POST-INJURY)

The anterior and posterior cruciate ligaments were reconstructed with allografts approximately 1 month after the first surgery. A bone-patellar tendon-bone allograft was used for the ACL and an Achilles' tendon allograft was used for the PCL. Allograft materials were used in this surgical procedure secondary to both cru-

Table 20-1

REHABILITATION FOLLOWING LATERAL SIDE REPAIR

Clinical Goals

- Maintain joint integrity
- Control swelling
- ROM: 10 to 120 degrees knee flexion (prior to the ACL/PCL reconstruction)

Exercises

- CPM: to tolerance (up to 10 to 120 degrees knee flexion)
- Quad isometrics (in 20 to 30 degrees of knee flexion)
- Nonweightbearing (NWB) (no closed kinetic chain activities)
- Active/active assist/passive ankle ROM

ciates being involved. In using allografts, the thinking was that there would be less soft tissue disruption to the involved and uninvolved knee with the surgical procedure. Utilization of an Achilles' tendon allograft could closely approximate the strength of the PCL and, therefore, more closely approximate normal knee function postoperatively.[4] A surgical assistant prepared the allografts while the surgeon was arthroscopically evaluating and preparing the graft tunnels.

The ACL/PCL reconstruction was performed with a femoral nerve block. A tourniquet was used to decrease bleeding and improve visualization of the knee. The reconstructions were performed with arthroscopic assist and fluoroscopy to ensure proper graft tunnel placement. The grafts were sized to 1 cm in diameter so as to fit into the 10 mm tibial and femoral tunnels. The PCL was reconstructed prior to the ACL. For the PCL, the bone plug from the Achilles' tendon was placed in the femoral tunnel and secured with an interference screw. The soft tissue end of the Achilles' tendon was then fixed to the tibia via a soft tissue screw with the knee in approximately 80 degrees of flexion. The ACL allograft was fixed first on the femoral side and then on the tibia with interference screws at both ends.[4-7] The ACL graft was tensioned at 20 degrees of knee flexion.

Following the ACL/PCL graft fixation, the knee had full ROM and was tested for stability. There was a 0+/3 Lachman, and anterior and posterior drawer. The knee was stable to varus and valgus testing at all degrees of knee flexion/extension. Total tourniquet time was 126 minutes at 300 mmHg. Following surgery, the athlete had normal distal pulses and the neurologic exam was unchanged from the preoperative findings (drop foot was present). The athlete was placed in a sterile, bulky, compressive dressing and a postoperative hinge brace set at 0 to 70 degrees. He received a femoral nerve block postoperatively so as to decrease the immediate postoperative pain. The athlete was admitted to the hospital following surgery and discharged 1 day later.

REHABILITATION FOLLOWING THE ACL/PCL RECONSTRUCTIONS

Phase I

Rehabilitation following the ACL/PCL reconstructions was designed to take into consideration both of these structures with emphasis on the PCL. Because rehabilitation following PCL reconstruction is more con-

Table 20-2

ACL/PCL RECONSTRUCTIONS

Passive ROM

0 to 4 weeks	Zero to 70 degrees (watch for proximal tibial sag). Tibia should be supported proximally when the patient is supine with the knee in full extension.
4 to 6 weeks	Proceed with PROM as tolerated, keeping in mind that the proximal tibia should be supported to prevent posterior sag.

Weightbearing

0 to 3 weeks	Once full extension is obtained, the patient may begin weight-bearing as tolerated with the knee in an a postoperative knee brace (locked in full extension).
3 to 6 weeks	Postoperative brace is unlocked to provide for more normalized weightbearing (if there is quad control).
6 to 8 weeks	Removal of the postoperative brace and crutches. Application of an ACL/PCL functional brace for ADLs and exercise.

servative in terms of ROM and strength training than ACL rehabilitation, it was felt that PCL rehabilitation should predominate.[8,9] Prior to beginning the ACL/PCL rehabilitation, a literature review of ligament biomechanics and existing postoperative care was performed.[2,5-21] With this in mind, the initial program guidelines were established (Table 20-2). It is important to recognize that the rehabilitation program was altered according to the athlete's response to the forces placed on the knee during rehabilitation and functional activities throughout this process.

During the initial postoperative period for the second surgery, emphasis was placed on avoidance of forces that could disrupt the healing ACL/PCL grafts. The posterior/lateral repair was not considered to limit the rehabilitation process beyond the guidelines outlined for the ACL/PCL during the early phases of rehabilitation. Particular consideration was placed on keeping the tibial-femoral relationship intact so as to limit the forces placed on the PCL graft. If the tibia is free to "drop back" into a position that is posterior to the femur, the PCL graft will tend to stretch out or creep.[5] Therefore, whenever the athlete was supine there was a mechanical block placed under the proximal tibia so as to avoid this "drop back" in the tibia as it relates to the femur (Figure 20-1). Full extension could be obtained but not at the expense of the tibial-femoral relationship. The tibial-femoral relationship was evaluated frequently by placing the knee in approximately 80 degrees of flexion and observing the tibial position in relationship to the femur. In this position, the tibia should be in front of the femur. The rehabilitation process was in part progressed based upon this evaluation.

ROM was limited to 0 to 70 degrees during the first 3 weeks after the second surgery to limit the forces on the PCL.[9] After approximately 70 degrees of knee flexion, tension on the PCL graft is increasing.[1,13] Since PCL reconstructions have an increased incidence of stretch, it was felt that any unnecessary forces on the PCL graft should be avoided or at least limited during the initial postoperative period.[9] Weightbearing was limited until the athlete could achieve full extension. Once full extension was obtained, the athlete was then able to weightbear to tolerance with the knee locked in a hinge brace in full extension. During gait, the athlete was instructed to avoid knee recurvatum or external tibial rotation. By locking the knee in full extension, forces on the ACL/PCL grafts could be reduced by sharing the loading with the other knee ligaments, the brace, and the knee articulation. The hinge brace was adapted in order to utilize the AFO for weightbearing

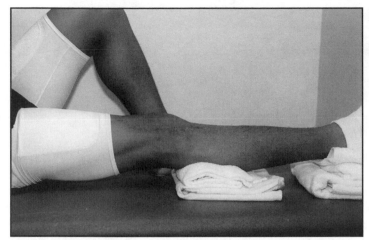

Figure 20-1. Supine props.

activities. The athlete was able to achieve the necessary ROM within the first 3 weeks after the second surgery. He began one-fourth weightbearing at this time with progression to full weightbearing over the next month. He had significant difficulty in obtaining a quad contraction with a loss of proximal patellar glide, also noted during this time frame. Regular and more forceful patellar glides were performed beginning in the third week postoperatively. Cocontraction of the quadriceps and hamstrings was performed during this time frame. There was no change in the peroneal nerve function during this period.

Once full extension and quad control were achieved, the athlete could weightbear with the postoperative brace unlocked while using the AFO. Passive ROM was progressed as tolerated after the first 4 weeks of the second surgery keeping in mind that the tibial-femoral relationship should be maintained. The athlete's ROM was measured at 0 to 80 degrees at 3 weeks postoperatively with no increase in the posterior sag following the second surgery. The knee was stable with anterior/posterior as well as valgus/varus motions. The quad contraction was still quite poor (3-/5) and there was significant quad atrophy on observation. The athlete was referred for an EMG/nerve conduction velocity and found to have a femoral nerve injury of unknown origin. It is possible that the nerve block utilized postoperatively resulted in a neurapraxia to the femoral nerve and subsequent quad atrophy. For this reason, it was decided that weightbearing would be limited to that which could be performed with the hinge brace locked in full extension. Patellofemoral joint glide appeared to be normalizing at 4 weeks post ACL/PCL reconstruction secondary to the increased emphasis on mobilization. Leg press was initiated (while in the hinge brace) in a 20- to 40-degree ROM so as to enhance the quadriceps recovery. The 20- to 40-degree ROM was chosen so as to decrease the posterior shear and therefore cause the least amount of stress on the PCL graft.[20] The leg press was performed with two legs utilizing a 25-repetition maximum. When the athlete was able to perform 100 consecutive repetitions (100 repetition rule), an increase in resistance was obtained. Cocontraction of the quadriceps and hamstrings was also performed during this time frame. The athlete was unable to walk in the AFO without the hinge brace locked in full extension during this period due to the quad atrophy. Table 20-3 summarizes rehabilitation during Phase I.

Phase II

At 6 weeks post ACL/PCL reconstruction, the athlete had 0 degrees of extension to 120 degrees of knee flexion. The anterior/posterior stability was unchanged with no posterior sag noted. Varus laxity was graded at 1+/3. The quadriceps muscle tone was improving with the quad set graded at 3+/5. Patellofemoral joint motion was now within normal limits. There was a mild knee effusion noted possibly secondary to an increase in the activity level. ROM continued to be progressed as tolerated in flexion. Open kinetic chain (OKC) knee extension exercises in a range of 70 to 30 were initiated. This ROM was utilized to increase the quad activity while keeping the forces on the ACL/PCL at minimal levels.[1,8,10,11,15-18,20,21] The OKC knee

Table 20-3

REHABILITATION FOLLOWING ACL/PCL RECONSTRUCTIONS

Phase I: 0 to 6 weeks

Clinical Goals

Maintain joint/ligament integrity, improve quad control: 3+ to 4-/5, progress to WBAT (in postoperative brace locked in full extension/AFO), ROM: 0 to 120 degrees knee flexion.

Exercises

CPM: up to 0 to 120 degrees knee flexion, supine props (see Figure 20-1) for knee extension, wall slides (knee flexion), cocontraction of the quads/hams, leg press (20 to 40 degrees), knee flexion (25-repetition maximum progressing to 100 repetitions prior to adding resistance), and patellar mobilization (superior glide particularly).

Testing

Observe the posterior sag and EMG (femoral nerve).

Phase II: 6 to 16 weeks

Clinical Goals

Maintain joint/ligament integrity, improve quad control to 3+ to 4-/5, progress to WBAT with the brace unlocked (in the AFO), and ROM to full motion.

Exercises/Treatment

Open kinetic chain (OKC): no isolated hamstring activity, quads, knee extension machine/Orthotron (70 to 30 degrees initially progressing to 90 to 30 degrees by 9 weeks) 25 repetition maximum (two to four sets).

Closed kinetic chain (CKC) (in the functional brace/AFO): leg press (60 to 30 degrees), squats (60 to 30 degrees), 100-repetition rule for the first 8 weeks postoperatively, after 8 weeks postoperatively two to four sets of 25 repetitions were utilized, no single limb activities

Aqua Ark (walking only), DC electrical stimulation to the anterior tibialis/peroneals, ROM: as tolerated in knee flexion/knee extension to 0 degrees only, WBAT (functional knee brace [unlocked]/AFO), four-way hip machine.

Testing

No posterior sag, varus stress test (1+/3), quad set: 3+/5, peroneal nerve was unchanged (0/5).

Phase 3: 16 to 32 weeks

Clinical Goals

Maintain joint/ligament integrity, improve quad control to 4/5, and improve leg control to allow for ambulation without the functional brace.

Table 20-3 continued

Exercises/Treatment

OKC: quads, knee extension machine/Orthotron (90 to 10 degrees), emphasize eccentrics for the patellar tendonitis, 15-repetition maximum (two to four sets).

CKC: leg press/squats: 80 to 10 degrees, 15-to 25-repetition maximum (two to four sets), emphasize proper alignment, cycling/stair machine/Aqua Ark, agility drills (as tolerated), and no single leg activities.

DC electrical stimulation: to the anterior tibialis/peroneals

Testing

One to 2 mm of posterior sag at 80 degrees knee flexion, varus stress test: 1+/3, and quad set (4+/5).

extension was performed on a standard knee extension machine and an Orthotron (Cybex International, Inc, Medway, Mass). The athlete was able to walk for short periods with the hinge brace unlocked due to improved quad tone. The athlete remained in the AFO for all weightbearing activities.

The peroneal nerve dysfunction had not changed since the time of injury. It was concluded that a direct current electrical stimulation could be used to limit the muscle fiber morbidity. DC electrical stimulation was initiated at this time. Chronaxie measurements were attained initially and used as the minimum pulse duration for stimulation. Electrodes were placed over the peroneal muscles using a bipolar technique with intensity increased to achieve a grade 3/5 muscle contraction of the dorsiflexors. The patient received 50 contractions per visit with a 10-second rest between contractions, two to three times per week.[22,23]

The athlete went home for the college term break for approximately 4 weeks (2 to 3 months after the ACL/PCL reconstructions). During this time, he was followed several times a week by another clinician that adhered to the postoperative guidelines outlined by our staff. ROM was progressed to 0 to 130 degrees with no changes in the posterior sag of the tibia. The athlete remained stable in both the frontal (valgus/varus) and sagittal (anterior/posterior) planes. The quad tone was graded at 4-/5, but quad atrophy was still apparent. Closed kinetic chain leg press was performed at 30 to 60 degrees, while open kinetic chain was utilized in a 90 to 30 degree ROM. Two-legged squats and leg presses were utilized, but no single-limb closed kinetic chain strength training activities were allowed due to the posterolateral repair. Squats were performed in front of a mirror so as to improve feedback to the athlete and, therefore, provide improved neuromuscular training. Neuromuscular training was enhanced by multiple repetitions performed with proper form. The 100-repetition rule continued to be utilized during the first 8 weeks post ACL/PCL reconstruction. Walking in an Aqua Ark (Therapeutic Systems, Inc, Doylestown, Pa) was also initiated during this period. The athlete was now walking in an AFO and a functional knee brace that was opened up to full ROM. Rehabilitation during this period was unremarkable with the exception of an eversion ankle sprain while walking at home without the functional brace or the AFO. There was a slight increase in lateral knee joint pain following the ankle injury, but no swelling or knee instability could be elicited. Table 20-4 outlines rehabilitation during phase II of rehabilitation.

Phase III

At the 4-month evaluation following the ACL/PCL reconstruction, the athlete did not have any motor changes in his peroneal nerve function. There was a "burning" sensation noted in the dorsum of the foot, but no changes were observed in the anterior or lateral compartments of the lower leg. ROM was now within normal limits. He was noting improved lower extremity strength and the knee remained stable. A minimal posterior sag was observed for the first time when the athlete was evaluated in the 80-degree knee flexed position. The varus stress test remained at the 1+/3 level. There were firm end points with the ACL, PCL, MCL, and LCL. The quad tone was graded at 4/5 with a good vastus medialis oblique (VMO) contraction observed. The athlete was remaining stable, resisted training, was progressed to 20 to 70 degrees for open kinetic chain knee extension, and 10 to 70 degrees for closed kinetic chain activities (squats and leg press). Isolated hamstring activity was not initiated secondary to good hamstring muscle tone and the PCL reconstruction.[20] The athlete remained in the functional knee brace and the AFO for all weightbearing activities, including the closed kinetic chain exercises.

Secondary to the increase in rehabilitation and functional activity, the athlete began to develop a patellar tendonitis at approximately 5 months postoperatively. The athlete also noted some persistent lateral knee pain in the area of the lateral epicondyle. This appeared to be secondary to the functional knee brace condyle pad slipping in this area. A new condyle pad was obtained and the symptoms resolved within several weeks. There was essentially no change in the level of stability with approximately 1 to 2 mm of increased posterior sag noted on the involved side when compared to the uninvolved knee when the knee was flexed to 80 degrees. Cycling, Stair machine, and the Aqua Ark were continued or initiated to assist with neuromuscular integration and aerobic training. Cycling was initially performed at higher rates of speed (150 RPM) and progressed to 90 RPM prior to 6 months post ACL/PCL. Open and closed kinetic chain activities remained relatively constant at this time. It was observed that the athlete was aligning himself in a varus attitude during his squats. A valgus producing lateral heel wedge was used to assist the athlete to stay out of varus when performing squats. Modalities and an increase in OKC eccentric exercise were used to treat the patellar tendonitis. Table 20-3 outlines the rehabilitation for postoperative ACL/PCL phase three.

By month 6, the athlete had reached his rehabilitation potential until there were further changes in the peroneal nerve. The knee remained stable, but further closed kinetic chain strength training and a functional progression toward return to football could not be performed. The athlete continued to work on open kinetic chain activities for the lower extremity, including isolated knee extension and hip flexion, extension, abduction, and adduction. In an effort to improve proprioception and balance, the athlete was asked to perform stepping activities in the frontal and sagittal planes. The athlete remained apprehensive about activities of daily living (ADL) due to a feeling of "instability." He continued to wear a functional brace due to this instability until 8 months postoperatively. By 9 months post ACL/PCL, the athlete was ambulating without a functional brace but with an AFO.

Further improvement remained limited for the next several months. It was decided that a baseline of outcome data would be taken at 9 months post-injury. The athlete was given a KT-1000 test, the Cincinnati Knee Rating System (overall rating scheme), and an isokinetic test. The KT-1000 results showed 2 mm of difference between the right and left sides with manual maximum (30 lb) total drawer. This test was performed at 25 degrees of knee joint flexion. Daniel, et al has validated the use of the KT-1000 as a reliable research tool.[24]

The athlete was also given the Cincinnati Knee Rating System consisting of a self-reported assessment of the athlete's symptoms, activity level, and objective data.[9,25] The numerical score was 77 out of a possible 100. Due to an inability to perform functional testing secondary to the peroneal nerve dysfunction, the final rating was poor. In the Cincinnati Knee Rating System, any part of the scale graded as poor will cause an overall poor rating. Table 20-4 outlines the results of the Cincinnati Knee Rating System for this athlete. Validation of this outcome measure has been previously performed.[9,25,26]

A kin-com was used to test the athlete's knee strength isokinetically. The athlete was tested concentrically at 180 degrees per second for both the quadriceps and the hamstrings in a ROM of 20 to 80 degrees. An initial test was performed at 9 months postoperatively with the athlete wearing the functional brace. The athlete had a right/left quadriceps deficit of 55%, and a 19% hamstring deficit. One month later, the athlete was retested without the functional brace. He had a 39% quadriceps deficit and a 14% hamstring deficit.

Table 20-4

SUMMARY OF RESULTS FROM THE CINCINNATI KNEE RATING SCHEME

Subjective

Pain (8/10), swelling (8/10), partial giving way (10/10), and full giving way (10/10)

Activity Level

Walking (3/3), stairs (2/3), running (1/3), jumping (1/3), twists/cuts (1/3), examination, effusion (4/5), lack of flexion (4/5), lack of extension (4/5), tibiofemoral crepitus (5/5), and patellofemoral crepitus (5/5).

Instability

Anterior (10/10) and pivot shift (10/10).

Radiographs

Medial tibiofemoral (10/10), lateral tibiofemoral (10/10), and patellofemoral (10/10).

Functional testing

One-legged hop (0/10)

CONCLUSIONS

The final outcome of this case can be viewed in one of several ways. First, it is important to compartmentalize the results by observing the knee in an isolated fashion and, second, by assessing function of the limb in a more general sense. Physical examination of the knee showed good stability, ROM, and a lack of profound crepitus or effusion. Radiographically, the knee appeared to be normal. Isolated strength testing for the involved knee was still weak, but improving. All of the available signs regarding knee function showed a trend toward normality. Therefore, it may be concluded that isolated knee function has improved to near normal limits.

Overall limb function is another way of assessing this case. This is best observed by an outcome measure—the Cincinnati Knee Rating System. This method of rating the case showed that the athlete was unable to return to his previous level of activity. The reason for this loss of function was the loss of the peroneal nerve, not an impaired knee joint. The poor rating by the Cincinnati scale is more of an indication of the loss of limb function, due to the peroneal nerve, rather than the restoration of a knee to near normal function. In that there is still the possibility of peroneal nerve regeneration, this athlete's final outcome rating remains in doubt. A final rating of this athlete is not possible at the time of this publication.

This case outlines a method by which clinicians may optimize the results following a complex knee injury. Due to the infrequency of these injuries, specific protocols are not available. When presented with cases such as this the clinician must perform a thorough review of the current literature pertinent to the topic and proceed carefully through all phases of rehabilitation. Careful planning prior to the surgery and frequent examination of the athlete is necessary for an optimal outcome. Even with the best plans, perfect outcomes may not occur.

REFERENCES

1. Barber-Westin SD, Noyes FR. Rigorous statistical reliability, validity, and responsiveness testing of the Cincinnati Knee Rating System in 350 subjects with uninjured, injured, or anterior cruciate ligament-reconstructed knees. *Am J Sports Med.* 1999;4:402.

2. Beynnon BD, Fleming BC, Johnson RJ, et al. Anterior cruciate ligament strain behavior during rehabilitation exercises in vivo. *Am J Sports Med.* 1995;23:1,24-34.

3. Beynnon BD, Fleming BC, Pope MH, et al. The measurement of anterior cruciate ligament strain in vivo. In: Jackson DW, ed. *The Anterior Cruciate Ligament: Current and Future Concepts.* New York, NY: Raven Press Ltd;1993:9.

4. Brosky JA, Nitz AJ, Malone TR, et al. Intrarater reliability of selected clinical outcome measures following anterior cruciate ligament reconstruction. *J Orthop Sports Phys Ther.* 1999;29:1,39-48.

5. Cole BJ, Harner CD. The multiple ligament injured knee. *Clin Sports Med.* 1999;18(1):241-262.

6. Covey DC, Sepega AA.Current concepts review: injuries of the posterior cruciate ligament. *J Bone Joint Surg Am.* 1993;75:1376-1386.

7. Daniel DM, Stone ML. T-1000 anterior-posterior displacement measurements. In: Daniel DM, ed. *Knee Ligament: Structure, Function, Injury, and Repair.* New York, NY: Raven Press Ltd; 1990:24.

8. Fu FH, Harner CD, Johnson DL, et al. Biomechanics of knee ligaments. *J Bone Joint Surg Am.* 1993;75(11):1716-1727.

9. Green RB, Noble PC, Woods GW, et al. Rehabilitation of the posterior cruciate deficient knee: a biomechanical simulation. *Ortho Trans.* 1989;13:319-320.

10. Grood ES, Noyes FR, Butler DL, et al. Ligamentous and capsular restraints preventing straight medial and lateral laxity in intact human cadaver knees. *J Bone Joint Surg Am.* 1981;63(11):1257.

11. Harner CD. Multiple ligament injuries of the knee. Paper presented at: The AOSSM annual meeting; July 13, 1998; Vancouver, BC.

12. Harner CD, Xerogeanes JW, Livesay GA, et al. The human posterior cruciate ligament complex: an interdisciplinary study. *Am J Sports Med.* 1995;23(6):736-745.

13. Jenkins WL, Munns SW, Loudon J. Knee joint accessory motion following anterior cruciate ligament allograft reconstruction: a preliminary report. *J Orthop Sports Phys Ther.* 1998;28(1):32-39.

14. Kannus P, Bergfeld J, Javinen M, et al. Injuries to the posterior cruciate ligament of the knee. *Sports Medicine.* 1991,12(2):110-131.

15. Lutz GE, Palmitier RA, Chao EYS. Comparison of tibiofemoral joint forces during open-kinetic-chain and closed-kinetic-chain exercises. *J Bone Joint Surg Am.* 1993;75(5):732-739.

16. Markolf KL, Gorek JF, Kabo M, et al. Direct measurement of resultant forces in the anterior cruciate ligament. *J Bone Joint Surg Am.* 1990;72(4):557-567.

17. Nelson RM, Hayes KW, Currier DP. *Clinical Electrotherapy.* 3rd ed. Norwalk, Conn: Appleton and Lange; 1999.

18. Noyes FR, Schipplein OD, Andriacchi TP. The anterior cruciate deficient knee with varus alignment: an analysis of gait adaptations and dynamic joint loadings. *Am J Sports Med.* 1992; 20(6):707-716.

19. Noyes FR, Barber-Westin SD. Surgical restoration to treat chronic deficiency of the posterolateral complex and cruciate ligaments of the knee joint. *Am J Sports Med.* 1996;24(4):415-426.

20. Ohkoshi Y, Yasuda K, Kaneda K, et al. Biomechanical analysis of rehabilitation in the standing position. *Am J Sports Med.* 1991;19(6):605-611.

21. Robinson AJ, Snyder-Mackler L. *Clinical Electrophysiology.* 2nd ed. Baltimore, Md: Williams & Wilkins; 1995.

22. Shelbourne KD, Nitz P. Accelerated rehabilitation after anterior cruciate ligament reconstruction. *Am J Sports Med.* 1990;18(3):292-299.

23. Shelbourne KD, Patel DV. Timing of surgery in ACL injured knee. *Knee Surgery, Sports Traumatology, and Arthroscopy.* 1995;3:148-156.

24. Veltri DM, Warren RF. Posterolateral instability of the knee. *J Bone Joint Surg Am.* 1994;76(3):460-472.

25. Wascher DC, Becker JR, Dexter JG, et al. Reconstruction of the anterior and posterior cruciate ligaments after knee dislocation. *Am J Sports Med.* 1999;27(2):189-196.

26. Wojtys EM, Loubert PV, Samson SY. Use of a knee-brace for control of tibial translation and rotation. *J Bone Joint Surg.* 1990;72(9):1323-1329.

27. Wilk KE, Escamilla RF, Fleisig GS, et al. A comparison of tibiofemoral joint forces and electromyographic activity during open and closed kinetic chain exercises. *Am J Sports Med.* 1996;24(4):518-527.

28. Yack HJ, Collins CE, Whieldon TJ. Comparison of closed and open kinetic chain exercises in the anterior cruciate ligament-deficient knee. *Am J Sports Med.* 1993;21(1):49-54.

Chapter Twenty-One

OATS Procedure for an Osteochondral Lesion of the Patella

Thomas V. Gocke III, MS, ATC/L, PA/C, Robert G. Jones, MD

INTRODUCTION

Injuries to the patella range from simple overuse syndromes to more complicated chondral injuries. In the majority of cases, injury to the patella will not result in loss of the thick hyaline articular cartilage that is found on the multiple facets of the patella. In the unlikely event of a significant chondral injury, several treatment options are available, including arthroscopic debridement of devitalized areas of articular cartilage, subchondral drilling to stimulate fibrous cartilage development in the defect area, patellectomy, and patellar resurfacing. However, the only method that allows for replacement of native hyaline cartilage is osteoarticular transplantation, which allows the defect to be filled with true hyaline cartilage surrounded by a small halo of fibrocartilage. One major concern following transplantation of the osteochondral graft is bony healing and minimizing adjacent injury to the surrounding articular cartilage of the femoral condyle and the femoral sulcus. A period of nonweightbearing helps facilitate healing and reduce sheer forces at the site of implantation. Our goals in the rehabilitative phase were to achieve full range of motion (ROM), reduce swelling, improve strength, and allow this high school athlete to return to his primary athletic position as a baseball catcher. The athlete demonstrated he was able to complete his rehabilitative program on an independent basis without sequela.

SUBJECT

This patient was a 15-year-old male who was a multisport high school athlete. His primary sport was baseball in which he was a catcher, but he also participated in football and basketball.

MECHANISM OF INJURY

He was playing high school basketball at the time of injury and stated that he jumped and landed on an extended right knee. He was unable to recall if he twisted his knee on landing. He described feeling a popping sensation but could not recall a specific location where he felt this pop. He was unable to continue playing basketball but was able to fully bear weight on the affected extremity. Within several hours of the injury, he developed minimal swelling and had only mild soreness to his knee. By the next morning, he noticed an increased amount of swelling to his knee. He stated, however, that it "loosened up" after a shower. He was able to resume basketball practice and games within 2 to 3 days. He continued to complain of pain after increased activity. Approximately 1 week after the onset of his symptoms, he noticed a catching sensation in his knee with certain motions. He reported no specific frequency or consistency associated with this catching sensation. He described a sensation of something "floating around in my knee." He denied any other traumatic episodes regarding his knee, but his symptoms were consistent with those of osteochondral lesions.

CLINICAL EXAMINATION

The athlete was examined in the office by the orthopedic surgeon 1 week after the onset of his symptoms. He had diminished active and passive ROM secondary to joint effusion. He had a 2+ joint effusion that was suspected to be a hemarthrosis. We requested permission to aspirate this effusion, but the patient declined. He had some mild patellofemoral pain with palpation of his articular patellar facets and increased pain with patellar apprehension in the medial patellar ligament and retinaculum. The Q-angle was normal (<15 degrees) and there was no excessive patellar tethering or lateral tracking. Medial and lateral joint lines were not tender. A loose body was palpated in the medial gutter and later felt in the lateral gutter and suprapatellar pouch. Two separate loose bodies were found at the time of arthroscopy. The medial and lateral collateral ligaments were stable to stress test at both 0 and 30 degrees respectively. Lachman and posterior drawer tests were negative for instability. A pivot shift test and KT 1000 measurements were not performed. The patient had difficulty firing his quadriceps for isometric contraction secondary to weakness and pain about his knee, and muscle strength could not be graded. His calf was supple and his pulses and sensation were intact for the right lower extremity.

Further diagnostic testing consisted of obtaining a magnetic resonance imaging (MRI) scan to further delineate the loose body, its origin, and to assess ligaments and cartilaginous structures in the knee. We explained that even if the origin of the loose body was defined, it would not change the outcome and necessity for surgical intervention and would add a medical expense that would not enhance the treatment of this condition. The question of waiting until the end of basketball season to undergo a knee arthroscopy to remove the loose body was discussed. We explained that the potential for further injury to the hyaline articular cartilage was great and could lead to further chondral injury. Advised that a course of rehabilitative exercise would be beneficial. A program of quadriceps sets and straight leg raises (SLR) prescribed. Immediate surgical intervention was recommended because of his known loose body, pain, and effusion.

DIAGNOSTIC IMAGING

Standard three-view plain radiographs (anterior-posterior, lateral, and tangential) were obtained and revealed no evidence of osteochondral defect in the medial or lateral femoral condyles, femoral trochlea, or patella. Likewise, there were no radiopacity loose bodies noted on plain radiograph (Figures 21-1 and 21-2).

A preoperative MRI scan was discussed with the patient and his family. Although this information might be of added benefit when determining the location of his loose body, especially in light of normal plain radiographs, it ultimately would not change the treatment plan for this patient. Based on his worsening symptoms, joint effusion, and obvious loose body on clinical exam, his best treatment option was arthroscopy and addressing the intra-articular pathology.

PREOPERATIVE REHABILITATION

During the patient's initial encounter with the orthopedic surgeon, he scheduled surgery and began a home exercise program. The program consisted of quadriceps sets, straight leg raises (SLR), and edema/swelling control measures. He was instructed to perform the strengthening exercises three to four times per day until the day of surgery. We encouraged the use of the Cryo/Cuff multiple times each day to reduce swelling/edema and to help with pain management. We also limited his activity to normal walking for school and eliminated basketball practice and games. The goals of our program were to increase muscle strength, increase ROM, and decrease edema/swelling and pain. Quadriceps sets were initiated at 25 repetitions each hour, holding each contraction for a 5- to 10-second count. Straight leg raises started at 10 repetitions, two times per day and increased as the patient could tolerate.[1-5] We did not strongly emphasize ROM exercises because of the loose body found on clinical examination. We feared that aggressive ROM exercises may cause further damage to the articular surfaces, therefore ROM exercises were confined to the patient's existing walking activity only. We believed that improvement in ROM would be better achieved postoperatively after the loose body had been removed. Also, the persistent joint effusions hampered drastic improvements in the patient's ROM.[4,5]

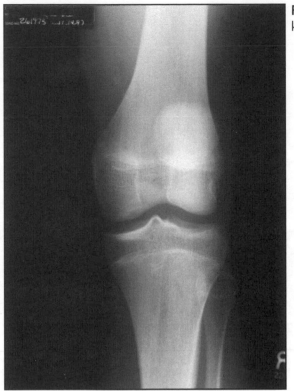

Figure 21-1. Anterior-posterior (AP) view of the knee.

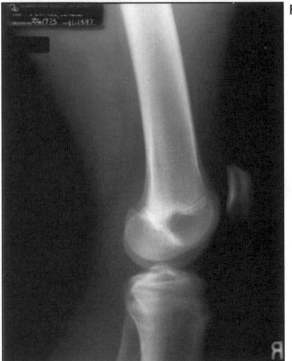

Figure 21-2. Lateral view of the knee.

It would be our goal to have the patient at near optimum quadriceps strength and ROM prior to undergoing any surgical intervention. However, time was of the essence because of the rather large loose body found on clinical exam and the amount of time that would be needed for graft healing and extensive rehabilitation prior to the spring baseball season. With all these factors in place, surgery was arranged at the earliest possible time.

SURGICAL PROCEDURE

On November 19, 1997, the patient underwent right knee arthroscopy with removal of two loose bodies and an open arthrotomy for repair of a patellar osteochondral lesion by means of an autogenous replacement graft from the nonweightbearing portion of the anterolateral femoral condyle. The athlete was taken to the operating suite and after adequate general endotracheal anesthesia was administered, the patient's knee was examined and the loose body located in the lateral gutter. A 22-gauge needle was introduced into the loose body through the skin to stabilize it, prevent its migration during the sterile prep, and allow easy retrieval during arthroscopy. The skin was prepped and draped in a sterile fashion and the arthroscope was introduced into the knee via a medial parapatellar incision. The lateral gutter was then entered and the loose body was identified by direct visualization. A small lateral incision was made in the skin and carried down into the joint. An arthroscopic grabber was introduced into the knee and the loose body was grasped and removed from the knee. It measured approximately 9 x 12 mm (Figure 21-3).

The knee was systematically examined and found to have pristine medial and lateral femoral and tibial articular surfaces through full ROM. Attention was then turned to the patellofemoral joint and the suprapatellar pouch. It was here that the chondral defect was noted and the origin of loose body was identified. It appeared to be localized in the lateral ridge of the patellar facet (Figure 21-4). The medial gutter was examined prior to withdrawing the arthroscope and another loose body was discovered that measured approximately 3 x 4 mm (Figure 21-5). The medial compartment was again examined through full ROM and no osteochondral defects were noted. It was believed that this fragment was part of the larger fragment removed from the lateral gutter by a separate arthrotomy incision. All arthroscopic instruments were removed from the knee. Secondary to the size of the loose body and the chondral patellar defect, the surgeon decided that an open osteochondral replacement graft for the patella would provide the best long-term results. A midline incision was made to expose the parapatellar deep structures, and a parapatellar incision was made to expose the joint. The patella was then everted and 12-mm hole was cored utilizing the OATS (Arthrex, Naples, Fla) system and a 9-mm coring reamer (Figure 21-6). This served as the recipient site for the autogenous articular cartilage graft. Following preparation of the recipient site, attention was turned to harvesting a donor articular cartilage graft. A 10-mm harvesting reamer was used to ream to a depth of 13 mm on the superior aspect of the anterolateral articular surface of the femoral condyle (Figure 21-7). The donor graft was removed. It was placed for size, fit, and articular surface contour, then impacted into its final position (Figure 21-8).

The arthroscope was again introduced into the knee and the joint was copiously irrigated. No debris or loose bodies were noticed. The fit and contour of the donor plug were well seated in the patella. Passive ROM showed that the donor plug was not impinging on the femoral trochlea. A wound drain was placed in the joint prior to completion of wound closure. A sterile compressive dressing and Cryo/Cuff were applied. He was discharged the day of surgery with instructions to use the Cryo/Cuff multiple times per day and to elevate his operative leg. He was made nonweightbearing and instructed in crutch-assisted ambulation.

CLINICAL FINDINGS

During the first postoperative visit, plain radiographs revealed that the transplanted osteochondral cylinder appeared to be "proud" with respect to the adjacent subchondral bone. It was decided that a postoperative MRI scan of the right knee was warranted. The purpose for this scan was to assess the status of the transplanted bony plug seated in the patella and the congruency of the chondral surface. The result revealed the osteochondral graft was well positioned and created a smooth overlying articular surface. There is a difference in cartilage thickness between the donor site (femur) and the recipient site (patella). The hyaline cartilage is

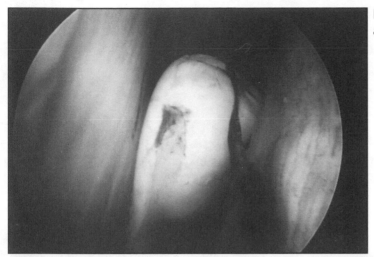

Figure 21-3. Arthroscopic view of a loose body lateral gutter.

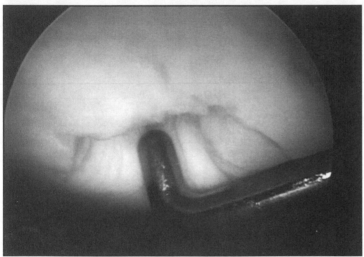

Figure 21-4. Arthroscopic view of a patellar chondral defect.

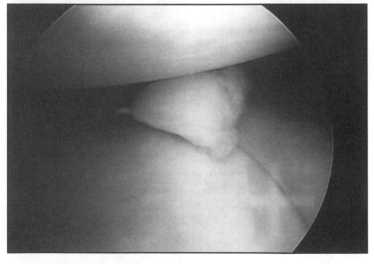

Figure 21-5. Arthroscopic view of a loose body joint surface.

Figure 21-6. Donor site osteochondral plug instrumentation.

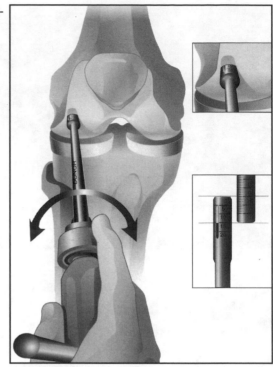

Figure 21-7. Recipient site instrumentation.

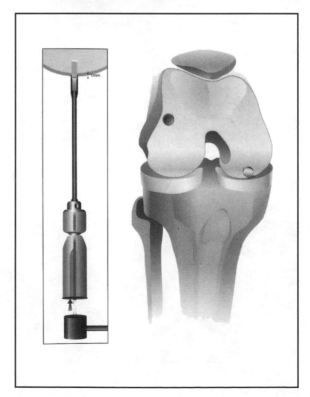

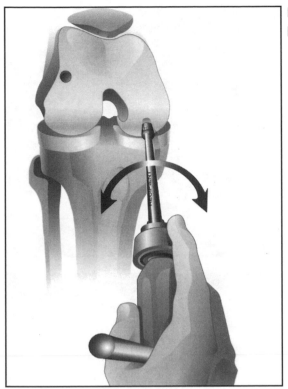

Figure 21-8. Example instrumentation of donor plug implantation.

thicker in the patella as compared to the femur and in order to create a congruent articular surface, the "proud" subchondral bone is inevitable (Figures 21-9 to 21-11).

POSTOPERATIVE REHABILITATION

The postoperative rehabilitation course was initiated on the first postoperative day. Prior to the patient's discharge from the hospital, he was instructed to resume the preoperative exercise program consisting of quadriceps sets, SLR, and cryotherapy for pain management and edema control. We encouraged him to ice and elevate his leg for 20 to 30 minutes each hour while awake during the first 10 to 14 days postoperatively. The postoperative dressing was removed for hygiene purposes, ROM exercises, and while awake during the day. The patient was nonweightbearing with crutch ambulation for the first 6 weeks postoperatively to allow the transplanted graft a chance to achieve bony healing, thus preventing the plug from becoming dislodged and in essence becoming another loose body. As in the preoperative rehabilitation program, our postoperative rehabilitation goals were to achieve normal ROM, improve strength, and reduce edema/swelling.[15]

Phase II: 0 to 14 Days

The patient was seen in the office to remove the wound drain on the second postoperative day. It was not removed prior to discharge because there was still a significant amount of bloody drainage. ROM was 0 degrees extension and 30 degrees flexion on the second postoperative day. He continued the quadriceps sets and SLR program at home and in therapy. He was instructed to work on active range of motion (AROM) and passive range of motion (PROM) exercises while at home. The Cryo/Cuff was used after all exercises.

Figure 21-9. MRI lateral view of the patella.

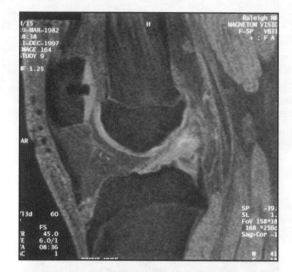

Figure 21-10. MRI of the donor site (femur).

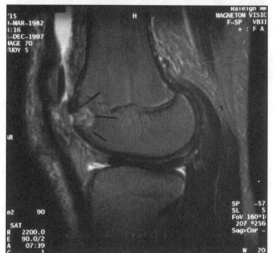

Figure 21-11. MRI tangential view of the patella.

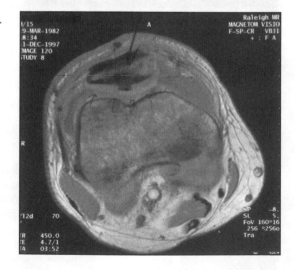

Phase III: 2 to 6 weeks

During the next 4 weeks, the patient continued to be nonweightbearing but was able to improve his strength and ROM. Knee ROM was 0 degrees extension to 130 degrees flexion by the 2-week postoperative visit. He had no complaints of pain and only minimal patellofemoral crepitation. Noticeable quadriceps atrophy was present, possibly secondary to 2+ effusion. We offered to aspirate the effusion with the hope of improving ROM, but the patient declined. Routine postoperative radiographs were obtained and revealed a possible unseating of the bony transplanted plug in the patella. A subsequent MRI determined that the transplanted bony plug was in proper position and had healthy hyaline articular cartilage surrounding its surface. The patient was placed in a hinged knee brace without ROM restrictions but was to continue with the nonweightbearing status. By the 6-week postoperative visit, AROM was 0 degrees extension to 145 degrees flexion, and he could perform a full squat without pain or difficulty. The patient had been walking without the crutches or brace for a "few" days prior to this follow-up visit. He had no complaints of pain or crepitation about his patellofemoral joint, and joint effusion was markedly decreased. His hinged brace and nonweightbearing status were discontinued. At much insistence by the patient, he was allowed to begin a walk/jog program on a very limited basis. He was restricted to straight ahead running and cautioned to avoid severe twisting and cutting type activities. Although he was restricted from these activities, he was permitted to swing a baseball bat in the controlled environment of the batting cage. He was not allowed to get into a catcher's squat, but he could sit on a bucket and simulate the catching position as long as it did not cause pain or swelling. We continued to encourage strength development, as it was noticed that his quadriceps still showed signs of atrophy. He was advised to continue cryotherapy after each exercise program and several times at home each night.

Phase III: 6 to 10 Weeks

The patient returned for his 9-week postoperative visit (January 27, 1998) and reported doing well. It should be mentioned that he was weaned to a home exercise program shortly after his 6-week postoperative visit to facilitate his desire to work out with his high school baseball team and because he traveled some distance to attend formal therapy sessions. He demonstrated limited clinical findings that would necessitate his continuance in formal therapy; however, he was instructed that if he failed to progress in his home exercise program, formal therapy sessions would be reinstituted. He was able to perform two sets of 20 repetitions of the leg press at 80 pounds and the leg extension at 50 pounds, rope jumping for 10 minutes two times per day, and jogging 1 to 2 miles three times per week. He also increased his intensity and time in the batting cage. He began to catch without the bucket in controlled situations. He was anxious to resume full, unrestricted baseball practice and games. He had been able to maintain his ROM and had no effusions. He did report some mild stiffness after exercise but noticed no popping pain or crepitation about the patellofemoral joint. He was released to full, unrestricted activity.

At his week 12 postoperative visit, he had no complaints of pain or swelling. He had resumed full activities without limitation/restriction. Repeat radiographs showed excellent healing of his transplanted bony plug and no evidence of failure. Clinical examination revealed some mild, nonpainful patellofemoral crepitation, negative effusion, and good patellofemoral mobility. He still had some persistent quadriceps atrophy despite his return to normal activity and continued exercise for quadriceps strengthening. The patient has had no limitations to any activity, including weightlifting, baseball, football, and basketball.

Follow-up examination 18 months postoperatively revealed that he was able to play baseball at the national and international Junior Olympic level without complaints of pain, swelling, or catching about his knee. He has had no episodes of patellofemoral pain. Examination revealed full ROM, improved quadriceps muscle girth, a negative patellar apprehension sign, no patellar facet pain, no ligamentous laxity, and no signs of meniscal pathology.

DISCUSSION

This case study represents an unusual circumstance of a patient who experienced a chondral injury following a patellar dislocation. Typically, the athlete experiences medial parapatellar pain, joint swelling, loss of normal ROM, and muscle atrophy.[1,2,4-7] It is uncommon to find a chondral injury to the patella, especially when it presents itself several days post-injury.

In most cases, the need for post-injury radiographs is a highly debated topic. Plain radiographs reveal only bony injuries. An osteochondral injury will reveal an osseous defect, while a chondral injury will reveal a normal radiograph. MRI is the most sensitive diagnostic study available to visualize cartilage injuries.[1-8] This added exposure allows clinicians to better understand injuries to the hyaline articular cartilage that can potentially go undetected. In our case, the most definitive diagnostic and therapeutic tool was arthroscopy. Arthroscopy allowed the surgeon to visually examine the affected joint to determine the location, origin, size, and nature of the loose body, and to assess the most appropriate method of treatment for this patient's chondral lesion.[2,9]

Until recently, there were no specific orthopedic or arthroscopic procedures that would allow for replacement of hyaline articular cartilage into a chondral lesion anywhere in the knee joint. Most arthroscopic procedures incorporated debridement (abrasion chondroplasty) of the osteochondral defect (OCD) lesion edges to remove any loose or devitalized edges of the hyaline cartilage adjacent to the chondral defect. However, it does not allow for stabilization of the defect or surrounding articular cartilage. Over time, the edges of a chondral defect expand, creating a larger defect area, potentially creating more loose bodies and possibly necessitating the need for future arthroscopies.[2,10-14] Newman[15] reported that articular cartilage is capable of withstanding repetitive stresses of great intensity. He found that hyaline cartilage does not possess any properties that would aid in its ability to heal after injury and attributed this to its avascular composition, immobility, and limited ability of the chondrocytes to reproduce after injury.

Cartilage is composed of a matrix and a ratio of protoglycans, collagen, noncollagenous proteins, and water. It is this matrix/ratio that researchers have been trying to reproduce in order to treat osteochondral lesions. Subchondral drilling of an OCD through an open arthrotomy incision, which was introduced by Ficat et al.[16] They theorized that this procedure would stimulate bleeding at the drill sites and ultimately lead to the development of a thick fibrocartilagenous layer overlying the affected area.[2,8,10,12-17] While Ficat et al reported good results in their study population, they stated that it took approximately 4 months for the chondral defect to fill. They described the new tissue to be thinner than normal articular cartilage but considered it to be viable. Moran, et al[19] performed a study of autogenous resurfacing of patellar articular cartilage defects in rabbits. They found the groups that were treated with a continuous passive motion machine and nonweightbearing had excellent healing rates. They demonstrated by electron microscopy and histologic examination that the cartilaginous materials in the transplanted articular cartilage stimulated proliferation of the chondrocyte matrix so that this new cartilage could not be differentiated from the existing native articular cartilage.[10,15,19,20] Lastly, patellectomy and artificial patellar resurfacing have been mentioned in the literature as possible treatments for severe patellar arthritis and injury. While this might relieve pain, these procedures are associated with problems such as loss of the biomechanical advantage in the extensor mechanism and polyethylene wear in the resurfaced patella.[2,11,21]

With the innovation of osteoarticular transplantation, the patient's native articular cartilage can be harvested and moved to another area, in this case from the anterolateral femoral condyle to the patella. This not only facilitates normal joint nutrition and protection, but greatly reduces arthritic changes that are commonly associated with chondral injuries. Buckwalter and Mankin[10] reviewed a variety of procedures that have recently been developed to address injuries to the weightbearing surfaces of the knee. While patellar injuries are not specifically addressed, the authors stated that transplanting an articular cartilage matrix will restore subchondral bone, improve normal articular joint contour, and alleviate joint pain and incongruity. Simonian et al[22] examined the donor sites for osteoarticular transplantation in the femoral condyle. They were particularly interested in the amount of contact pressure placed on any donor site during a normal ROM about the knee. The commonly recognized donor sites are the anterolateral border of the lateral femoral condyle (five sites) and the upper one-half of the femoral notch (two sites adjacent to the medial and lateral femoral

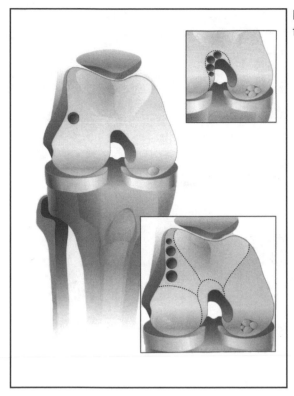

Figure 21-12. Sites on a femoral articular surface for donor plug harvesting.

condyles and one site at the apex of the notch) (Figure 21-12). They listed all 10 sites and reported that these sites were involved in significant contact pressures about the femoral articular condyles in 0 degrees extension and to 110 degrees flexion. They concluded that while there were some donor site areas with less contact pressure, none of these sites were completely free from pressure during normal knee ROM. Likewise, they mentioned concern for the long-term effects associated with articular cartilage harvest at these sites.[22]

CONCLUSION

Our case presents an elite high school athlete who injured his knee while jumping and suffered a significant chondral lesion to his patella. As a baseball catcher, the chondral injury to this weightbearing joint posed a significant problem that could have jeopardized his career. Knee arthroscopy and osteochondral transplant with the OATS instrumentation provided a viable option for treatment. Transplantation of an osteochondral plug, in our case, has provided this athlete with long-term, pain-free, and unlimited activity. A conservative approach to rehabilitation was instituted consisting of nonweightbearing activity for 6 weeks immediately postoperatively, to allow the transplanted osteochondral plug to heal. After completion of this phase, the athlete began a progressive ROM strengthening and general conditioning program. The patient continues to follow up with the surgeon and, to date, he is competing in high school baseball as a catcher with pain-free function in the involved knee.

REFERENCES

1. Mercier LR. *Practical Orthopedics*. St. Louis, Mo: Mosby-Year Book; 1995.
2. Lavelle DG. Acute dislocations: Campbell's operative orthopedics. In: Crenshaw AH, ed. St. Louis, Mo: Mosby-Year Book; 1992.
3. Snider RK. Essentials of musculoskeletal care. American Academy of Orthopedic Surgery; 1997.
4. Kisner C, Colby LA. *Therapeutic Exercise-Foundations and Techniques*. Philadelphia, Pa: FA Davis; 1987.

5.   Torg JS, Welsh RP, Shephard RJ. *Current Therapy in Sports Medicine*. Toronto, Canada: BC Decker; 1990.

6.   Galea AM, Albers JM. Patellofemoral pain. *The Physician and Sports Medicine*. 1994;22(4):48-58.

7.   Hughston JC. Subluxation of the patella. *J Bone Joint Surg Am*. 1968;50(5):1003-1026.

8.   Helms CA. *Fundamentals of Skeletal Radiology*. Philadelphia, Pa: WB Saunders Co; 1995.

9.   Bobic V, Morgan CD. *The Osteochondral Autograft Transfer Technique and Instrumentation*. Naples, Fla: Arthrex; 1998.

10.   Buckwalter JA, Mankin HJ. Articular cartilage repair and transplantation. *Arthritis Rheum*. 1998;41(8):1331-1342.

11.   Krajca-Radcliffe JB, Coker TP. Patellofemoral arthroplasty: a 2- to 18-year follow-up study. *Clin Orthop*. 1996; 330:143-151.

12.   Horton WA. *Bone and Joint Dysplasias: Primer on the Rheumatic Diseases*. Atlanta, Ga: Arthritis Foundation; 1997.

13.   Anderson AF, Pagnani MJ. Osteochondritis dissecans of the femoral condyles. *Am J Sports Med*. 1997;25(6):830-834.

14.   Ewing JW, Voto JS. Arthroscopic surgical management of osteochondritis dissecans of the knee. *Arthroscopy*. 1988;4:37-40.

15.   Newman AP. Current concepts. Articular cartilage repair. *Am J Sports Med*. 1998;26(2):309-324.

16.   Ficat RP, Ficat C, Gedeon P, et al. Spongialization: a new treatment for diseased patella. *Clin Orthop*. 1979;144:74-83.

17.   Childers JC, Ellwood SC. Partial chondrectomy and subchondral bone drilling for chondromalacia. *Clin Orthop*. 1979;144:114-120.

18.   Rae PJ, Noble J. Athroscopic drilling of osteochondral lesions of the knee. *J Bone Joint Surg Br*. 1989;71:534.

19.   Moran ME, Kim HK, Salter RB. Biological resurfacing of full-thickness defects in patellar articular cartilage of the rabbit. *J Bone Joint Surg Br*. 1992;74:659-667.

20.   Outerbridge HK, Outerbridge AR, Outerbridge RE. The use of lateral patellar autologous graft for the repair of a large osteochondral defect in the knee. *J Bone Joint Surg Am*. 1995;77:65-72.

21.   Rand JA, Gustilo B. Comparison of inset and resurfacing patellar prostheses in total knee arthroplasy. *Acta Orthop Belg*. 1996;62:1,154-162.

22.   Simonian PT, Sussman PS, Wickiewicz TL, et al. Contact pressures at osteochondral donor sites in the knee. *Am J Sports Med*. 1998;26(4):491-494.

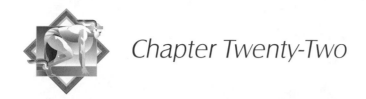 *Chapter Twenty-Two*

Primary Anterior Cruciate Ligament Reconstruction Using the Contralateral Autogenous Patellar Tendon: Separate Rehabilitation Programs for Each Knee

K. Donald Shelbourne, MD, Tinker Gray, MA, John Darmelio, ATC

INTRODUCTION

The contralateral autogenous patellar tendon has been used frequently as a graft source for revision anterior cruciate ligament (ACL) reconstruction. The use of the contralateral patellar tendon made it easier to determine its actual morbidity.[1] We observed that the postoperative rehabilitation seemed to progress more smoothly when the graft was harvested from the contralateral knee. Consequently, in 1994, we began offering patients the option of using a contralateral patellar tendon graft for primary ACL reconstruction. Since 1994, the specific rehabilitation programs for both knees have evolved through experimenting with the amount and intensity of exercises needed to rehabilitate the donor site. This case report illustrates the rehabilitation program as it was conducted in 1999.

RATIONALE FOR USING THE CONTRALATERAL PATELLAR TENDON AUTOGRAFT

Although there are other graft choices available for ACL reconstruction, the autogenous patellar tendon graft still appears to be the most reliable for obtaining good stability in the long-term after surgery.[2-6] While ACL reconstruction with hamstring grafts and allografts can obtain acceptable results, the postoperative rehabilitation programs to date do not allow functional activities as early as the rehabilitation programs for the autogenous patellar tendon graft.[2-8]

The concern about using a patellar tendon autograft has been related to the morbidity after harvesting approximately one-third of the patellar tendon. The reported morbidity problems include patellofemoral crepitus, donor site pain, and a permanent side-to-side quadriceps muscle strength deficit.[9-12] These morbidity problems, however, have been reported with the use of the hamstring grafts and allograft as well.[2,3,6,7,13,14]

We believe that the morbidity associated with ACL reconstruction surgery is a rehabilitation dilemma. The goals of rehabilitation after ACL reconstruction are to reestablish full knee range of motion (ROM), leg strength, and function without sacrificing the knee stability that is obtained by surgery. In athletics and with activities of daily living, full functional ability requires symmetrical ROM, strength, and endurance. It is the loss of symmetrical leg function that needs to be addressed with the postoperative rehabilitation program.

Figure 22-1. A hyperextension device can be used to assist the patient with regaining full normal hyperextension in the knee.

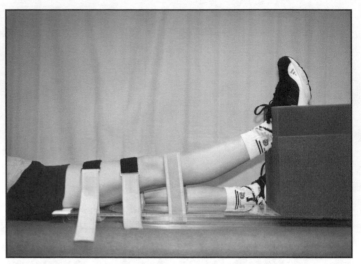

The rehabilitation exercises required to regain strength and full ROM are contradictory and are difficult to achieve simultaneously during the early postoperative period with the ipsilateral procedure. It would be ideal to be able to aggressively work quadriceps muscle strengthening for the graft donor site immediately after surgery. The ACL reconstructed knee, however, needs a period of rest to recover from the trauma of surgery and to prevent a painful hemarthrosis from occurring. Also, to strengthen the donor site and quadriceps muscles effectively after surgery, the patient must have adequate ROM and very little effusion.[15-17] When we performed revision ACL surgery using the contralateral patellar tendon graft, it became apparent that harvesting the graft itself did not limit the patient's ability to achieve almost full ROM, and there was no effusion in the graft knee the day of surgery. At the same time, when the graft was harvested from the contralateral knee, the ACL reconstructed knee seemed to regain ROM faster as well.

Therefore, we believed that by using a contralateral graft, we could more efficiently direct the postoperative rehabilitation programs by separating the conflicting goals of rehabilitation into both knees. Also, by harvesting the graft from the contralateral knee, the already weakened ACL injured knee is not weakened further. The rehabilitation program for the ACL reconstructed knee could focus upon controlling swelling and obtaining full ROM; the rehabilitation program for the grafted knee could focus on aggressive donor site strengthening immediately after surgery. The ultimate goals of the separate rehabilitation programs are to restore symmetrical function and strength to both legs; we believe these goals are not achieved as reliably with an ipsilateral graft.

SUBJECT

The patient was a 14-year-old high school freshman girl who injured her right knee while playing soccer on March 25, 1999. She was running down the field when she planted her right foot to change directions to go to the left. Her knee gave-way, she felt a pop, and fell to the ground. She grabbed her knee, thinking she had a major injury. An athletic trainer was at the game and told the patient to ice her knee throughout the night. When she went to practice the next day, she was not allowed to practice because her knee was swollen. She was seen by a local orthopedist who suspected that she had an ACL tear. The doctor ordered an magnetic resonance imaging (MRI) scan to confirm the diagnosis.

The patient was given a cold compression device to control swelling and pain. The doctor also gave her a hyperextension device (Figure 22-1) to assist with regaining full hyperextension equal to the opposite normal knee.

She was instructed to use the cold compression device as much as possible except when doing ROM exercises. For 1 week after the injury, she used the hyperextension device three times a day for 5 to 10 minutes at a time. She was referred to the senior author to discuss undergoing an ACL reconstruction and for subsequent rehabilitation. The patient's goal was to be able to play competitive soccer by August 1999.

Upon physical examination on April 20, 1999, the patient's knee had a mild effusion, a positive Lachman with a soft endpoint, a mild flexion rotation drawer, no posterior drawer, and no medial or lateral laxity. The ROM in her normal knee was 7/0/145; the ROM in her right injured knee was 7/0/138. The patient was able to walk full weightbearing with a normal gait.

The patient had a positive attitude toward surgery and rehabilitation. Because of the rehabilitation directions given by the local physician, her knee was physically ready to undergo surgery. The details of the surgery and postoperative rehabilitation were explained fully to the patient and her parents. The rationale for using the contralateral autogenous patellar tendon graft was also explained. The surgery date was set for April 28, 1999.

Preoperative Testing

The preoperative KT1000 arthrometer test revealed a side-to-side manual maximum difference of 6 mm. An isokinetic muscle strength test showed 66% strength in the quadriceps muscles and 83% strength in the hamstring muscles compared to the opposite normal leg.

Surgical Procedure

Pain prevention protocol utilizing intravenous ketorolac was begun.[18] The patient underwent an intraarticular ACL reconstruction using a miniarthrotomy technique as described by Shelbourne and Rask.[19] An arthroscopy was performed on the right knee to determine the status of the menisci and chondral surfaces. The patient had normal articular cartilage in all compartments. She had a vertical medial meniscus tear on the inferior surface, which puckered upon probing. The tear was near the periphery of the meniscus and was thought to be one that could heal without suture repair. The tear was abraded and trephinated to stimulate healing. The lateral meniscus was intact. Routine incisions and tibial and femoral bone tunnels were made in the involved knee. On the contralateral knee, a medial parapatellar incision was made, and a 10-mm autogenous patellar tendon graft with bone plugs on each end was harvested from a 26 mm-wide patellar tendon. Three sutures were placed in each bone plug. The patellar bone plug was placed into the tibial tunnel, and the tibial bone plug was placed into the femoral tunnel of the involved knee. The graft was secured tightly with the sutures tied over tibial and femoral buttons with the knee in 30 degrees of flexion. To prevent overtensioning the graft, the ACL reconstructed knee was moved through full ROM. This movement ensures that the graft placement has not captured the joint.

To eliminate a permanent patellar and tibial defect from harvesting the bone plugs, the bone shavings obtained from the notchplasty and drilling the femoral and tibial tunnels were packed into the defects on the contralateral knee. To reduce the tendon soreness that often occurs on the night of surgery, the graft knee was moved through full ROM after closure of the tendon and before the patient was brought to consciousness.

Routine closure was performed on both knees. Light dressings were applied to both knees and were secured into place with an antiembolism stocking on each leg. A cold compression device was applied immediately to the ACL reconstructed knee for pain control and to prevent postoperative hemarthrosis.

Postoperative Rehabilitation

The postoperative rehabilitation was designed to accomplish different goals for each leg. Rehabilitation for the ACL reconstructed knee focused on limiting activity during the first week postoperatively in order to prevent swelling, obtain full hyperextension and at least 110 degrees of flexion, and establish good leg control. One week after surgery, rehabilitation of the ACL reconstructed knee consisted of maintaining extension, increasing flexion, establishing a normal gait, and light quadriceps strengthening exercises. The rehabilitation for regaining tendon size and strength in the graft knee began immediately after surgery and focused on high repetitions of patellar tendon strengthening and maintaining full ROM.

Table 22-1

POSTOPERATIVE REHABILITATION PROGRAM FOR BOTH KNEES

Time	ACL Reconstructed Knee	Donor Knee
Preoperative Program		
Goals	Obtain full ROM, reduce swelling, achieve good leg control, achieve a normal gait, good mental attitude, and understand postoperative rehabilitation program.	Maintain leg strength
Exercises	Hyperextension device 3x/day, prone hang exercise, heel slides, active terminal extension, gait training, and explanation of postoperative rehabilitation goals and program.	
Surgery	IV ketorolac pain prevention program. Both knees are moved through a full ROM from full hyperextension to flexion (heel touches the buttocks) and a Cryo/Cuff is applied over light sterile dressings.	
Day of Surgery to 1 Week Postoperatively		
Goals	Full passive hyperextension, flexion to at least 110 degrees, independent straight leg raise, and weightbearing as tolerated for bathroom privileges only.	Full passive hyperextension, full flexion, independent straight leg raise, and weightbearing as tolerated for bathroom privileges only.
Exercises	CPM machine set to move from 0 degrees extension to 30 degrees of flexion, Cryo/Cuff for cold and compression (to remain on	Leg elevated on pillows, Cryo/Cuff for cold and compression (to remain on the knee at all times except during exercises), heel

Table 22-1 continued

Time	ACL Reconstructed Knee	Donor Knee
	the knee at all times except during exercises), heel props for extension (elevate the heel on the end of the bed frame or object to allow gravity to assist, 10 minutes every waking hour), knee flexion in CPM machine (move the setting to the highest flexion, leave the leg in 110 degrees flexion for 10 minutes), knee flexion out of CPM machine (passive flexion, pull heel toward buttocks), flexion in Shuttle machine (place leg in the machine and use the straps to pull the heel toward the buttocks), and leg control exercise (active quadriceps contractions, straight leg raises, and active terminal extension).	props for extension, maintaining extension is easy; the donor leg is used as a comparison for the other leg (10 minutes every waking hour), passive knee pull heel toward buttocks, and donor site strengthening with Shuttle machine (repetitions every waking hour, progressively increasing the resistance as tolerated).
Week 2 (7 to 14 Days Postoperatively)		
Goals	Maintain full extension, knee flexion to 125 degrees, minimal swelling, normal gait, and be able to lock knee straight bearing full weight.	Maintain full extension and flexion, no swelling, and normal gait.
Exercises	Extension, heel props, prone hangs, single leg stance (patient locks the knee in full extension with weight on the ACL reconstructed leg), flexion, heel slides in the shuttle machine, and gait training in front of the mirror.	Gait training in front of mirror, shuttle exercises (150 repetitions 2 x/day), and lateral step-down exercise (10 to 15 cm height, 50 repetitions, 6 to 8x/day).

	Table 22-1 continued	
Time	**ACL Reconstructed Knee**	**Donor Knee**
Week 3 to 4 (15 to 28 Days Postoperatively)		
Goals	Maintain full extension	Maintain full ROM
Exercises	Increase flexion to equal opposite knee and maintain minimal swelling.	
Goals	Agility drills and sport-specific activities.	Agility drills and sport-specific activities.
Exercises	Active terminal extension, heel slides, sit on heels, and stair machine (5 to 10 minutes).	Stationary bicycling 5 minutes, stair machine 5 to 10 minutes, weight training (unilateral), leg press (4 x 12), leg extensions (3 x 12), and lateral step-down exercises (10 cm height, 6x/day).
From 4 Weeks after Surgery		
Goals	Maintain full ROM, maintain minimal swelling, return of quadriceps strength, agility and sport-specific activities and progress to partial and full competition, adjust activities based on controlling swelling and maintaining ROM, and bike 15 to 20 minutes.	Maintain full ROM, maintain no swelling, return of quadriceps strength, agility and sport-specific activities and progress to partial and full competition, adjust activities based on controlling donor site soreness, and bike 15 to 20 minutes.
Exercises	Stair machine 10 to 12 minutes, soccer drills, 40 m sprints, group soccer drills, and playing competitive soccer.	Stair machine 10 to 12 minutes, leg press (body weight, four sets of 12 repetitions), leg extension (four sets of eight repetitions), forward step-down exercise (6 to 8x/day, repetitions to failure), soccer drills, 40 m sprints, group soccer drills, and playing competitive soccer.

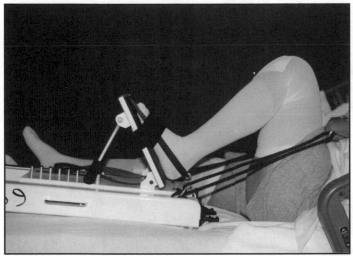

Figure 22-2. A shuttle device was used by the patient to perform multiple resistive leg press exercises for the graft knee, while at the same time allowing the ACL reconstructed knee to rest.

The rehabilitation progressed to higher intensity strengthening exercises and functional sport-specific drills before the patient was allowed to return to playing soccer. The specific exercise routine that the patient performed to obtain the rehabilitation goals is explained in Table 22-1.

The patient stayed in the hospital for one night and was discharged home the morning after surgery. The purpose of having the patient stay in the hospital was to make sure that the patient and her family had a full understanding of the postoperative routine that was to be followed for the first week at home. Even with a great deal of preoperative teaching and explanation of the postoperative routine, we have found that patients do not completely understand the specific rehabilitation exercises until they are performing them after the surgery. The overnight stay also allows for the use of an intravenous continuous drip of ketorolac. This preemptive pain management protocol of bedrest, elevation, cold/compression, and ketorolac has been effective for preventing a hemarthrosis, and eliminating the need for oral narcotics postoperatively.[18]

Upon arrival to the hospital room, the patient's ACL reconstructed leg was placed in a continuous passive motion (CPM) machine, and the machine was set to move from 0 degrees extension to 30 degrees of flexion. In the past, the CPM machine was used to put the knee through full ROM continuously, but we believed that the continuous motion to the extremes of knee extension and flexion contributed to swelling. We now use the CPM machine mainly for elevation and gentle motion. The patient's leg remained in the CPM machine at all times during the first week after surgery, except when she was performing specific ROM exercises. Although the rehabilitation program has been coined as "accelerated," the first week of rehabilitation focused on complete rest for the ACL reconstructed knee as a means to prevent swelling and allow for an easier return of knee motion.

A shuttle device (Contemporary Design Company, Glacier, Wash) was used during the first 2 weeks postoperatively to specifically rehabilitate the graft donor site. The machine is a small leg press unit that has six adjustable resistive cords that can be used to gradually increase resistance. It has two red cords (1 kg resistance each) and four black cords (3 kg of resistance each) (Figure 22-2).

The patient used the device every 2 hours (six times/day) during waking hours. Starting with two black cords, the patient did 100 repetitions per session. During the first week after surgery, she progressed to using all six cords (approximately 14 kg of resistance) with 100 repetitions per session.

At 1 week postoperatively, a step box was provided to the patient so several types of exercises to rehabilitate the graft donor site could be performed. The box was adjustable from 9 to 21 cm off the floor. Three step-box exercises were prescribed and the patient gradually progressed from the easier forward step-up exercise to the most difficult forward step-down exercise. All the step-box exercises should be performed under slow control to make sure that the quadriceps muscles are being used correctly (Figures 22-3a to 22-5b).

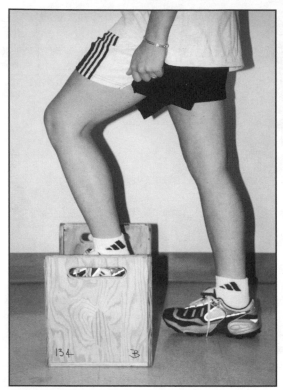

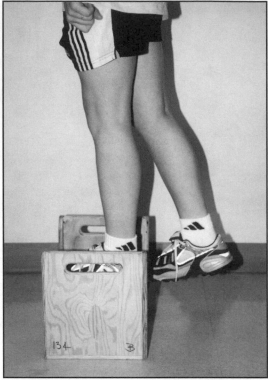

Figure 22-3a. The step box is placed in front of the athlete.

Figure 22-3b. Step up on the box with the involved leg without using the other leg to push off the floor. Keep the toes of the non-involved leg pointed toward the step box.

The patient was instructed to do as many step-up or step-down repetitions as she was able, but at least 25 repetitions at the selected height. If 25 repetitions could not be performed properly, the height was lowered. If more than 50 repetitions could be performed, the height was raised at the next session.

With the use of the shuttle device and the step-box, the patient was able to consistently and aggressively exercise the graft donor site while, at the same time, allow the ACL reconstructed knee to remain quiet. At 2 weeks postoperatively, additional weight training exercises were added to the routine to provide a period of increased resistance. The patient continued to perform the step-box exercise, however, as a means to provide additional stimulation to the healing graft site.

At 1 month postoperatively, the patient was tested for knee stability and leg strength. The rehabilitation program was advanced to include functional activities and increased weight resistance activities. These activities were increased according to her strength progress.

CLINICAL OUTCOMES

The patient progressed through the rehabilitation program smoothly. The clinical findings at each postoperative visit are summarized in Table 22-2. Four weeks after surgery, the patient had full symmetrical extension and flexion to 137 degrees in the ACL reconstructed knee. Because she had met the rehabilitation goals, she began agility drills and sport-specific activities in progressive order—jogging forward, jogging backward, figure-eight running, side-to-side movements, short sprints, and dribbling and passing a soccer ball.

At 6 weeks after surgery, the patient attended a soccer camp (from June 14 through June 18, 1999), during which she continued her specific donor site strengthening exercise with the step-box. She performed 50

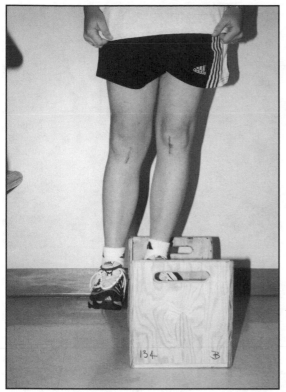

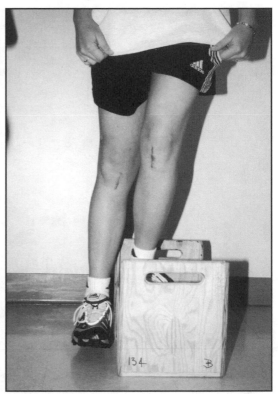

Figure 22-4a. Stand to the side of the step box on the involved leg so that the noninvolved leg is free to be lowered.

Figure 22-4b. Keep the shoulders level over the hips and bend the involved knee so that the noninvolved foot barely touches the floor. Straighten the involved knee without using assistance from the noninvolved leg.

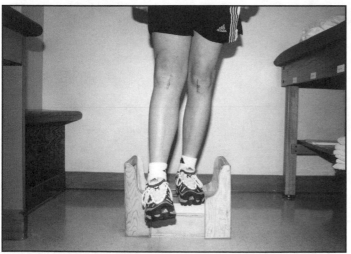

Figure 22-5a. Stand on the step box with the involved leg so that the noninvolved leg is free to be lowered to the front of the box.

Figure 22-5b. Keep the shoulders level over the hips and bend the involved knee so that the non-involved foot barely touches the floor. Straighten the involved knee while keeping the shoulders and hips level.

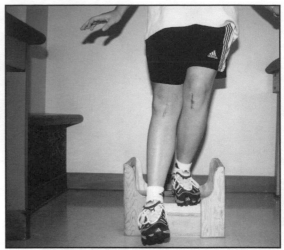

Table 22-2		
OBJECTIVE CLINICAL FINDINGS AFTER SURGERY		
Time after Surgery	**Physical Test**	**Finding**
Preoperatively		
April 20, 1999	ROM	Right knee: 5-0-145 Left knee: 5-0-145
	KT-1000	6 mm manual maximum difference
	Isokinetic evaluation 60 degrees/second 180 degrees/second	RQ/LQ: 80/96 = 83% RQ/LQ: 47/71 = 66%
	Isometric leg press Single leg hop	Left leg: 248 lbs Left: 110 cm
Postoperatively		
1 week	ROM	Right knee: 5-0-115 Left knee: 5-0-145
	Gait	Normal
2 weeks	ROM	Right knee: 5-0-129 Left Knee: 5-0-145
	Gait	Normal
4 weeks (May 27, 1999)	ROM	Right knee: 5-0-137 Left knee: 5-0-145
	KT-1000	2 mm manual/maximum difference
	Active heel height difference	0 cm

Table 22-2 continued

Time after Surgery	Physical Test	Finding
	Isokinetic evaluation 60 degrees/second	RQ/LQ: 66/56 (ACL reconstructed leg: 69% of preoperative normal leg; graft leg: 58% of normal leg)
	180 degrees/second	RQ/LQ: 50/47 (ACL reconstructed leg: 71% of preoperative normal leg; graft leg: 66% of preoperative normal leg)
	Leg press	ACL reconstructed leg: 254 lbs (102% of preoperative normal leg)
8 weeks (June 29, 1999)	ROM	Right knee: 5-0-145 Left knee: 5-0-145 Able to kneel and sit on heels
	KT-1000	2 mm manual/maximum difference
	Active heel height difference	0 cm
	Isokinetic evaluation 60 degrees/second	RQ/LQ: 82/76 (ACL reconstructed leg: 85% of preoperative normal leg; graft leg: 79% of normal leg; 7% side-to-side difference)
	180 degrees/second	RQ/LQ: 50/47 (ACL reconstructed leg, 71% of preoperative normal leg; graft leg, 66% of preoperative normal leg)
	Leg press	ACL reconstructed leg: 254 lbs (102% of preoperative normal leg) Graft donor leg: 210 lbs (85% of preoperative normal leg)

Figure 22-6. At 2 months postoperatively, the patient had full symmetrical knee ROM and she was able to sit on her heels comfortably.

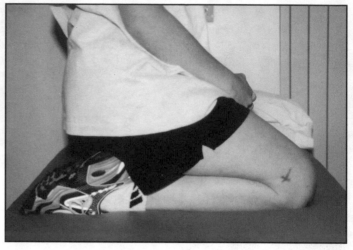

repetitions of the forward step-down exercise eight times a day. She participated in the team soccer drills but did not play in game or scrimmage situations. The camp activities consisted of several hours of soccer drills each day that included shooting, dribbling, passing, heading, trapping, and juggling. The patient was able to perform four to six 40-m sprints daily. During this period, she was aware of decreasing her activity level if she developed swelling, decreased knee motion, or persistent tendon soreness that was not relieved with ice therapy.

By 2 months postoperatively, she had greater than 90% quadriceps muscle strength in the ACL reconstructed knee and the donor knee, compared to the normal knee preoperatively. The side-to-side strength difference was 4% on the single leg hop test. The patient also had full ROM in both knees and she was able to sit on her heels (Figure 22-6).

The patient continued to perform small group controlled drills regularly through the month of June. Even though strength and full knee motion had been achieved, the patient needed to regain confidence and proprioception in both legs. To enhance this, the patient began playing basketball in July to help her with foot agility and speed, and to encourage her to not look down at her feet when performing skills.

The patient continued her leg strengthening exercises throughout July, during which time she increased the time involved with competitive soccer drills and games. At 12 weeks postoperatively the patient began playing soccer games and was able to compete for 20 to 30 minutes without rest. She was able to play in a complete game of soccer without substitution at 4 months postoperatively

DISCUSSION

The method of utilizing the contralateral autogenous patellar tendon for primary ACL surgery has been employed for over 850 patients since 1994. Although one of the reasons to use the graft source is to return athletes back to activities faster, the real advantages are seen during the early postoperative period when patients find that they are able to regain motion and leg control quickly and easily. A previous comparative study of ACL reconstruction using the contralateral or ipsilateral patellar tendon graft revealed that 75% of patients in the contralateral group achieved 110 degrees of flexion in the ACL reconstructed knee by 2 weeks postoperatively compared with only 47% of patients in the ipsilateral group.[20] The patient in this case study achieved flexion in the ACL reconstructed knee of 129 degrees by 2 weeks postoperatively and 137 degrees by 4 weeks postoperatively.

To minimize patellar tendon soreness, we have found that the patient needs to be committed to consistent and frequent leg strengthening repetitions with the shuttle device and step-box. When we first began using the contralateral patellar tendon in 1994, patients performed ROM exercises the day of surgery, but the strengthening exercises to stimulate regrowth of the patellar tendon donor site did not begin until a week after surgery. Also, the strengthening program was not as aggressive and did not include the routine of high-repetition exercises six times/day. We now believe that the hourly shuttle device and step-box routine is the key to minimizing and eliminating donor site soreness, and for regaining the patellar tendon size during the first month postoperatively. Once the patellar tendon size has increased, the high repetitions of the quadriceps exercise along with increased resistance between 1 and 2 months postoperatively advances the patient's quadriceps strength considerably.

It also appears that side-to-side quadriceps muscle strength differences, frequently found using the ipsilateral graft, are overcome using a contralateral graft. The patient in this case report not only had 92% of her preoperative strength at 2 months postoperatively, but also had only a 7% side-to-side difference between legs. By 3 months postoperatively, the patient had symmetrical quadriceps muscle strength as measured with isokinetic testing and with functional testing with the single leg hop test.

Most importantly, patients have been able to progress through the postoperative rehabilitation program and obtain comfortable motion and daily function quickly. Even patients who do not have an immediate goal of returning to athletics or work still would like to have a knee with full ROM, no swelling, and good strength as soon as possible after surgery. These goals can be achieved more reliably and quickly using the contralateral graft. Once the patient has a normal feeling knee with good function, he or she can decide if and when to resume preinjury activities without an increased risk of graft rupture.[4]

REFERENCES

1. Rubiunstein RA, Shelbourne KD, VanMeter CD, et al. Isolated autogenous bone-patellar tendon-bone graft site morbidity. *Am J Sports Med.* 1994;22:324-327.

2. Aglietti P, Buzzi R, Zaccherotti G, et al. Patellar tendon versus doubled semitendinosis and gracilis tendons for anterior cruciate ligament reconstruction. *Am J Sports Med.* 1994;22:211-218.

3. Marder RA, Raskind JR, Carroll M. Prospective evaluation of arthroscopically assisted anterior cruciate ligament reconstruction: patellar tendon versus semitendinosis and gracilis tendons. *Am J Sports Med.* 1991;19:478-484.

4. Shelbourne KD, Gray T. Anterior cruciate ligament reconstruction with autogenous patellar tendon graft followed by accelerated rehabilitation. *Am J Sports Med.* 1997;25:786-795.

5. Shelton WR, Papendick L, Dukes AD. Autograft versus allograft anterior cruciate ligament reconstruction. *Arthroscopy.* 1997;13:446-449.

6. Stringham DR, Pelmas CJ, Burks RT, et al. Comparison of anterior cruciate ligament reconstruction using patellar tendon autograft or allograft. *Arthroscopy.* 1996;12:414-421.

7. Lephart SM, Kocher MS, Harner CD, et al. Quadriceps strength and functional capacity after anterior cruciate ligament reconstruction. *Am J Sports Med.* 1993;21:738-743.

8. Noyes FR, Barber SD, Mangine RE. Bone-patellar ligament-bone and fascia lata allografts for reconstruction of the anterior cruciate ligament. *J Bone Joint Surg Am.* 1990;72:1125-1136.

9. Engebretsen L, Benum P, Fasting O, et al. A prospective, randomized study of three surgical techniques for treatment of acute ruptures of the anterior cruciate ligament. *Am J Sports Med.* 1990;18:585-590.

10. Graf B, Uhr F. Complications of intra-articular anterior cruciate reconstruction. *Clin Sports Med.* 1990;7:835-848.

11. Rosenberg TD, Franklin JL, Baldwin GN, et al. Extensor mechanism function after patellar tendon graft harvest for anterior cruciate ligament reconstruction. *Am J Sports Med.* 1992;20:519-525.

12. Sachs RA, Daniel DM, Stone ML, et al. Patellofemoral problems after anterior cruciate ligament reconstruction. *Am J Sports Med.* 1989;17:760-765.

13. Jackson DW, Grood ES, Goldstein JD, et al. A comparison of patellar tendon autograft and allograft used for anterior cruciate ligament reconstruction in the goat model. *Am J Sports Med.* 1993;21:176-185.

14. Yasuda K, Tsujino J, Ohkoshi Y, et al. Graft site morbidity with autogenous semitendinosis and gracilis tendons. *Am J Sports Med.* 1995;23:706-714.

15. Gryzlo SM, Patek RM, Pink M, et al. Electromyographic analysis of knee rehabilitation exercises. *J Orthop Sports Phys Ther.* 1994;20:36-43.

16. Leib FJ, Perry J. Quadriceps function: an anatomical and mechanical study using amputated limbs. *J Bone Joint Surg Am.* 1968;50:1535-1548.

17. Jensen K, Graf BK. The effects of knee effusion on quadriceps strength and knee intra-articular pressure. *Arthroscopy.* 1993;9:52-56.

18. Shelbourne KD, Liotta FJ, Goodloe SL. Preemptive pain management program for anterior cruciate ligament reconstruction. *Am J Knee Surg.* 1998;11:116-119.

19. Shelbourne KD, Rask BP. Anterior cruciate ligament reconstruction using a mini-open technique with autogenous patellar tendon graft. *Techniques in Orthopedics.* 1998;13:221-228.

20. Shelbourne KD, Urch S. Primary anterior cruciate ligament reconstruction using the contralateral autogenous patellar tendon. *Am J Sports Med.* In press.

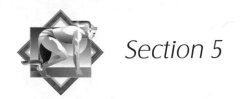

Section 5

Foot, Ankle, and Lower Leg

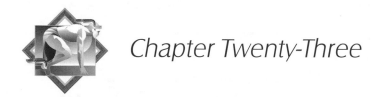

Chapter Twenty-Three

Ankle Sprain and Proximal Fibular Fracture in a Professional Football Player

J. Scott Woodward, MS, PT, SCS, ATC, Martin Boutblik, MD,

Stephen L. Antonopulos, MS, ATC

INTRODUCTION

The most frequently injured peripheral joint encountered by the physically active population has proven to be the ankle.[1,2] Ankle injuries are among the most prevalent injuries sustained in both amateur and professional athletes.[3,4,5] The incidence of ankle injuries has been reported from 14.2% to as high as 33% in various athletic populations.[4,6]

Lateral ankle sprains are the most common of these injuries.[1,7,8] Anatomic factors, including osseous mechanics, small ligamentous mass, and weak tensile strengths of lateral supporting ligaments predispose the lateral ankle to injury.[3,8,9] However, these are not necessarily the most serious or debilitating ankle injuries incurred. While much less common, injuries involving the stronger tensile ligamentous structures such as the deltoid ligament, tibiofibular ligaments, and the interosseous membrane can complicate and slow recovery time significantly.[10,11,12] Several studies have shown that an ankle injury complicated with syndesmosis involvement can increase the time of return to competition by as much as 50%.[13,14] The mechanism of injury is commonly ankle dorsiflexion with simultaneous forced external rotation of the foot and internal rotation of the tibia/fibula (Figure 23-1).[2,8,15-17]

Anatomically, the talocrural joint is formed by the distal tibia and fibula, which create the roof/mortise of the joint superiorly, articulating with the talus inferiorly. Superiorly, the tibia/fibula articulations are bound together by three supporting structures: the proximal tibiofibular syndesmosis, the interosseous membrane, and the distal tibiofibular syndesmosis.[7,18,19] The distal tibiofibular syndesmosis is stabilized by four ligaments: the inferior interosseous ligament, the anterior inferior tibiofibular ligament, the posterior inferior tibiofibular ligament, and the inferior transverse tibiofibular ligament.[8,18] Osteokinematically, the superior surface of the talus is wider anteriorly than posteriorly. This creates a wedge-shaped articulating surface that moves between the medial tibial malleolus and the lateral fibular malleolus.[7,8,19] During dorsiflexion of the ankle, the distal tibia/fibula articulation composing the ankle mortise is forced to separate slightly to accommodate the wider talus and allow for this motion to occur.[7,20,21] The distal tibiofibular syndesmosis, while providing a great deal of stability to the ankle mortise and talocrural joint, allows this accessory give or separation for normal dorsiflexion and plantarflexion to occur in the normal stable ankle.[8,13]

While not common, injury to the syndesmosis not only delays recovery time but can also be the sign of a much more serious injury.[3,8] Reviewing the mechanics of injury to these structures leads to a better understanding of the potential for severe injury. Forced external rotation of the talus with internal rotation of the

Figure 23-1. Mechanism of injury with anatomical inset.

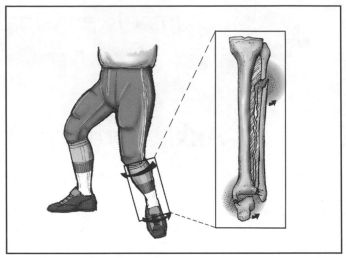

lower extremity can result in a series of pathological events in the ankle joint.[8] First, if the force is of adequate intensity, the deltoid ligament may tear or the tibial malleolous may be avulsed. This can be followed by a fracture of the fibula. If the distal syndesmotic ligament remains intact, the fracture will occur distal to the ligament. If the syndesmotic ligaments are disrupted, the fracture will occur more proximally. The higher the fibular fracture, the greater the damage to the anterior tibiofibular ligament. The Maisonneuve fracture occurs at the proximal fibula and is associated with disruption of the ankle mortise and tearing of the interosseous membrane up to the level of the fracture. The fracture pattern results in a grossly unstable ankle joint and requires operative treatment.[8] This case study describes the treatment of an elite athlete who sustained a Maisonneuve fracture. The patient presented is a National Football League (NFL) running back who was injured in a game situation. The purpose of this case study is to present a rehabilitation approach following such an injury and the potential complications that may arise.

SUBJECT

The patient was a 25-year-old running back/special teams player in the NFL who injured his right ankle in a preseason football game in 1994. While running down field on a special teams play, the player was upended by an opposing player and landed awkwardly on his right ankle. The patient felt that he had sustained an external rotation type injury to his ankle, which was subsequently confirmed by a review of game films. The patient had significant pain, especially on the lateral side of his ankle, and was not able to bear weight.

Onfield examination revealed swelling along the anterolateral aspect of the ankle. Active and passive range of motion (ROM) was mildly restricted by lateral ankle pain, especially passive dorsiflexion. The patient was moderately tender over the anterior syndesmosis of the lateral ankle. He was mildly tender medially over the deltoid ligament and minimally tender over the lateral ankle ligaments and the malleoli. He had a positive compression test with pain in the area of the syndesmosis on-side-to side compression of the leg at mid calf.[22,23] The patient had lateral pain in the area of the syndesmosis on passive external rotation of the ankle.[11,22] The ankle was grossly unstable with anterior drawer and talar tilt testing. The patient was tender over the proximal fibula. He had a partial peroneal nerve injury with 4/5 weakness of the extensor halluces longus (EHL) and mildly decreased sensation over the first web space. The patient ambulated to the sideline with assistance, nonweightbearing through the right lower extremity. The sideline examination confirmed the findings on the field.

Radiographs of the ankle and leg showed minimal medial widening of the clear space between the medial malleolus and the talus, mild widening of the syndesmosis, and an oblique fracture of the proximal fibula (Maisonneuve fracture) (Figure 23-2).

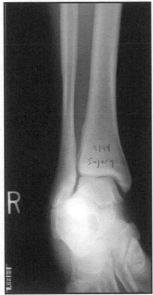

Figure 23-2. X-ray of injury before surgery showing syndesmosis instability.

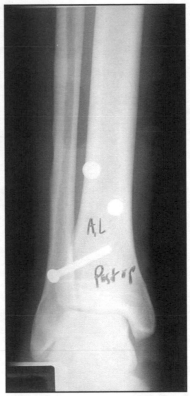

Figure 23-3. X-rays after surgical repair with cortical screw.

The patient was initially treated with RICE (rest, ice, compression, elevation) and placed into a well-padded plaster splint with the ankle at neutral position. He was placed on crutches, nonweightbearing, in preparation for the return trip home, as the game was an away contest.

Re-examination upon return home showed the swelling to be diminished. The partial peroneal nerve injury was resolving with near normal first web space sensation and improved 4+/5 EHL strength. The nerve injury subsequently resolved fully. The remainder of the examination was essentially unchanged from the initial evaluation. Repeat radiographic evaluation showed increased widening of the ankle joint. The patient was taken into the operating room for examination under anesthesia and fixation of the syndesmosis. Under anesthesia, the ankle joint was grossly unstable with external rotation and there was widening of the medial clear space between the medial malleolous and the talus. An incision was made laterally over the distal fibula. Large boney forceps were used to provide side-to-side compression between the tibia and the fibula and to reduce the ankle mortise anatomically. A large fragment AO cortical screw was placed across both cortices of the fibula and one cortex of the tibia to maintain an anatomic relationship between the distal fibula and the tibia. The screw was placed without compression and with the ankle held in mild dorsiflexion to prevent overtightening the tibiofibular joint (Figure 23-3). Repeat external rotation stress testing with the syndesmotic screw in place showed the ankle mortise to be stable with no evidence of widening.

POSTOPERATIVE REHABILITATION

Postoperatively, the patient was initially immobilized in a short leg cast nonweightbearing for 4 weeks and given a home exercise program consisting of proximal hip strengthening. At week 5, the cast was removed, and the patient's formal rehabilitation was started. The goals of this phase were to regain ankle ROM and begin controlled strength training. The patient displayed considerable soft tissue scarring over the anterior

Table 23-1

ACTIVE RANGE OF MOTION AND MANUAL MUSCLE TESTING AT VARIOUS TIME INTERVALS

	Week 4	Week 8	Week 12	Week 16	Week 20
Dorsiflexion					
ROM	15 degrees	-4 degrees	10 degrees	8 degrees	14 degrees	14 degrees
MMT	5/5	3-/5	4-/5*	4/5*	5-/5	5/5
Plantarflexion					
ROM	40 degrees	10 degrees	20 degrees	31 degrees	35 degrees	43 degrees
MMT	5/5	3-/5	4-/5*	4/5*	4+/5*	5/5
Inversion					
ROM	28 degrees	6 degrees	24 degrees	30 degrees	30 degrees	30 degrees
MMT	5/5	3-/5	4/5*	4/5	5-/5	5/5
Eversion					
ROM	14 degrees	2 degrees	14 degrees	15 degrees	14 degrees	14 degrees
MMT	5/5	3-/5	4/5	5-/5	5/5	5/5

syndesmotic region, considerable limitations in ROM and strength (Table 23-1), as well as moderate gastrocnemius and soleus tightness.

The patient was initially treated with soft tissue mobilization, joint mobilization of the talocrural joint, and passive and active ROM for dorsiflexion, plantarflexion, eversion, and inversion. In addition, an exercise program consisting of proximal hip strengthening, low intensity stationary biking, and upper extremity isotonics in the weight room was initiated. This program was progressed with the addition of resistive band linear ankle exercises, intrinsic foot strengthening, single plane wobble board proprioception, and a pool program. The pool program included weightbearing and nonweightbearing exercises, utilizing the buoyancy and viscosity properties of the water to facilitate controlled resistive exercise, and to control the ground reaction forces during weightbearing.[24] By week 7, the patient was utilizing the passive setting on the Biodex (Biodex Corp, Shirley, NY) isokinetic dynamometer for active/assistive ROM and performing manually resisted exercises (MREs) for linear ankle patterns. At the eighth week, the patient had progressed to proprioceptive neuromuscular facilitation (PNF) patterns for MREs. Toe-touch weightbearing was continued until 8 weeks after surgery, at which time the syndesmotic screw was removed.

At week 8, the patient began weaning from the crutches. ROM had progressed to 10 degrees of dorsiflexion, 20 degrees plantarflexion, 24 degrees inversion, and full eversion. The patient continued his rehabilitation program with increases in repetitions, sets, and intensity as tolerated. By week 10, the patient had progressed to full weightbearing. He began an intermediate exercise program, including the Plyosled (Topaz

Medical, Englewood, Colo), bilateral heel lifts, isokinetic ankle (dorsiflexion, plantarflexion, inversion, and eversion) exercises, a treadmill walking program, elastic cord resisted walking exercises, and aerobic conditioning on a stair machine. By the 11th week postoperatively, ROM and strength measures were increased enough to allow a low intensity walk/jog treadmill program to be instituted.

At week 12, the patient continued to display soft tissue thickening over the anterior tibiofibular ligament. He displayed ROM deficits of approximately 30% with dorsiflexion and plantarflexion secondary to talocrural joint mobility restrictions; however, he displayed full inversion and eversion ROM measures. Manual muscle test strength values were 4/5 for the tibialis posterior, 5-/5 for the peroneals, and 4/5 for the gastrocnemius and soleus; however, he was unable to perform a full unilateral toe raise. He continued to possess minimal to moderate tightness in his gastrocnemius and soleus. The patient continued to perform progressive isotonic exercises for not only the ankle, but also the entire lower extremity to aid in increasing total lower extremity strength. A basic supportive taping routine consisting of a basketweave, figure eight, and heel locks was initiated during the athlete's running activities to assist with stability during these activities.[1,9,20] He continued a low-intensity running routine on the treadmill; however, he began to complain of tenderness over the plantar surface of the first ray.

Observation and analysis of running mechanics revealed reduced dorsiflexion at the talocrural region during late stance phase, with a compensatory increase in pronation and external rotation of the foot. In addition, the patient had a significant reduction in stride length/flight time following the push-off phase of the right lower extremity. A bone scan was ordered and confirmed a stress fracture in the first cuneiform. The rehabilitation program was modified to decrease the aggravating activities; the running program was also discontinued at this time. The pool program was progressed to help reduce pain and the stresses of ground reaction forces. Joint mobilizations and stretching activities were continued to lengthen capsular and musculotendinous restrictions to improve talocrural mechanics in an attempt to restore normal dorsiflexion. In addition, the patient had progressed beyond single plane wobble boards to activities using the Kinesthetic Ability Trainer (Breg Inc, Vista, Calif). The patient progressed from bilateral and unilateral balancing and ROM/control exercises, to balance with the challenge of throwing and catching various balls in random patterns.

At 16 weeks, the patient's first ray symptoms had subsided significantly. In addition, active dorsiflexion had progressed to within normal limits, and plantarflexion to 35 degrees, which was approximately a 10% deficit compared to the noninjured ankle. Strength values improved to 5-/5 for tibialis anterior and posterior, 5/5 for peroneals, and 4+/5 for the gastrocnemius and soleus, although the patient still could not perform a full unilateral toe raise with the injured ankle. Minimal gastrocnemius and soleus tightness was evident at this phase of his rehabilitation. The exercise program continued with isotonic and proprioceptive progression, as well as a full spectrum isokinetic program for ankle plantarflexion, dorsiflexion, inversion, and eversion. The isokinetic program was utilized to strengthen those muscle groups acting on the ankle, progressing to fast velocity contractile speeds in an attempt to increase neuromuscular control and speed of muscular initiation. This follows the principles of specificity of training in an attempt to train the muscular components as closely as possible to the angular velocities experienced during activities such as running.[25] The patient also continued his pool program two to three times per week while adapting to increasing ground reaction forces necessary to resume running activities for full return to his desired activity. The patient performed resistive cord exercises in all planes two to three times per week, beginning with walking and progressing to running, to improve gait mechanics and prepare for more difficult functional activities.

The patient continued to be relatively pain-free at 18 weeks with respect to the first ray and returned to a treadmill walk/jog program. In addition, a functional progression was initiated beginning with low-level basketball court activities, focusing on light cutting and pass catching activities. The patient also began a plyometric progression at this time to help improve ballistic strength and control needed for acceleration and jumping, etc. In addition, he continued with isotonic, proprioceptive, isokinetic, and pool activities. Supportive taping was continued throughout this phase to help stabilize the patient's ankle during progression to more aggressive rehabilitative exercises. The patient noted being more comfortable and having increased confidence wearing the supportive tape during his functional and running exercises, as he had used supportive taping throughout his college and professional career.

At 20 weeks, the patient demonstrated full active ROM of all ankle motions including plantarflexion, as well as 5/5 manual muscle test values for all muscle groups. The patient continued to be unable to perform a unilateral toe raise on the injured lower extremity. The plyometric routine progressed in both intensity and height, and the functional progression advanced to acceleration/deceleration work with an increase in intensity and velocity of cutting activities. The running program progressed to indoor track surfaces for which he was able to jog approximately 1 mile pain-free; however, the patient displayed significant difficulty and antalgia when attempting to accelerate beyond a normal jogging cadence. Much time and effort was spent refining gait/running mechanics to alleviate this with verbal and manual cueing techniques, as well as the aid of a mirror for visual feedback.

At week 22, the patient began working approximately two times per week on endurance and form running with a track/running coach. He began to complain of decreased ankle ROM into dorsiflexion with slight increase in first ray pain shortly after this time. Again, the talocrural joint was found to be hypomobile into dorsiflexion, with a measure of 11 degrees. Aggressive joint mobilization and stretching were resumed. The patient was also fitted with semirigid orthotics to help provide better support and contact to the foot during running activities. By week 24, the patient had full return of dorsiflexion, as well as minimal complaints of first ray discomfort despite increasing his running time significantly and resuming full sprinting activities. The patient was now able to perform full unilateral toe raises with the injured ankle. In addition, the patient completed his full functional progression on grass, including acceleration, deceleration, cutting motions/change of direction, and sport-specific activities including pass routes and blocking technique. In order for the patient to progress to the next phase, he had to complete the prior level without difficulty or limitation.

Follow-up radiographs revealed proper healing and stability of the talocrural joint. The patient was able to return to professional football the following season without any subsequent symptoms related to his right ankle.

DISCUSSION

Syndesmosis injuries are much less common than lateral ankle sprains and can be more complex with respect to treatment and rehabilitation. Secondary to the fracture and instability present with this patient's ankle, surgical repair was required to provide the necessary stability. The fixation was then removed following proper healing to allow normal talocrural mechanics to be restored. Several authors have reported the necessity of a fixation procedure secondary to the soft tissue damage and potential instability, as well as the removal of the hardware for restoration of mobility.[15,26-29]

For this athlete, the primary goal was to return to play in the NFL as soon as was physically possible. The first goal of treatment following the surgical procedure was related to restoring proper mechanics and normal motion of the ankle while allowing the time necessary for normal soft tissue healing. Immobilization has been shown to produce dense connective tissue changes, which are accelerated after trauma secondary to the presence of inflammatory exudates.[30-32] These periarticular connective tissue changes can affect joint capsule and ligamentous structures, promoting marked soft tissue thickening and fibrosis.[33] In a study testing dorsiflexion stiffness after nontraumatic immobilization of rats, a significant increase in both time and torque were required to restore full dorsiflexion.[34] Similarly, Chesworth and Vandervoort reported that patients immobilized by casts following traumatic malleolar fractures displayed significant decreases in maximum passive dorsiflexion when compared to nonimmobilized fractures.[35] While the healing process is basically uncontrollable, the phases of modeling and remodeling can be influenced through the rehabilitation procedure.[36,37] For this patient, much time was devoted to the restoration of proper talocrural mobility with joint mobilization, deep tissue mobilization, and a stretching regime all designed to affect the connective tissue involved.

Initially, ROM progressed well; however, complications developed with recovery when the athlete began to experience pain in the first ray of the injured lower extremity. When the symptoms did not resolve in a reasonable time frame, further diagnostic testing revealed a stress fracture of the first cuneiform. Stress fractures are the result of forces that are repetitive as well as in excess of the bone's structural limitations. If the forces are allowed to continue long enough, the bone will fatigue and then fail, producing the stress fracture.[38] The first priority when treating a stress fracture is to identify and alleviate the source of injury.[8,23,39]

Normal walking mechanics require a minimum of 10 degrees of dorsiflexion.[23] When increasing the cadence to running, a greater degree of dorsiflexion has been demonstrated to occur at the late mid-stance phase.[40,41] With this athlete, proper talocrural mechanics had not been completely restored prior to beginning a jog/running program. While the athlete had achieved the minimum 10 degrees of dorsiflexion, he had not reestablished the baseline value set by his noninjured ankle. In compensation for the lack of full talocrural dorsiflexion necessary during the midstance and push-off phases of running, it is likely that the patient experienced an increase in stress on the first ray transmitted through midtarsal and MTP joint extension.[19,42,43]

Studies of ground reaction forces (GRFs) help to explain the distribution and quantity of pressures experienced during the various phases of ambulation. With normal level surface walking, the first ray/great toe has been shown to experience forces comparable to the peak pressure placed on the foot during the gait cycle. When increasing the cadence to running, the late stance and push-off phases of the gait cycle have been shown to produce the greatest loading of forces on the forefoot, particularly the first ray.[20,44-46]

This increase in MTP extension, combined with the high pre-existing GRF of the forefoot, could easily surpass normal osseous load limits of the first ray, resulting in a stress-related injury. After a brief active-rest phase with emphasis placed on restoration of proper mechanics and full dorsiflexion of the ankle, the patient was able to return to running with much less difficulty and pain.

Other goals for return of an athlete to activity include strengthening, proprioceptive training, and proper functional progression. This patient demonstrated good return of strength and proprioception after full return of ankle dorsiflexion and was able to begin and tolerate a functional progression with much less difficulty. The functional progression was initiated indoors on a wood basketball court to aid in controlling the activity. However, the patient continued to have difficulty with ballistic strength activities such as plyometrics and those requiring acceleration secondary to the inability to push off of his toes and forefoot adequately. The push-off phase has been identified by several authors as a limiting factor in return to activity secondary to pain following a syndesmosis sprain.[12,47] When examining the normal ground reaction forces of gait, a characteristic increase in pressure is experienced at push-off.[48] With running, vertical GRF has been found to increase greater than two times those experienced by the foot when walking. In a study of ground reaction forces following syndesmotic sprain and fixation, Spaulding demonstrated that both vertical and horizontal force values did not approach normal levels until 4 months, and he suggested that this recovery time indicated the necessity of syndesmosis stability for the stresses imposed during the stance and push-off phases of gait.[47] This limitation is consistent with our patient and is suggestive of the healing parameters necessary for withstanding the excessive stresses experienced during athletic activities following this procedure.

Once full plantarflexion was restored passively, attention was focused on improving end range and ballistic plantarflexor strength, incorporating the stretch-shorten cycle. This progression must be implemented at the appropriate time interval secondary to the significant GRF experienced with jumping, which has been reported in excess of 16 times body weight.[49] With plantarflexion, the gastrocnemius and soleus are the primary muscular components involved. During the mid and late-stance phases of gait, these muscles act to control dorsiflexion, storing elastic energy during an eccentric contraction. At push-off, these same muscles concentrically contract, providing propulsion.[50,51] This principle is the basis of plyometric exercise, incorporating both musculotendinous and neural training.[36] Training the stretch-shorten cycle has been suggested to increase power and strength while improving the quickness and speed of muscular responses necessary for athletic activities, in addition to providing for specificity of training.[36,52] After this phase, the patient's running mechanics improved significantly, particularly with regard to stride length and cadence.

To regain full functional ability, rehabilitation must usually incorporate the SAID principle (specific adaptations to imposed demands).[9] The functional progression is one of the most efficient means of providing these forces, progressing from low intensity/simple skills to high intensity/difficult skills that simulate the activities required of the athlete in his particular environment.[9] Tissue healing limitations must be considered when designing this program, and the athlete must be proficient in the less taxing skills before progressing to the more difficult. In this way, the functional ability of the athlete can be accurately assessed prior to returning to the practice environment. No exercise can truly simulate the speed and volatile environment of a collision sport such as professional football, but it does allow both the clinician and athlete to assess physical abilities, and gain confidence before returning to full contact. While a judgment must be made in order to return to full activity, the functional progression allows for a greater knowledge of the individual's capabilities and limitations prior to the actual event.

SUMMARY

This case presentation emphasized returning a 25-year-old athlete to full NFL participation following a Maisonneuves fracture. The injury occurred during the second week of training camp during the first exhibition game, requiring surgical stabilization and more than 5 months of rehabilitation. This case study shows how rehabilitation can be affected by other factors, such as a stress fracture, and how changes must be made to the rehabilitation program to allow for proper healing and progression. In this case, the patient developed first ray symptoms that were diagnosed as a stress fracture of the first cuneiform. Treatment was altered to allow proper healing of the cuneiform to occur but was also directed at the possible cause—restricted talocrural joint mobility. Once proper motion was restored and adequate healing time was allowed, the patient was able to return to full rehabilitation activities, including an extensive functional progression. The athlete was then able to return to full NFL participation, where he continues to be employed.

REFERENCES

1. Arnheim DD. *Modern Principles of Athletic Training*. 7th ed. St. Louis, Mo: Times Mirror/CV Mosby; 1989.

2. Jackson R, Wills RE, Jackson R. Rupture of the deltoid ligament without involvement of the lateral ligaments. *Am J Sports Med*. 1988;16:541-543.

3. Boruta PM, Bishop JO, Braly WG, Tulos HS. Acute lateral ankle ligament injuries: a literature review. *Foot Ankle Int*. 1990;11:107-113.

4. National Athletic Trainers' Association. Participation/injury overview. *NATA News*. 1996; April:17-23.

5. Zelisko JA, Noble HB, Porter M. A comparison of men's and women's professional basketball injuries. *Am J Sports Med*. 1982;10:297-299.

6. Perry J. *Gait Analysis: Normal and Pathological Function*. Thorofare, NJ: SLACK Incorporated; 1992.

7. Moore KL. *Clinically Oriented Anatomy*. 2nd ed. Baltimore, Md: Williams & Wilkins; 1989.

8. Wilson FC. Fractures and dislocations of the ankle. In: Rockwood CA, Green DP, eds. *Fractures in Adults*. Vol 2. Philadelphia, Pa: JB Lippincott Company; 1984.

9. American Academy of Orthopedic Surgeons. *Athletic Training and Sports Medicine*. 2nd ed. Rosemont, Ill: American Academy of Orthopedic Surgeons; 1991.

10. Attarian DE, McCrackin HJ, DeVito DP, et al. Biomechanical characteristics of human ankle ligaments. *Foot Ankle Int*. 1985;6:54-58.

11. Boytim MJ, Fischer DA, Neuman L. Syndesmotic ankle sprains. *Am J Sports Med*. 1991;19:294-298.

12. Taylor DC, Bassett FH. Syndesmosis sprains of the ankle. The influence of heterotropic ossification. *Am J Sports Med*. 1992;20:146-150.

13. Inman VT. *The Joints of the Ankle*. Baltimore, Md: Williams & Wilkins; 1976.

14. Hopkinson WJ, St. Pierre P, Ryan JB, et al. Syndesmosis sprains of the ankle. *Foot Ankle Int*. 1990;10:325-330.

15. Ebraheim NA, Mekhail AO, Gargasz SS. Ankle fractures involving the fibula proximal to the distal tibiofibular syndesmosis. *Foot and Ankle Int*. 1997;18(8):513-521.

16. Guise ER. Rotational ligamentous injuries to the ankle in football. *Am J Sports Med*. 1976;4:1-6.

17. Pankovich AM. Fractures of the fibula proximal to the distal tibiofibular syndesmosis. *J Bone Joint Surg*. 1978;60:221-229.

18. Gray H. *Gray's Anatomy*. Philadelphia, Pa: Running Press; 1974.

19. McGee DJ. *Orthopedic Physical Assessment*. 2nd ed. Philadelphia, Pa: WB Saunders Company; 1992.

20. McPoil TG, McGarvey TC. The foot in athletics. In: Hunt GC, ed. *Physical Therapy of the Foot and Ankle*. New York, NY: Churchill Livingstone; 1988.

21. Ogilvie-Harris DJ, Reed SC, Hedman TP. Disruption of the ankle syndesmosis: biomechanical study of the ligamentous restraints. *Arthroscopy*. 1994;10(5):558-560.

22. Brosky T, Nyland J, Nitz N, et al. The ankle ligaments: consideration of syndesmotic injury and implications for rehabilitation. *J Orthop Sports Phys Ther.* 1995;21(4)197-205.

23. McPoil TG, Brocato RS. The foot and ankle: biomechanical evaluation and treatment. In: Gould JA, Davies GA, eds. *Orthopedic and Sports Physical Therapy.* St. Louis, Mo: CV Mosby Company; 1985.

24. Thein JM, Brody LT. Aquatic-based rehabilitation and training for the elite athlete. *J Orthop Sports Phys Ther.* 1998;27(1):32-41.

25. Davies, GJ. *A Compendium of Isokinetics in Clinical Usage.* Onalaska, Wis: S & S Publishers; 1987.

26. Hughes JL, Weber H, Willenegger H, et al. Evaluation of ankle fractures: nonoperative and operative treatment. *Clin Orthop.* 1979;138:111-119.

27. Kaye RA. Stabilization of ankle syndesmosis injuries with a syndesmotic screw. *Foot Ankle Int.* 1989;9:290-293.

28. Olerud C. The effect of the syndesmotic screw on the extension capacity of the ankle joint. *Arch Orthop Trauma Surg.* 1985;104:299-302.

29. Peter RE, Harrington RM, Henley MB, et al. Biomechanical effects of internal fixation of the distal tibiofibular syndesmotic joint: comparison of two fixation techniques. *J Orthop Trauma.* 1994;8(3):215-219.

30. Enneking WF, Horowitz M. The intra-articular effects of immobilization on the human knee. *J Bone Joint Surg Am.* 1972;54(5):973-985.

31. Gamble JG, Edwards DD, Max SR. Enzymatic adaptation in ligaments during immobilization. *Am J Sports Med.* 1984;12(3):221-228.

32. Noyes FR. Functional properties of knee ligaments and alterations induced by immobilization. *Clin Orthop.* 1977;123:210-242.

33. Ouzounian TJ, Kabo JM, Grogan TJ, et al. The effects of pressurization on fracture swelling and joint stiffness in the rabbit hind limb. *Clin Orthop.* 1986;210:252-256.

34. Reynolds CA, Cummings GC, Andrew PD, et al. The effect of nontraumatic immobilization on ankle dorsiflexion stiffness in rats. *J Orthop Sports Phys Ther.* 1996;23(1):27-33.

35. Chesworth BM, Vandervoort AA. Range of motion in uninvolved and involved ankle joints of patients following ankle fractures. *Phys Ther.* 1995;75:253-261.

36. Voight ML, Draovitch P. Plyometrics. In: Albert M, ed. *Eccentric Muscle Training in Sports and Orthopedics.* New York, NY: Churchill Livingstone; 1991.

37. Staniitski CL. Common injuries in preadolescents and adolescent athletes. recommendations for prevention. *Sports Med.* 1989;7:32.

38. Devas M. *Stress Fractures.* Edinburgh, UK: Churchill Livingstone; 1975.

39. Roy S, Irvin R. *Sports Medicine: Prevention, Evaluation, Management, and Rehabilitation.* Englewood Cliffs, NJ: Prentice Hall, Inc; 1983.

40. Scranton PE. Forces under the foot: a study of walking, jogging, and sprinting force distribution under normal an abnormal feet. In: Bateman JE, Trott AW, eds. *The Foot and Ankle.* New York, NY: Brian C. Decker, Thieme-Stratton, Inc; 1980.

41. Slocum DB, James SL. Biomechanics of running. *JAMA.* 1968;205:97.

42. Brown HE, Mueller MJ. A "step-to" gait decreases pressures on the forefoot. *J Orthop Sports Phys Ther.* 1998;28(3):139-145.

43. Mueller MJ. Use of an in-shoe pressure measurement system in the management of patients with neuropathic ulcers and metetarsalgia. *J Orthop Sports Phys Ther.* 1995;21(6):328-336.

44. Birke JA, Cornwall MA, Jackson M. Relationship between hallux limitus and ulceration of the great toe. *J Orthop Sports Phys Ther.* 1988;10:172-176.

45. Hutton WC, Dhanendran M. A study of the distribution of loads under the normal foot during walking. *Int Orthop.* 1979;3:153-157.

46. Stott JRR, Hutton WC, Stokes IAF. Forces under the foot. *J Bone Joint Surg Br.* 1973;55:335-344.

47. Spaulding SJ. Monitoring recovery following syndesmosis sprain: a case study. *Foot Ankle Int.* 1995;16(10):655-660.

48. Winter DA. *The Biomechanics and Motor Control of Human Gait.* Waterloo, Canada: University of Waterloo Press; 1987.

49. Hay JG. Citius, altius, longius (faster, higher, longer): the biomechanics of jumping for distance. *J Biomech.* 1993;26(Suppl1):7-21.

50. Jackson DW, Ashley RD, Powell JW. Ankle sprains in young athletes. *Clin Orthop.* 1974;101:201-214.

51. Mann R, Sprague P. Kinetics of sprinting. In: Terauds J, ed. *Biomechanics in Sports.* Del Mar, Calif: Research Center for Sports; 1982.

52. Thurman C, Braun B, Halpern AA, et al. Effectiveness of pulsed eccentric loading exercise. *Med Sci Sports Exerc.* 1991;23:S118.

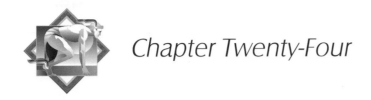

Chapter Twenty-Four

Medial Ankle Sprain: Deltoid Ligament Rupture in the Collegiate Athlete

Ned Shannon, ATC

INTRODUCTION

When an athlete sprains an ankle, the percentage is high that it is a lateral injury. In basketball, ankle sprains comprise more then 50% of major injuries, and in soccer and volleyball more then 25%. Occasionally, however, there is the event of an eversion or medial ankle sprain. Eversion sprains occur less frequently due to the anatomy of the ankle and the strength of the deltoid ligament. The injury is caused by an excessive valgus stress to the ankle, causing the foot to pronate and slightly dorsiflex (Figure 24-1). The deltoid ligamentous structure is stretched and may rupture if the force is great enough. Severe eversion forces may involve the spring ligament along with the deltoid ligament (see Figure 24-1). The athlete will complain of pain and stiffness into the longitudinal arch area and have difficulty during the push-off phase of the walking gait.

SUBJECT

The athlete in this case study was a 19-year-old male basketball center in his sophomore year. He was rebounding during an intercollegiate practice and landed off balance on his right ankle. The athlete reported feeling a sharp pain on the inside of his foot/ankle that radiated up the medial lower leg. He was able to walk off the practice court after a few minutes of rest. As he walked, he indicated that the pain seemed to decrease in intensity.

INITIAL EVALUATION

Upon initial evaluation, the medial ligaments were intact but had sustained moderate damage. The deltoid ligament was tender to touch and there was mild swelling about the medial aspect of the ankle and arch. Strength through inversion/eversion was weak (2/5), as was plantarflexion and dorsiflexion. No discoloration was noted, nor was there any joint deformity. The eversion test was positive, producing mild laxity (2/5) and significant pain (5/5). The anterior drawer test produced pain but no laxity, and the talar tilt test was negative. Palpation of the spring ligament and the sustentaculum tali produced tenderness (4/5).

INITIAL TREATMENT AND REHABILITATION

Acute sprain care consisted of rest, ice, compression, and elevation (RICE) for the first 72 hours, along with a course of nonsteroidal anti-inflammatory medication (NSAIDs). Crutches were used for the first 24 hours to facilitate proper ambulation and decrease pain and the likelihood of reinjury. Ultrasound was initiated 3 days after the injury at 1.0 watts (W), 50%, for 6 minutes. A cold whirlpool for 12 minutes was fol-

Figure 24-1. Mechanism of an eversion ankle sprain: palpation of the spring ligament.

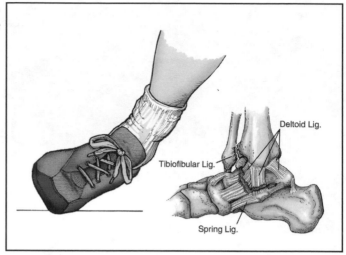

lowed by 5 minutes of ankle dorsiflexion and plantarflexion stretches using a towel in a nonweightbearing position.

Approximately 4 days post-injury, pain had decreased to 1/5 and swelling was dramatically reduced with no ecchymosis. Ultrasound was increased to 1.0 W at 100% for 6 minutes. Gastrocnemius/soleus stretch on a slant board was added along with inversion/eversion and plantarflexion/dorsiflexion exercises on the multiaxial machine. Strengthening exercises were added and included towel crunches and toe raises. Ice and continuous high-voltage electrical muscle stimulation were applied for 20 minutes after each therapy session.

The athlete continued to complain of mild pain over the calcaneonavicular ligament and navicular tuberosity 10 days after the injury. Weightbearing had been established and flat-footed drills were tolerable. Application of medial longitudinal arch taping with ankle strapping emphasizing foot pronation was provided. Off-the-shelf arch supports were also added to his basketball shoes.

Activity increased as rehabilitation progressed over the next three practices. Approximately 2 weeks after the initial injury, the athlete landed, crushing his arch on another player's ankle. The following day the team orthopedist evaluated the athlete. X-rays showed no fracture or disruption along the midfoot or navicular. There was evidence of an osteochondritis on the talus. On exam, there was significant swelling along the anterior deltoid ligament down to the navicular. The tibialis posterior sheath was tender and quite swollen. When the athlete was standing flat-footed, there was a noticeable reduction in arch contour compared to the left foot. He had a great deal of difficulty establishing an arch. The physician diagnosed a severe deltoid ligament sprain of the medial ankle. Upon completion of the orthopedic exam, an Aircast walking boot was prescribed and a magnetic resonance imaging (MRI) scan was scheduled for the next day.

The MRI confirmed significant disruption of the deltoid ligament. The tibialis posterior tendon was intact with significant tendonitis distally. The osteochondritis was intact and no loose bodies were noted. Management of symptoms was continued as before with a combination of cryotherapy and electrotherapy to manage pain. Range of motion (ROM) work with towel exercise limiting inversion movements of the ankle was continued.

SURGERY

The orthopedic surgeon discussed the circumstances with the athlete and explained that repair of the ruptured deltoid ligament with medial ankle exploration and excision of loose osteochondritis of the talus would provide better stabilty than waiting for the ligament to heal itself. Due to the clinical findings and the potential positive outcome of the procedure, the athlete decided to pursue aggressive treatment. Surgery was scheduled for November 17, 23 days after the initial injury.

Visual inspection of the entire foot/ankle joint ensured that there was no unforeseen damage. Once inside the joint, the defect to the deltoid ligament was located near the tibialis posterior crossing on the anterior segment. Three sutures were placed in each bone plug. The ankle was slightly dorsiflexed, the heel was brought into slight varus, and the deltoid was repaired by sewing the sutures to one another and approximating the deltoid appropriately. The medial osteochondritis was located and appeared loose. The fragment was removed in one piece to open the medial ankle and promote increased function without pain. The area was curetted to stimulate a new layer of healing. The entire site was closed with 3-0 nylon vertical mattress sutures.

POSTOPERATIVE REHABILITATION

A well-molded fiberglass cast was applied to immobilize the ankle and foot in neutral and provide comfort and protection. The device was used for approximately 5 weeks. Along with the cast, crutches for non-weightbearing ambulation were provided. Once postsurgical swelling decreased, the athlete was fitted for orthotic devices. Nonweightbearing passive ROM exercises began by the 11th day after surgery and included general dorsiflexion and plantarflexion movements. Towel crunches with a light sand weight and inversion and eversion motion were also initiated. Ultrasound at 100%, 1.0 W for 6 minutes, followed by ice pack application for 20 minutes finished therapy on a daily basis. About 3 weeks after surgery, the athlete complained of a burning sensation inside the fiberglass cast. A 3M (3M Healthcare, St. Paul, Minn) short leg cast replaced the fiberglass cast and relieved the symptom, which allowed the athlete to continue with therapy.

The cast was removed after 6 weeks. Weightbearing was established and good medial soft tissue tension on the medial arch was noted. Orthotics were added with instructions to wear them in basketball shoes around the house. Crutches were continued for partial weightbearing and balance. Therapy progressed to weightbearing dorsiflexion on a slant board. This position was held for 5 seconds with a 10-second rest and repeated 10 times. Partial weightbearing gait training was initiated with shoe and orthotic on. Strengthening of dorsiflexion and plantarflexion continued using manual resistance (three sets of 8 to 10 repetitions). Cold whirlpool replaced ice pack, and ultrasound was discontinued.

Ten weeks after surgery, the athlete was able to walk in the hall with no support under his foot. Some soft tissue thickness was noted around the medial deltoid and surgical site but caused no pain or loss of ROM. The athlete demonstrated limited plantarflexion and dorsiflexion compared to the unaffected side. Force applied by the athlete to his arch in a standing position caused no collapse of the arch. Therapy was elevated to full weightbearing movements such as walking forward one-half to one-fourth of a mile. Stair machine for 10 to 15 minutes, followed by cold whirlpool for 10 minutes, tissue mobility massage for 5 minutes, and dorsiflexion stretching for 2 to 3 minutes were initiated. Light basketball shooting drills produced mild pain over the Achilles' tendon, which was treated symptomatically. The left foot had become irritated and inflamed over the lateral side of the calcaneous. It was diagnosed as possible bursitis and treated with a circular pad to relieve pressure on the site.

At 5 months post-surgery, ankle alignment looked excellent and all arch collapse was eliminated. X-rays showed that the osteochondritic area where the fragment was removed was well healed. Pain was only over the anteromedial deltoid area when the foot was plantarflexed. A lack of about 8 degrees of plantarflexion was noted. Dorsiflexion was slightly less, with approximately 5 degrees lacking.

Along with the physical rehabilitation, the athlete was going through mental trials as well. He was discouraged with the seemingly slow progress of therapy. Emotional support from the surgeon and team athletic trainer helped, but a second athletic trainer provided additional motivation.

Addition of an Ankle Stabilizing Orthosis (ASO) (Medical Specialties Inc, Charlotte, NC) lace-up ankle brace for stability during light to moderate drills aided the athlete mentally and physically (Figure 24-2). This brace was chosen because of its added side stabilization and figure eight strapping, which provided an additional heel lock on either side of the ankle joint. The comfort that the brace provided increased patient compliance.

Figure 24-2. Ankle lace-up brace used to give the athlete increased stabilization when returning to functional and athletic activity.

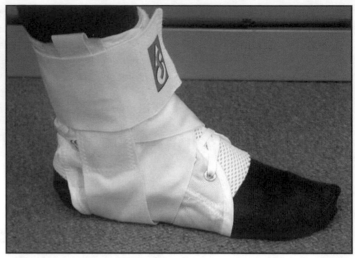

RETURN TO SPORT ACTIVITY

Sport-specific drills were added at this time and included 10 half-court laps of forward and backward running. The athlete was tender with push-off and deceleration on both movements, but after approximately four half-court laps, the joint warmed up and the mild discomfort dissipated. Next, the athlete performed 10 laps of a half-court side shuffle in a basketball defensive position, after which a short aerobic recovery was provided. The athlete then took a position under the back board and was instructed to jump using both feet and touch a spot 6 inches above the bottom of the back board. This was repeated 10 times. To test the involved ankle, the athlete hopped on that foot 10 times attempting to touch only the bottom of the backboard. This was repeated on the unaffected side. To finish, the athlete was given passes at different points around the basket and performed jump shots. Usually 20 to 25 shots were attempted with encouragement to jump and lift as high as possible.

The athlete returned to play in the summer of 1996 without restriction. The following basketball season was successful with minimal symptoms. Recurrent, mild swelling and pain were treated symptomatically with RICE and antiinflammatory medications. ROM was off by 1 to 2 degrees in both dorsiflexion and plantar flexion. This was acceptable due to the addition of tape and brace for support and protection. The ASO ankle brace and athletic tape provided prophylactic support bilaterally.

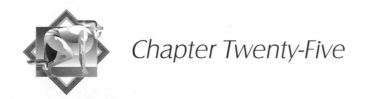

Chapter Twenty-Five

Displaced Distal Tibiofibular Fracture in a High School Football Player

Kecia E. Sell, MS, PT, ATC

INTRODUCTION

Combined fractures of the tibia and fibula occur most often in contact sports such as soccer and football. Many types of mechanisms can be responsible for the etiology of tibial fractures. The energy required to fracture the average tibia is about 1/10,000 of the kinetic energy of an 80 kilogram skier traveling at 24 miles per hour. Because the distal portion of the tibia is closer to the neutral axis, torsional loads typically cause fractures to this portion of the bone.[1] The middle third of the tibia is the strongest and least often fractured, and the proximal and middle thirds of the fibula are the strongest.

While there is little literature available on the incidence of tibiofibular fractures in football, several studies outline the incidence in soccer. Boden et al[2] studied 31 soccer players who sustained a fracture of the lower leg from a direct blow and reported that 42% of the injuries occurred while slide tackling. Athletes with combined tibia and fibula fractures averaged 40 weeks to return to soccer and those with isolated tibia fractures average 35 weeks. Soccer players with isolated fibula fractures returned to their sport the quickest at 18 weeks.[2] In a study of 74 soccer players who sustained tibial fractures, Shaw et al[3] reported that 93% were able to return to soccer, but only 74% said that their function was unimpaired. The average time for these athletes to return to active soccer was 40 weeks.

This case study will outline the course of treatment for a distal tibia/fibula fracture in a high school football player. Initial treatment was unsuccessful and the fracture remained unstable. Resultant surgery included tibial shaft rodding with a closed interlocked intramedullary nail. The course of rehabilitation through physical therapy will be discussed and summarized.

SUBJECTIVE HISTORY

The athlete was a male high school football player at a suburban Minneapolis school. At the time of injury, he was 17 years old and weighed 240 lbs. He played defensive end and was also active in basketball and track. He had no previous injuries and his health status was good with no significant past medical history.

INJURY MECHANISM

The injury occurred in the third quarter of a football game in the fall of 1996. The subject recalls only that a player landed on his left leg as he was trying to tackle an opponent. He states that he felt the lower part of his leg buckle and crack. The mechanism was further viewed from a game video. The athlete was playing left defensive end and the offensive team ran a sweep around his side. He was pursuing the running back when one of his teammates fell in front of him. The athlete planted his left leg as his teammate rolled on the ground into his left lower extremity. The athlete attempted to leap over the player, but his left foot stayed

Figure 25-1. Example of typical tibiofibular injury mechanism in football.

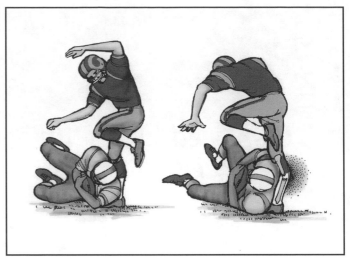

planted, resulting in a torsional injury with the tibia being forced into a varus and posterior position. As the athlete jumped over the player with his right lower extremity, his left leg eventually continued over the player. The subject landed first on his arms and then rolled onto his left side, clutching his left lower leg. The mechanism is further depicted in Figure 25-1.

Typically, the foot is forcibly abducted on the leg, producing a transverse fracture of the distal tibia and fibula. A foot that is planted in combination with an internally rotated leg can also produce a fracture of both the tibia and fibula.[4] Ankle fractures typically occur in three situations:

1. When the foot is forcibly abducted or adducted.
2. When the foot is fixed to the ground and the lower leg is forcibly internally or externally rotated.
3. When the lateral or medial malleolus is forcefully avulsed.[4] When the injury occurs with the foot planted, a long, oblique, spiral fracture of the distal tibia and possibly proximal fibula may occur.[5]

ONFIELD EVALUATION

The athletic trainer did not directly observe the injury mechanism, but as she approached the injured athlete on the field, it was obvious he was in extreme pain. When the athlete removed his hands from the site of injury, the deformity was apparent. There was a varus deformity of the distal portion of the leg, causing the plantar aspect of the foot to face a cephalomedial direction. Additional inspection revealed a closed fracture site. Distal pulse and sensation to light touch were intact. The athletic trainer signaled to the sidelines to call for an ambulance since the athlete was in extreme pain and would require careful splinting and transport. An orthopedic surgeon was present for the initial on-field evaluation. He concurred with the athletic trainer that transportation to the emergency room was appropriate. The athlete was able to actively flex his toes a small amount, but was unwilling to move the knee or the ankle. The paramedics arrived and stabilized the left lower leg with a splint, and the athlete was transferred to a stretcher and taken to the ambulance.

DIAGNOSTIC TESTING

Radiographs were taken in the emergency room revealing a fracture of the distal tibia and fibula at the junction of the middle and distal thirds with a transverse fracture of both components with angulation. Growth plates were closed and neurovascular status was intact.

SURGICAL TREATMENT

Initial Reduction

The athlete was admitted to the hospital and prepared for surgery. With the athlete under anesthesia, the surgeon performed a closed manual reduction of the fracture and applied a long leg cast. Post-reduction x-rays revealed proper position in the anterior-posterior and lateral planes. The anterior portion of the cast was cut out to allow for swelling. The athlete was discharged the following day. He was placed on crutches and instructed to remain nonweightbearing.

The athlete returned for his first postoperative visit 5 days after initial reduction. At this time, he was still having significant pain and difficulty with transfers and ambulation secondary to the long leg split cast. Anterior-posterior views of x-rays revealed that the leg was starting to drift into a valgus alignment. The lateral views showed good alignment. The orthopedic surgeon determined that the fracture was unstable and stated that the patient would benefit from a closed interlocked intramedullary rod. He believed that this would free up the athlete's knee for improved range of motion (ROM) and would allow for improved control of the alignment of the fracture. Continued long-leg casting would require multiple cast changes and wedging, and given the size of the patient, it would be a more difficult way to manage the injury. Because of the ease of mobilization in the cast leading to angulation, the surgeon decided to attempt the intramedullary fixation.

Open Reduction with an Intramedullary Rod

The following surgical procedure is described according to operative notes. The subject received a general endotracheal anesthetic. An entry portal was made into the tibia through a vertical incision just medial to the patellar tendon. The tibia was cleared of subcutaneous tissue to allow an awl to enter the canal, and a guide rod was placed across the fracture site. Nine millimeters was reamed for placement of an 8 mm rod. The guide wire was exchanged and the rod impacted across the fracture site, which was confirmed on the anterior-posterior and lateral plane x-ray. The fracture was stabilized and the guide wire was removed. The surgeon discovered that the fracture was noncomminuted and elected to interlock distally with two interlocking screws. Radiographs were once again taken and the fracture was found to be adequately reduced with an anatomically correct appearance. The fracture was impacted manually and the incisions were closed with sutures at the retinaculum layer, and with staples on the external skin closure. Dressings were applied underneath a posterior plaster splint. The subject was discharged the following day with no complications.

The literature discusses several methods for reduction of tibial shaft fractures. The most common include closed reduction with immobilization in a cast, open reduction with internal fixation, or fixation with an intramedullary rod.[6] External fixation is mainly used for the treatment of severe compound tibial fractures. Conservative management of tibial fractures leads to unacceptable deformity, with shortening or rotational malunion in up to 31% of patients. Ankle and subtalar stiffness are also common complications. Open reduction and plate fixation is associated with a high incidence of soft-tissue problems.[7]

The benefits of using an intramedullary rod are becoming more apparent and more supported. It is reported that this method decreases the duration of external immobilization, maintains alignment, and lowers the rate of infection.[6] The use of an intramedullary rod after reaming has become an attractive alternative now that image intensification makes closed intramedullary technique possible. The addition of interlocking proximal and distal bolts has broadened the indications for use of the technique.[8] Court-Brown et al[9] presented the results of 114 closed and 11 type I open tibial fractures using intramedullary nailing with an interlocking nail system. The mean time to union was 16.7 weeks and no fracture required bone grafting. The authors suggested that intramedullary nailing was an excellent way to treat both closed and open tibial fractures.[9] Bone and Johnson[8] treated 112 fractures of the tibia by manipulative reduction, reaming of the medullary canal, and fixation of the fracture fragments with an intramedullary nail. Follow-up of 100 fractures showed union in all but one. They concluded that using the intramedullary nail was excellent for unstable, acute fractures and for secondary procedures in fractures that are not associated with infection.[8] Robinson et al[7]

Table 25-1

INITIAL PHYSICAL THERAPY EVALUATION FINDINGS

Evaluation Category

Pain	4/10—symptoms increase with weightbearing
Swelling	Figure of eight measured 2 cm larger on involved ankle
Functional deficits	Unable to participate in athletics, unable to perform work as a dishwasher, some difficulty sleeping
Gait	Antalgic, decreased step length, decreased push-off, decreased ankle dorsiflexion
Knee ROM	Within normal limits
Ankle ROM	DF: -5 degrees; PF: 30 degrees
Knee strength deficits	4+/5 knee extension, mild quad atrophy
Ankle strength deficits	3/5 DF, 3+/5 PF, 3/5 inversion and eversion, unable to toe raise on involved leg
Joint mobility	Hypomobile distal tibia-fibula and tibial rotation
Flexibility	Moderately tight gastrocnemius/soleus complex

reviewed 63 patients with fractures of the distal tibial metaphysis with or without minimally displaced extension into the ankle. All fractures were managed by statically locked intramedullary nailing. At a mean of 46 months, all but five patients had a satisfactory functional outcome. The authors discussed that the advantage of intramedullary nailing was that it allowed immediate weightbearing and early movement. They concluded that closed intramedullary nailing was a safe and effective method of managing these fractures.[7]

POSTOPERATIVE TREATMENT

The subject began physical therapy 7 weeks after surgery. Progressive resistive exercises of the quadriceps and ankle, stationary biking, and weightbearing as tolerated (WBAT) were prescribed. Initial evaluation findings are summarized in Table 25-1.

Initial physical therapy evaluation findings were consistent with postsurgical ankle fractures. The area most frequently causing gait and functional deficits included lack of ankle dorsiflexion and weakness of the calf musculature. The athlete's goals included returning to work as a dishwasher and returning to basketball participation. His exercises were progressed as tolerated and he made rapid improvement. Rehabilitation exercises are summarized in.

FUNCTIONAL PROGRESSION

Initial functional activities were introduced 8 weeks postoperatively and included lateral movements, shuffles, and carioca drills. The athlete tolerated all functional activities well. At week 9, double leg jumping activities were initiated. The patient began jump shots and slowly progressed to leaping activities. At 12 weeks, he performed specific basketball drills to further simulate his return to competition. These included progression from running to sprinting, stopping and starting drills, single leg jumping, and easy zig-zag movements that progressed into full-speed cutting. The athlete was advised to progressively increase the intensity of these

Table 25-2
FUNCTIONAL STATUS QUESTIONNAIRE LEVELS

Index	Initial Level	Discharge Level
Work	9/10	10/10
Home	18/20	20/20
Recreation	0/10	9/10
Social	4/10	9/10

Table 25-3
OBJECTIVE CLINICAL OUTCOMES

Objective Test		
ROM	Initial Visit	Discharge Visit
Dorsiflexion	-5 degrees	10 degrees
Plantarflexion	30 degrees	45 degrees
Strength		
Dorsiflexion	3/5	4+/5
Plantarflexion	3+/5	5/5
Inversion	3/5	4+/5
Eversion	3/5	5/5

drills. He was instructed to wear a lace-up ankle brace and to ice after functional activities. The athlete reported no difficulty with this progression of functional activities. He returned to full basketball practice and competition 14 weeks postoperatively.

CLINICAL OUTCOMES

The sports medicine clinic where the athlete attended physical therapy used a functional status questionnaire for pre- and postsubjective outcome data. The results of these scores are summarized as general functional levels in Table 25-2. In addition, objective clinical data were collected at initial and discharge visits. Summaries of objective clinical outcomes are summarized in Table 25-3.

SUMMARY

This case study indicates the importance of communication between athletic trainer/physical therapist and the surgeon. The choice of surgical technique can greatly affect the speed of return to functional activity. In this case, a more invasive surgical procedure was chosen so that return to activity could more easily be accomplished in the shortest amount of time. This athlete was able to return to full functional athletic activities 14 weeks after surgery.

REFERENCES

1. Gould JA. *Orthopedic and Sports Physical Therapy.* St. Louis, Mo: CV Mosby; 1990.

2. Boden BP, Lohnes JH, Nunley JA, et al. Tibia and fibula fractures in soccer players. *Knee Surg Sports Traumatol Arthrosc.* 1999;7(4):262-266.

3. Shaw AD, Gustilo T, Court-Brown CM. Epidemiology and outcome of tibial diaphyseal fractures in footballers. *Injury.* 1997;5(6):365-367.

4. Arnheim DD. *Modern Principles of Athletic Training.* St. Louis, Mo: Times Mirror/Mosby College Publishing; 1985.

5. American Academy of Orthopedic Surgeons. *Athletic Training and Sports Medicine.* Rosemont, Ill: American Academy of Orthopedic Surgeons; 1991.

6. Littenberg B, Weinstein LB, McCarren M, et al. Closed fractures of the tibial shaft: a meta-analysis of three methods of treatment. *J Bone Joint Surg Am.* 1998;80(2):174-183.

7. Robinson CM, McLauchlan GJ, McLean IP, et al. Distal metaphyseal fractures of the tibia with minimal involvement of the ankle. *J Bone Joint Surg Br.* 1995;77(5):781-787.

8. Bone LB, Johnson KD. Treatment of tibial fractures by reaming and intramedullary nailing. *J Bone Joint Surg Am.* 1986;68(6):877-887.

9. Court-Brown CM, Christie J, McQueen MM. Closed intramedullary tibial nailing. *J Bone Joint Surg Br.* 1990;72(4):605-611.

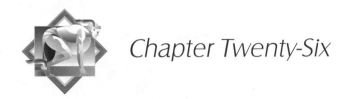

Chapter Twenty-Six

Acute Peroneal Tendon Dislocation in a Collegiate Baseball Player

David A. Porter, MD, PhD, Erin Barill, PT, ATC

INTRODUCTION

Peroneal tendon dislocation/subluxation is an uncommon injury that is often misdiagnosed as an ankle sprain. The dislocation/subluxation can almost always be traced to a single traumatic event. Snow skiing is the most common sport of injury (71%), while football is a distant second (7%).[1,2]

Anatomically, the peroneal tendons are restrained posteriorly to the distal end of the fibula in the retrofibular sulcus. The tendons are contained in the retrofibular sulcus, with the superior peroneal retinaculum as the most important stabilizing soft tissue structure.[1,3] The peroneal muscles function primarily to evert and plantarflex the ankle. They are much more responsible for eversion than plantarflexion. They also are the main dynamic lateral stabilizer of the ankle joint. Injury to these structures may involve a strain, dislocation/subluxation, rupture, or tendonitis. The following is a case presentation of an acute peroneal tendon dislocation.

SUBJECT

The patient is a 23-year-old male centerfielder for a Division I university baseball team. He is 6'1" and 195 lbs, and injured his right ankle April 16, 1998 during an intercollegiate baseball game. He described turning on a small incline and hyperdorsiflexing his foot as he was heading toward the wall to catch a fly ball. He felt a pop in his ankle and experienced immediate pain along the outside of his ankle. The popping and snapping continued over the lateral side of his ankle when he tried to run, but he played the remainder of the inning. At the end of the inning, the athletic trainer evaluated the athlete and was concerned about an acute peroneal tendon dislocation. The athlete was taped heavily and allowed to participate in the remainder of the game.

MECHANISM OF INJURY

This patient's mechanism of injury was typical for peroneal tendon dislocation, with a sudden dorsiflexion stress accompanied by a violent reflex contraction of the peroneal musculature.[4] The patient is often unsure of exactly what happened when the injury occurred.

CLINICAL EVALUATION

The athlete was evaluated the day after the injury by the orthopedic surgeon. He was evaluated the next day by the team's orthopedic surgeon, who diagnosed an acute peroneal tendon dislocation. Range of motion (ROM) and gait were normal. Strength was normal except for a slight decrease in eversion. When his foot

Figure 26-1. Diagram depicting a stress fracture of L-5 pars interarticularis.

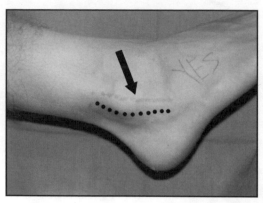

was placed in plantarflexion and slight eversion to take tension off the peroneal tendons, the examiner could passively dislocate the peroneus longus over the posterior lateral fibula (Figure 26-1).

Extreme discomfort or apprehension during resisted eversion of the foot during exam is a distinguishing characteristic of peroneal tendon dislocation or subluxation.[1,5,6] Examination of the patient with a peroneal tendon dislocation will reveal the greatest tenderness and swelling posterior to the fibula or along its posterior border (or both).

In the chronic setting, the athlete complains primarily of instability or a potential giving way or slippage around the ankle. The foot and ankle can, and often do, appear entirely normal in the chronic case. Asking the athlete to maximally dorsiflex and evert the ankle will often reproduce the subluxation or dislocation, confirming the diagnosis.

DIAGNOSTIC IMAGING

Diagnostic imaging included only plain radiographs and was normal, showing no fractures or dislocations. Plain radiographs with peroneal tendon dislocations can often show an avulsion fracture of the posterior rim of the fibula.[7]

DIFFERENTIAL DIAGNOSIS

Signs and symptoms of various ankle injuries are sometimes quite similar, making a thorough clinical exam essential in differentially diagnosing ankle pathology. Peroneal tendon tears, acute lateral ankle sprains, lateral process fractures of the talus, and osteochondral lesions of the lateral dome of the talus should all have signs and symptoms similar to peroneal tendon dislocations. Final diagnosis in this case was acute peroneal tendon dislocation.

TREATMENT

Treatment of acute peroneal tendon subluxations is controversial. While excellent results have been reported for surgical treatment of acutely dislocated tendons, not all patients with subluxed tendons are symptomatic or disabled.[8] The predictability of recurrence and ankle instability is difficult to determine, therefore many authors favor surgical treatment. In addition, the effect of ankle instability and recurrent subluxation on the integrity of the peroneal muscles is undetermined.

Results of nonoperative treatment for peroneal tendon dislocations are poor, typically resulting in an unacceptable rate of redislocation.[1] This patient's history and case are complicated by the fact he was an inseason athlete in his senior year of competition. We discussed with him that he would need operative intervention for definitive treatment. However, operative intervention at the time of initial presentation would have precluded his participation in collegiate baseball. He had about 1 month remaining in his senior year of sports eligibility.

We agreed to treat him nonoperatively to get him through the rest of the season. He was placed in an AirCast walking boot with built-in Cryo/Cuff for immobilization, ice, and compression. A U-shaped felt splint was placed over the fibula to hold the peroneal tendons in their anatomic position. Heavy taping and wrapping was then utilized to allow him to participate without further dislocation. He completed the season, then underwent operative intervention. He had some difficulty with pain and occasional popping during the season, but he was able to participate at the high level of Division I sports.

Surgical treatment after the season involved a lateral incision to expose the posterior lateral fibula and peroneal tendons. With the patient in a lateral decubitus position, a 6 to 8 cm incision was made over the posterior distal border of the fibula. The peroneal tendon sheath was then incised in line with our incision, leaving about a 1 cm tuft at the area of the posterior fibula. At the time of surgery, a longitudinal tear was noted in the peroneus longus tendon. The peroneus brevis tendon was normal. The peroneus longus tendon could be easily dislocated into a false pocket where the lateral periosteum and superior peroneal retinaculum were avulsed off the posterior lateral border of the fibula. The posterior lateral fibula was roughened with a bur, and the posterior "cancellous window" removed from the distal fibula in order to allow deepening of the fibular groove. A small bur was used to deepen the groove, then cortical cancellous bone was replaced in the depth of the groove. This was secured with permanent sutures through drill holes, then tied over the anterior lateral aspect of the fibula. The peroneal tendons were able to sit completely within the groove at this time. The superior peroneal retinaculum was reattached through drill holes in the fibula. The superior peroneal retinaculum was then imbricated to give a tight fit over the peroneal tendons. We were able to get normal, full ROM to his ankle and hind foot in the operating room. The skin was closed in a typical fashion. The patient was placed in an AirCast removable walking boot with an ankle Cryo/Cuff inside the boot. This allowed for immediate cold compression, edema control, and pain control.

POSTOPERATIVE REHABILITATION

The patient followed our postoperative rehabilitation program, which emphasized protection for the first 2 weeks, full normal weightbearing with the AirCast walking boot, pain modulation, inflammatory control, and active ROM (plantarflexion and dorsiflexion with foot internal rotation) (Table 26-1).

Phase I (0 to 21 days)

During the first week after surgery, the patient was placed in the walking boot with a built in Cryo/Cuff. He used crutches for the first week. For the first 5 days, the patient stayed off of his feet as much as possible and continued to minimize swelling by wearing the Cryo/Cuff in the walking boot. He was allowed to take his walking boot off three to four times per day to wiggle his toes.

During the second and third week after surgery, the patient began to wean off of the crutches and ambulate with just the walking boot. He started light ankle ROM including plantarflexion, dorsiflexion, and inversion with the foot in internal rotation. We emphasized that the patient should avoid dorsiflexion with eversion to prevent contracting the peroneals and stressing the surgery site. He also began biking while wearing the walking boot and desensitization massage was initiated.

Phase II (3 weeks to 2 months)

By 3 weeks, we believed the patient had a stable right fibular osteotomy with groove deepening and peroneal retinacula reconstruction. Rehabilitation was designed to restore ROM, wean out of the walking boot into active ankle brace, increase subtalar joint strength, and improve proprioception.

Rehabilitation emphasized ROM exercises in all directions. Resistive tubing exercises were initiated in all directions, including plantarflexion, dorsiflexion, inversion, and eversion. He began stair machine activity 4 to 5 days per week while wearing his ankle brace. Two weeks later, he began performing double leg calf raises progressing to single leg calf raises as tolerated. Proprioception activities included one-foot balance and biomechanical ankle platform system (BAPS) board training.

The patient was given a program for weaning out of the walking boot into the active ankle brace. During the first week, he wore the walking boot during the day and the brace at home in the evening. During the

Table 26-1

Initial Assessment

Time After Surgery	Activity
Phase I	
(0 to 3 weeks)	
Clinical goals	Immobilize peroneal reconstruction with walking boot, control swelling, partial weightbearing with axillary crutches, and active ROM (dorsiflexion with foot internally rotated, plantarflexion, inversion; no eversion).
Testing	Ankle ROM and ankle strength.
Exercises	Ankle ROM (dorsiflexion with foot internally rotated, plantarflexion, inversion; hold for 5 seconds and repeat 10 to 15 times, three to four times per day). During the first week, the patient remained down as much as possible. However, when getting up to go to the bathroom the patient was encouraged to use crutches. After the first week, the patient was weaned off crutches and began weightbearing with walking boot. Desensitization massage (5 minutes, 3 x to 4 x per day) and bike with boot.
Phase II	
(3 weeks to 2 months)	
Clinical goals	Restore full ROM, increase ankle strength, normal gait with active ankle brace, and improve proprioception.
Testing	Ankle ROM and ankle strength.
Exercises	ROM (all directions), resistive band (all directions; three sets of 15, 2 x per day), calf stretching, double leg toe raises at 5 weeks and progressed to single leg (three sets of 15, two times per day), bike/stair machine (10 minutes 4 x 5 x per day), and proprioception (one foot balance with eyes open and closed, biomechanical ankle platform system).
Phase III	
(2 months onward)	
Clinical goals	Full ROM, no swelling, normal gait with active ankle brace, subtalar ankle strength 5/5 with manual muscle testing, and early return to agility and sport-specific drills including functional progression drills.
Testing	Ankle ROM, isokinetic strength test at 3 months, and subjective questionnaire.
Exercises	Sport-specific drills (batting, throwing, and fielding), functional progression for return to baseball (Table 26-2), and calf flexibility (stair stretch).

Table 26-2

FUNCTIONAL PROGRESSION FOR BASEBALL OR SOFTBALL

Activity	Repetitions
Heel raises on injured leg	10 times
Walking at a fast pace	To first base
Jumping on both legs	10 times
Jumping on the injured leg	10 times
Jogging straight ahead	To first base
Jogging straight ahead and curves	Two laps around the bases
Sprinting (½, ¾, and full speed)	To first base
Running figure of eights	Rounding first base
Running backward	Home plate to pitcher's mound
Throwing	Simulate fielding fly ball
Hitting	Short toss to long toss
Position drills	Progress from hitting off tee, to batting cage, and finally to live hitting as directed by athletic trainer

second week he wore the walking boot Monday, Wednesday, and Friday, and the ankle brace on the other days and during the evenings. During the third week, he discontinued wearing the walking boot and only wore the ankle brace.

Phase III (2 months onward)

This phase of rehabilitation emphasized a balance program of musculoskeletal flexibility, Stair machine training, strength training, and functional progression for return to sports. The main goal was to return to full sports and recreational activity.

Rehabilitation still focused on ROM in all directions. Aggressive Achilles' tendon/calf stretching was implemented. Strengthening continued with resistive tubing exercises and weighted toe/calf raises. Sport-specific activity was started. The patient began batting and throwing the baseball and worked on a functional progression for return to full field sports (Table 26-2). Once the patient completed the functional progression, he began fielding activities. All functional progression activities were performed while wearing the ankle brace.

CLINICAL OUTCOMES

The patient had normal ROM and excellent strength on Cybex testing at 3 months postoperatively (Table 26-3). He was able to be involved in a summer baseball program. American Academy of Orthopedic Surgeons' Foot and Ankle Module (American Academy of Orthopedic Surgeons, Rosemont, Ill) score at 13.3 months postoperatively demonstrated no stiffness, limitation of function, giving away, or locking of the foot or ankle. He indicated he had mild pain and difficulty walking on uneven surfaces. He returned to his pre-injury level of activity, but at a lower competitive level because he had completed his college career.

SUMMARY

This case presentation focused on returning an NCAA Division I collegiate baseball player to full activity level as quickly and safely as possible following an acute dislocation of the peroneal tendon. The injury occurred during the middle of his senior baseball season. Conservative management was the choice initially

Table 26-3

POSTOPERATIVE CLINICAL OUTCOMES

	Left Uninvolved Ankle	1 Week	3 Weeks	2 Months	3 Months
ROM					
Dorsiflexion	15 degrees	-5 degrees	3 degrees	10 degrees	12 degrees
Plantarflexion	70 degrees	40 degrees	55 degrees	65 degrees	70 degrees
Inversion	18 degrees	N/T	8 degrees	13 degrees	16 degrees
Eversion	6 degrees	N/T	3 degrees	5 degrees	6 degrees
Gait		Slight antalgia with walking boot and crutches	Normal with walking boot	Normal with active ankle brace	Normal
Strength					
Dorsiflexion	5/5				
Plantar flexion	5/5	N/T	N/T	4/5	Isokinetic
Inversion	5/5	N/T	N/T	4/5	
Activity		N/T	N/T	4/5	
		N/T		Sport-specific exercise and functional progression	Return to full activity level and participation in sports

in order to allow him to complete the season. Following the baseball season, he underwent a right fibular osteotomy with groove deepening and peroneal retinacular reconstruction.

A progressive rehabilitation program that included ROM, strengthening, and gait training was implemented immediately following surgery, and was continually modified throughout the postoperative period. In this case the patient was cleared for full activity 3 months after surgery. The patient did not return to collegiate baseball because his eligibility was already used up however, he would have been cleared to do so otherwise. This surgical option would be appropriate for other athletes who want to return to athletics.

REFERENCES

1. Clanton TO, Porter DA. Primary care of foot and ankle injuries in the athlete. *Clin Sports Med.* 16(3):435-466, 1997.

2. Clanton TO, Shon LC. Athletic injuries to the soft tissues of the foot and ankle. In: Mann RE, Coughlin M, eds. *Surgery of the Foot and Ankle.* 6th ed. St. Louis, Mo: Mosby; 1993:1095-1224.

3. Orthner E, Wagner M. Peroneussehnenluxation (dislocation of the peroneal tendon). *Sportverletz Sportschaden.* 1989;3:112-115.

4. Eckert WR, David EA. Acute rupture of the peroneal retinaculum. *J Bone Joint Surg Am.* 1976;58:670-673.

5. Mason RB, Henderson IJP. Traumatic peroneal tendon instability. *Am J Sports Med.* 1996;24(5):652-658.

6. Martens MA, Noyez JF, Mulier JC. Recurrent dislocation of the peroneal tendons. Results of rerouting the tendons under the calcaneofibular ligament. *Am J Sports Med.* 1986;14(2):148-150.

7. Rask MR, Steinberg LH. The pathognostic sign of tendoperoneal subluxation: report of a case treated conservatively. *Orthop Rev.* 1979;8:65-68.

8. Zaltz I, Icheli LJ. Peroneal tendon dislocation. In: Torg JS, Shephard RJ, eds. *Current Therapy in Sports Medicine.* 3rd ed. St. Louis, Mo: Mosby; 1995:277-280.

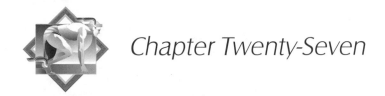

Chapter Twenty-Seven

A Middle Distance Runner with Chronic, Bilateral, Multicompartment Syndrome

Michael A. Shaffer, MSPT, ATC, Mary Meier, MS, ATC,

Thomas A. Greenwald, MD

INTRODUCTION

A compartment syndrome is a clinical condition that involves increased pressure within a contained space such as an osseofascial compartment in the forearm or lower leg.[1-5] Athletic trainers may be more familiar with the acute type of this disorder, whereby there is an initial injury to the musculature of the lower leg through direct blow, fracture, or overexertion.[6-7] Profuse edema follows this acute insult gradually increasing pressure within an unyielding fascial envelope. The result is progressive tissue necrosis necessitating emergent fasciotomy.[8]

Chronic compartment syndrome (CCS) of the lower leg typically affect the anterior and deep posterior compartments (Figure 27-1) in endurance athletes—most often runners—between the ages of 20 and 30. Bilateral complaints have been identified in as many as 80% of patients in some series.[1,3,4,8] In general, athletes with chronic compartment syndromes complain of a cramping or aching over the involved compartments that worsens with exercise. While the onset of symptoms is variable among athletes, a particular athlete will experience symptoms at roughly the same exercise duration/intensity.[3] Prolonged rest improves symptoms only until athletic activity is resumed. Other means of conservative treatment including stretching, modalities, and orthotics.[1]

Several mechanisms have been postulated to account for the production of symptoms in individuals diagnosed with CCS. Muscular compartment volume increases by as much as 20% during vigorous exercise.[9-12] As compartmental volume increases, microtears are created as the fascial envelope is stretched. The result is inflammation and scarring of the fascia. Over time, scar tissue gradually retracts and the fascia will hypertrophy in response to repetitive stress, resulting in a less compliant fascial envelope. Detmer, et al[1] found hypertrophied fascia in 25 of 36 fascial biopsies taken from a series of patients with CCS. They hypothesized that the gradual onset and progressive nature of symptoms in patients with CCS may be due to the progressive changes in fascial structure. They further theorized that fascial thickening may be irreversible with conservative treatments. Thus, symptoms will return once an athlete resumes activity unless the fascia is surgically released.[1,13-15]

Skeletal muscle is not perfused during an active contraction.[16] Instead, blood flow into the muscle occurs only between contractions.[17] As compartment pressure increases, the muscle relaxation pressure may rise to levels that will not allow adequate perfusion of muscle or nervous tissue.[18] Although new technology has questioned the relationship between ischemia and CCS,[19] most authors agree there is a link between increased compartmental pressures and the sequelae of ischemia (Figure 27-2).[3,5,18]

Figure 27-1. Anatomical cross section of the left lower leg (reprinted with permission from Dimanna DL, Buch PG. Chronic compartment syndromes in athletes: recognition and treatment. *Athletic Training.* 1990; 25:28-32).

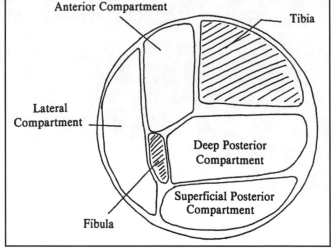

Figure 27-2. Pathophysiology of chronic compartment syndrome and relation to examination findings (reprinted with permission from Styf J. Chronic exercise-induced pain in the anterior aspect of the lower leg: an overview of diagnosis. *Sports Medicine.* 1989;7:331-339).

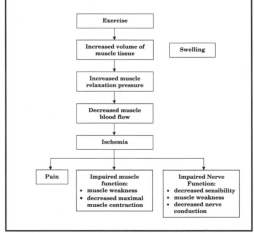

Because the symptoms associated with CCS tend to be directly related to physical activity, the physical examination at rest provides little information in the diagnosis of chronic compartment syndrome.[2,12-13] Following a brief period of exercise, clinical examination may provide signs and symptoms similar to the acute condition: excessive and progressive pain, pain with passive stretching, decreased muscle function, hypoesthesia of the associated nerve, and tenseness of the fascial boundaries.[12, 20] However, because these signs and symptoms are nonspecific, particularly in the lower legs of runners, the differential diagnosis can be quite difficult. Elevated intracompartmental pressures at rest and following exercise are the hallmarks of the diagnosis of chronic compartment syndrome.[12,14-15, 21-26]

SUBJECTIVE HISTORY

The patient was a 20-year-old male middle distance runner for a university track team. He first noticed discomfort bilaterally in his lower legs during high school. His symptoms were located primarily medially and would only occur when running distances greater than 5 miles. The symptoms increased noticeably as a freshman when he first began practice with the university track team in the fall of 1997 and were brought on with 400 or 800 m interval training during practice. He was treated with modalities without resolution of his symptoms. He was also evaluated in our physical therapy clinic, presenting with signs and symptoms consistent with tibialis posterior tendonitis. In addition, he demonstrated a mild pes planus foot with pronation in midstance. Custom molded orthotics were made to control pronation with medial posting at both the hindfoot and forefoot. The athlete was also instructed in ankle strengthening exercises using Theraband.

Throughout the spring of his freshman year and the fall of his sophomore year, the athlete continued to complain of medial "tendonitis" symptoms and "tightness" in his legs with longer runs. He continued treatments as symptoms arose and cross-trained in the SwimEx Aqua Therapy Pool (SwimEx, Warren, RI). He ceased all running over the winter break of his sophomore year and was entirely symptom free. Symptoms recurred immediately with training during the spring semester of 1999. Although he was performing well in his time trials, the athlete felt his symptoms were preventing him from training at a sufficient level to reach his full athletic potential.

CLINICAL EXAMINATION

Physical examination at rest in the athletic training room demonstrated diffuse tenderness bilaterally along the upper half of the lateral shaft of the fibula extending over the peroneal muscles. The athlete was point tender just posteromedial to the distal shaft of the tibia. Range of motion (ROM) and strength assessment was normal for all motions bilaterally. The athlete had no complaints of pain with resisted motion testing. Gait assessment demonstrated mild pronation in midstance. Shoe wear was normal.

MECHANISM OF INJURY

Chronic compartment syndromes most commonly affect the anterior and deep posterior compartments of the lower leg as a direct result of the biomechanics of human gait. Although typically thought of as a prime mover for open chain ankle dorsiflexion, the tibialis anterior's most important function may be as it contracts eccentrically to slowly lower the foot onto the ground after initial contact at the heel.[27,28] Likewise, the tibialis posterior and other muscles of the deep posterior compartment function eccentrically to control subtalar pronation as the hindfoot moves from a supinated position at heel contact to a more pronated position in midstance.[29,30] During running, ground reaction forces can approach three times body weight,[31] and the muscles of these compartments become susceptible to overuse injuries or compartment syndromes, particularly in distance runners with pes planus feet, as was the case with this athlete.

DIAGNOSTIC SETTING

The team orthopedic surgeon evaluated the athlete with similar findings. Although the athlete presented with diffuse tenderness and a chronic history, a bone scan was ordered to rule out stress fracture. Pre- and post-exercise scans were both negative.

Five days later, the athlete returned to the physician's office for intracompartmental pressure measurements. The Stryker intracompartmental pressure monitor system (Stryker, Kalamazoo, Mich) was used to record the athlete's pre-exercise compartment pressures. The athlete then ran on a treadmill until he was able to recreate his symptomatology (10 to 15 minutes). Pre- and post-exercise pressures in all compartments of the left leg were found to be indicative of compartment syndrome, as was the post-exercise measurement for the anterior compartment of the right leg.[22] In addition, there was a significant increase in pressure of the deep posterior compartment of the right leg following exercise (Table 27-1).

DIAGNOSIS

The patient was diagnosed with chronic, bilateral, multicompartment syndrome.

PREOPERATIVE EXERCISES

Given the chronicity of his symptoms, the athlete decided to redshirt for the 1999 indoor and outdoor seasons. After confirmation of the diagnosis of multicompartment syndrome with intracompartmental pressure measurement, the athlete scheduled surgery for February 26, 1999. The athlete continued low-level independent workouts until the time of surgery, letting his symptoms guide exercise intensity. Modalities

Table 27-1				
COMPARTMENT PRESSURE PRE- AND POST-EXERCISE				
	Right		Left	
Compartment	Pre	Post	Pre	Post
Anterior	10	30	40	40
Lateral	8	15	15	37
Deep posterior	5	18	30	34

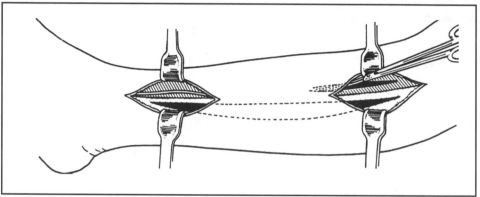

Figure 27-3. Fasciotomy of the anterior compartment. The lateral compartment release has been completed (reprinted with permission from Rorabe CH, Bourne RB, Fowler PJ. The surgical treatment of exertional compartment syndrome in athletes. *J Bone Joint Surg Am.* 1983;65:1245-1251).

were continued as needed. The patient was also referred to a local podiatrist for consultation of foot mechanics and molding of semirigid custom orthotics.

SURGICAL PROCEDURES

After standard orthopedic preparation and draping of the athlete's legs, 2-inch-long incisions were made at the junction of the mid and proximal thirds, and mid and distal thirds of the left lower leg consistent with the techniques of Rorabeck[24] and Mubarak et al[32] (Figure 27-3). Incisions were made halfway between the fibula and anterior crest of the tibia. The superficial peroneal nerve was identified and protected. Fascia of the anterior and lateral compartments was released through the distal incision. This process was repeated through the proximal incision releasing the entire fascial compartment. Next, a 4-inch long medial incision was made just posterior to the posterior crest of the tibia at the midcalf level. The saphenous nerve and vein were identified and retracted posteriorly. Using this incision, the deep posterior compartment was released throughout its entirety. The superficial posterior compartment was palpated and found to be soft and pliable. Wounds were irrigated with saline and antibiotic solution. Subcutaneous tissues were closed with sutures while surgical staples were chosen to close the skin. Postoperative dressings and a compressive wrap were applied. This process was then repeated on the right leg. The patient was discharged from the short stay unit, given two axillary crutches, and instructed to bear weight as tolerated. Analgesics and nonsteroidal anti-inflammatories were prescribed.

Postoperative Rehabilitation

Week 1

Immediate postoperative rehabilitation consisted of wound care, ice, and elevation to decrease postoperative discomfort and edema.[33-34] These treatments began the week after surgery and were conducted on a daily basis in the athletic training room. Three to 4 days after surgery, the athlete achieved full, pain-free weight-bearing and discontinued his crutches.

Week 2

Ten days postoperatively, the athlete returned to the physician's office. Staples were removed and the athlete was referred to physical therapy.

Three days later, on March 11, 1999, he presented to physical therapy with ecchymosis and edema around his surgical incisions, right greater than left and posteriorly greater than anteriorly (Figure 27-4). Symptoms had increased secondary to walking to and from classes, but he was hesitant to return to using crutches. Gait evaluation demonstrated a decreased overall rate, decreased right step length, and the athlete made initial contact in foot flat on the right. Active ROM for dorsiflexion was 0 to 7 degrees on the left and only 0 degrees on the right. Passive ROM and manual muscle testing values are listed in Table 27-2.[35,36] The athlete complained of decreased sensation over the lateral lower legs and feet. Light touch sensation testing confirmed that neurological facilities were intact but diminished in the left superficial peroneal nerve distribution.

Supervised therapy began with a warm whirlpool for 15 minutes. Although this modality placed the athlete's lower extremities in a dependent position, a whirlpool was felt to provide the most effective pre-exercise warm-up, with pain relief, increased hydrostatic pressure for edema reduction, the opportunity for light active ROM exercises (ankle alphabet), and cleansing of his surgical incisions.[37,38] Next the athlete was instructed in active assisted dorsiflexion stretching with a towel, to be completed four to five times a day. Stretching was completed with the knee extended to stretch the gastrocnemius, and with the knee flexed to bias the stretch to the soleus and posterior capsule of the ankle joint.[39] Very light passive stretching was also completed for ankle plantarflexion/toe flexion and ankle dorsiflexion/toe extension. All stretches were completed for three repetitions of 10 seconds. Although previous authors have advocated stretching for longer durations,[40,41] we tend to begin passive stretching for a shorter duration, particularly when rehabilitating acutely injured or postsurgical areas.

In addition to the rehabilitation program just described, the athlete was also exercising in the SwimEx therapy pool performing ankle ROM and working on gait pattern for a total of 15 minutes, two to three times per week. The patient performed these exercises in chest-deep water at approximately 35% weight-bearing.[42]

Week 3

Three weeks postoperatively, the patient returned home during the university's spring break (March 14 to March 21, 1999). He continued with independent active ROM exercises, self-stretching, and independent modality use.

Week 4

The athlete was re-evaluated after the break and demonstrated 0 to 15 degrees of dorsiflexion passive ROM on the left and 0 to 10 degrees on the right. Plantarflexion ROM was measured at 0 to 30 degrees bilaterally. The athlete reported he was symptom-free when walking and climbing stairs.

Given the decrease in the athlete's symptoms and his objective improvement, several modifications were made to his program. The warm whirlpool was discontinued and the athlete completed an active warm-up on a stationary bicycle with low resistance and no use of toe clips, which may have encouraged use of the dorsiflexors and toe extensors, unduly stressing the anterior compartment. Without the toe clips it was hoped

Figure 27-4. Weightbearing photograph of athlete at the time of initial physical therapy evaluation (13 days postoperatively).

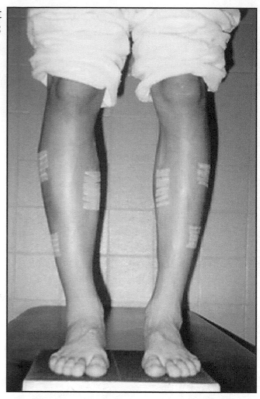

Table 27-2				
PASSIVE RANGE OF MOTION AND MANUAL MUSCLE TESTING				
	Right		Left	
Motion	ROM	MMT	ROM	MMT
Dorsiflexion	0 to 10 degrees	3/5	0 to 7 degrees	3/5
Plantarflexion	0 to 25 degrees		0 to 20 degrees	
Inversion	0 to 20 degrees	4/5	0 to 30 degrees	4/5
Eversion	0 degrees	3/5	0 to 5 degrees	3+/5

ROM = range of motion; MMT = manual muscle test

that burden would be assumed by the contralateral quadriceps and plantarflexing muscles of the superficial posterior compartment. Independent dorsiflexion stretching was progressed to a standard weightbearing position using a wall for support, and the athlete began to stretch for three repetitions of 30 seconds. In addition, the athlete began strength training exercises with a Theraband for dorsiflexion, inversion, and eversion for two sets of 10 repetitions. Theraband was employed to allow the athlete to continue with resistance exercises as part of a home exercise program. The athlete also began proprioceptive retraining on the biomechanical ankle platform system (BAPS). The BAPS was completed in a weightbearing position at level 3 on the right and level 4 on the left for one set of 10 repetitions in the straight planes of ankle plantar- and dorsiflexion, inversion and eversion, and clockwise and counterclockwise circles.

When he returned later that week, the athlete had no new complaints despite the increase in his program. He continued with the exercises of the previous session, plus began manually resisted ankle strengthening, bilateral heel raises, and unilateral plantarflexion strengthening in a nonweightbearing position on the Cybex leg press machine. Because the athlete's right leg had trailed the recovery of the left following surgery, it was felt that bilateral weightbearing heel raises may not be a challenge for the left leg. Toe raises on the leg press were added so the athlete could choose a resistance level appropriate for each leg and contract through the full, available ROM. Manual resistance exercises were performed during the athlete's rehabilitation sessions in lieu of Theraband to provide variety, accommodating resistance, and continual reassessment of the athlete's muscle performance. Once it was demonstrated the athlete was symptom-free with resistance training, repetitions were advanced to a standard three sets of 10 repetitions.[43]

Week 5

The surgeon re-evaluated the athlete on March 29, 1999 and was pleased with his recovery. The athlete was permitted to begin elliptical stair climbing and gradually increase the intensity of his SwimEx workouts. If this progression was well tolerated, the athlete was to begin running the following week. No new rehabilitation exercises were added in physical therapy, although the athlete did progress his resistance levels.

The athlete began nonweightbearing running in the SwimEx for 15 minutes, and elliptical stair climbing for 10 minutes on alternate days. Stationary bicycling with toe clips was also performed on his stair climbing days for cardiovascular retraining.

Week 6

The athlete was symptom-free with activities of daily living and all workouts. He began running for 10 minutes on an indoor track at a slow speed twice a week. The athlete had achieved the physical therapy goals of full, pain-free ROM and ankle strength > 4+/5, and was discharged after a total of six visits. He continued with independent treatments such as stretching, ankle strengthening with Theraband, cardiovascular work on the bike, elliptical stair climber, or the SwimEx on a daily basis. The athlete used cryotherapy on an as-needed basis following his workouts.

Week 8

The athlete was now running for approximately 15 minutes, three times a week. When questioned in the training room after a run, he admitted that he had become inconsistent with Theraband exercises. He continued to cross train on the elliptical stair climber and bike, but had ceased the SwimEx workouts.

Week 10

On May 6, 1999, the athlete returned to the physician's office for normal postsurgical follow-up. He reported he was able to run for 20 minutes at moderate intensity (2.5 to 2.75 miles) without symptoms. He continued to complain of hypoesthesia into the superficial peroneal nerve distribution of the left leg but was otherwise without complaint.

FUNCTIONAL PROGRESSION

Overall, the athlete's rehabilitation followed a step-wise progression. Initially, the focus was on reducing edema and postoperative pain with passive modalities. As these problems were addressed, the primary goals became the restoration of ROM and muscle function. The final step of supervised rehabilitation was a progression of cardiovascular exercises that culminated in running. When he resumed running, the athlete independently advanced his workouts with informal contact with the athletic training and physical therapy staffs.

Although the progression from rehabilitation exercises to running is often thought of as one of the final rehabilitation goals, preparation for this step began during the second postoperative week. At this point, the athlete began working on his gait pattern in a reduced weightbearing medium in the SwimEx. Our clinical experience has shown us the importance of re-establishing a normal gait pattern early on in the rehabilitation program. We have found a normal gait pattern helps to decrease pain, restore muscle function, and anecdotally corresponds to an early return to athletic activity.

By the fourth postoperative week, the athlete had demonstrated sufficient improvement (decreased pain and edema, improved gait pattern) to progress to stationary bicycling. Initially, the athlete was protected by removal of the toe clips. Later, the toe clips were replaced and the time and resistance of cycling was gradually increased. The elliptical stair climber allowed for progression to a full weightbearing exercise. The elliptical stair climber and running in the SwimEx allowed us to simulate running early on during the rehabilitation process while limiting the amount of pounding the recovering muscles had to absorb. The athlete resumed running around the sixth postoperative week. Since then, he has been gradually increasing his workload in terms of running frequency, duration, and intensity.

Although a thorough rehabilitation program has not been described in the literature, this athlete's rehabilitation program and progression appears consistent with previous authors.[2,13,14,24,32,44]

CLINICAL OUTCOME

This athlete returned to campus for the start of his junior year and was re-examined by his surgeon. At the time of that appointment on August 26, 1999, the athlete was approximately 6 months postoperatively. He reported that he had been able to resume his normal summer training regimen, running approximately 3 to 5 miles a day, 3 to 4 days a week. In addition, he had been playing basketball 2 to 3 days a week, all without any recurrence of preoperative symptomatology. He continues to complain of hypoesthesia in the superficial peroneal nerve distribution distal to his incision. He denies that there has been any significant change in this symptom since surgery, although he admits that it is not limiting in any way.

The recovery of this athlete appears consistent with reports of other individuals with CCS treated with fasciotomy. Many authors have reported near total resolution of symptoms in 90% of patients undergoing surgical decompression.[1,14,32] Elevated intracompartmental pressures are the hallmarks of the diagnosis of CCS and tend to be the best predictors of surgical outcome.[1,14,24,32] Reported failures are almost always the result of incomplete release of the deep posterior compartment.[13,14,24] The return of symptoms is usually noted within the first 6 months postoperatively and has been successfully treated with a second fasciotomy.[1,14]

We remain cautiously optimistic about this athlete's outcome until he resumes his typical inseason workout regimen. Supervised track practice will begin within the next week, and only after the athlete resumes interval training and distance runs over 5 miles will his true outcome be known.

SUMMARY

This report illustrates a case of chronic bilateral multicompartment syndrome in a college-aged middle distance runner. For 3 years the athlete battled symptoms of "tightness" in his legs with longer distance runs. Intracompartmental tissue pressures were recorded before and after exercise to confirm the diagnosis. The athlete continued to experience symptoms despite modality treatments, supervised rehabilitation, foot orthotics, and rest. After the fasciotomies were performed, the athlete was able to resume running by 6 weeks and has since resumed his normal summer training regimen. We are all anxious to see how the athlete will tolerate the beginning of fall track practice, but there is no indication thus far that he will not have an excellent outcome.

REFERENCES

1. Detmer DE, Sharpe K, Sufit RL, et al. Chronic compartment syndrome: diagnosis, management, and outcomes. *Am J Sports Med.* 1985;13:162-170.

2. Dimanna DL, Buck PG. Chronic compartment syndromes in athletes: recognition and treatment. *Athletic Training.* 1990;25:28-32.

3. Martens MA, Moeyersoons JP. Acute and recurrent effort-related compartment syndrome in sports. *Sports Med.* 1990;9:62-68.

4. Moeyersoons JP, Martens M. Chronic compartment syndrome: diagnosis and management. *Acta Orthop Belg.* 1992;58:23-27.

5. Ross DG. Chronic compartment syndrome. *Orthop Nursing.* 1996;15:23-27.

6. Klodell CT, Pokorny R, Carrillo EH, et al. Exercise-induced compartment syndrome: case report. *The American Surgeon.* 1996;62:469-471.

7. Pearl AJ. Anterior compartment syndrome: a case report. *Am J Sports Med.* 1981;9:119-120.

8. Pedowitz RA, Gershuini DH. Pathophysiology and diagnosis of chronic compartment syndrome. *Operative Techniques in Sports Medicine.* 1995;3:230-236.

9. D'Ambrosia R, Drez D. *Prevention and Treatment of Running Injuries.* Thorofare, NJ: SLACK Incorporated; 1989:22-24, 89-108.

10. Hunter-Griffin LY. *Clinics in Sports Medicine: Overuse Injuries.* Philadelphia, Pa: WB Saunders; 1987:273-290,405-426.

11. Mubarak SJ, Hargens AR. *Compartment Syndrome and Volkmann's Contracture.* Philadelphia, Pa: WB Saunders; 1981:117-122, 209-226.

12. Touliopolous S, Hershman EB. Lower leg pain: diagnosis and treatment of compartment syndromes and other pain syndromes of the leg. *Sports Med.* 1999;27:193-204.

13. Abramowitz AJ, Schepsis AA. Chronic exertional compartment syndrome of the lower leg. *Orthopedic Review.* 1994;March:219-225.

14. Schepsis AA, Martini D, Corbett M. Surgical management of exertional compartment syndrome of the lower leg. *Am J Sports Med.* 1993;21:811-817.

15. Styf JR, Korner LM. Chronic anterior-compartment syndrome of the leg: results of treatment by fasciotomy. *J Bone Joint Surg Am.* 1986;68:1338-1347.

16. Barcroft H, Millen JL. The blood flow through muscle during sustained contraction. *J Physiol.* 1939;97:17-31.

17. Folkow B, Gaskell P, Waaler BA. Blood flow through limb muscle during heavy rhythmic exercise. *Acta Physiol Scand.* 1970;80:61-72.

18. Styf J. Chronic exercise-induced pain in the anterior aspect of the lower leg: an overview of diagnosis. *Sports Medicine.* 1989;7:331-339.

19. Balduini FC, Shenton DW, O'Connor KH, Heppenstall RB. Correlation of compartment pressure and muscle ischemia utilizing 31P-NMR spectroscopy. *Clin Sports Med.* 1993;12:151-165.

20. Matsen FA, Winquist RA, Krugmire RB. Diagnosis and management of compartmental syndromes. *J Bone Joint Surg Am.* 1980;62:286-291.

21. Genuario SE. Differential diagnosis: exertional compartment syndromes, stress fractures, and shin splints. *Athletic Training.* 1989;24:31-34.

22. Pedowitz RA, Hargens AR, Mubarak SJ, et al. Modified criteria for the objective diagnosis of chronic compartment syndrome of the leg. *Am J Sports Med.* 1990;18:35-40.

23. Puranen J, Alavaikko A. Intra-compartmental pressure increase on exertion in patients with chronic compartment syndrome in the leg. *J Bone Joint Surg Am.* 1981;63:1304-1309.

24. Rorabeck CH, Bourne RB, Fowler PJ. The surgical treatment of exertional compartment syndrome in athletes. *J Bone Joint Surg Am.* 1983;65:1245-1251.

25. Rorabeck CH, Bourne RB, Fowler PJ, et al. The role of tissue pressure measurement in diagnosing chronic anterior compartment syndrome. *Am J Sports Med.* 1988;16:143-146.

26. Styf J, Korner L, Suurkula M. Intramuscular pressure and muscle blood flow during exercise in chronic compartment syndrome. *J Bone Joint Surg Br.* 1987;69:301-305.

27. Michaud TC. *Foot Orthoses and Other Forms of Conservative Foot Care.* Baltimore, Md: Williams Wilkins; 1993.

28. Winter DA. *The Biomechanics and Motor Control of Human Gait: Normal, Elderly, and Pathological.* 2nd ed. Ontario, Canada: University of Waterloo Press; 1991:63.

29. Sarrafian SK. *Anatomy of the Foot and Ankle: Descriptive, Topographical, Functional.* 2nd ed. Philadelphia, Pa: JB Lippincott Company; 1993.

30. Inman VT, Ralston HJ, Todd F. *Human Walking.* Baltimore, Md: Williams & Wilkins; 1981:52-53.

31. Sarrafian SK. *Anatomy of the Foot and Ankle: Descriptive, Topographical, Functional.* 2nd ed. Philadelphia, Pa: JB Lippincott Company; 1993.

32. Mubarak SJ. Surgical management of chronic compartment syndromes of the leg. *Operative Techniques in Sports Medicine.* 1995;3:259-266.

33. Michlovitz SL. *Thermal Agents in Rehabilitation.* Philadelphia, Pa: FA Davis Company; 1986.

34. Prentice WE. *Therapeutic Modalities in Sports Medicine.* 4th ed. Boston, Mass: WCB McGraw-Hill; 1999.

35. Norkin CC, White DJ. *Measurement of Joint Motion—A Guide to Goniometry.* Philadelphia, Pa: FA Davis Co; 1985.

36. Kendall FP, McCreary EK, Provance PG. *Muscles Testing and Function.* 4th ed. Baltimore, MD: Williams & Wilkins; 1993.

37. Michlovitz SL. *Thermal Agents in Rehabilitation.* Philadelphia, Pa: FA Davis Company; 1986.

38. Prentice WE. *Therapeutic Modalities in Sports Medicine.* 4th ed. Boston, Mass: WCB McGraw-Hill; 1999.

39. Kisner C, Colby L. *Therapeutic Exercise.* 2nd ed. Philadelphia, Pa: FA Davis Co;1990.

40. Kisner C, Colby L. *Therapeutic Exercise.* 3rd ed. Philadelphia, Pa: FA Davis Co;1999.

41. Bandy WD, Irion JM. The effect of time on static stretch on the flexibility of the hamstring muscles. *Phys Ther.* 1994;74:845-850.

42. Thein JM, Brody LT. Aquatic-based rehabilitation and training for the elite athlete. *J Orthop Sports Phys Ther.* 1998;27:32-41.

43. Kisner C, Colby L. *Therapeutic Exercise.* 2nd ed. Philadelphia, Pa: FA Davis Co; 1990.

44. Rampersaud YR, Amendola A. The evaluation and treatment of exertional compartment syndrome. *Operative Techniques in Sports Medicine.* 1995;3:267-273.

Chapter Twenty-Eight

Syndesmotic Ankle Sprain in an Elite High School Volleyball Player

Robert S. Gray, MS, ATC

INTRODUCTION

Subject

The patient was a 17-year-old high school volleyball player who injured her left ankle on August 25, 1998 while participating in the first interscholastic volleyball game of the season. Her position on the team was that of outside hitter. She reported that while attempting to hit a cross court "kill" shot, she landed on the foot of one of her teammates and sustained an inversion-type injury to her left ankle. She experienced immediate pain and swelling but did not report the sensation of a pop.

The certified athletic trainer performed the initial evaluation immediately after the injury occurred. The athlete immersed her ankle in a bucket of ice water for approximately 10 minutes, a compressive wrap was applied, and she was placed on crutches and referred to the nearest medical facility for x-rays to rule out a fracture to the left ankle.

The athlete's parents transferred her to the nearest medical facility. After examination by the emergency room physician, standard x-ray views were taken of the ankle including anterior/posterior, lateral, and oblique. The x-ray report stated that bony structures were intact, there was no evidence of fracture or dislocation, and the ankle mortise was well maintained. Soft tissue swelling was present adjacent to the lateral malleolus. The patient's left ankle was placed in an AirCast, compressed with an elastic bandage. She was instructed to remain on her crutches and was referred to the team physician at the high school for continued care. The team physician evaluated the athlete the next day in the clinic. The results of this evaluation are given in Table 28-1. Following this evaluation, the athlete was placed in a posterior plaster splint with stirrups, instructed to be nonweightbearing on her crutches, and continue to use her anti-inflammatory medication.

DIFFERENTIAL DIAGNOSIS

Treatment

The athlete was a senior cocaptain of the volleyball team and had aspirations of returning to competition as soon as possible. She was instructed to return to the team physician's office in 2 days for a follow-up evaluation. At the follow-up evaluation, it was noted that the plaster splint was broken in several places and not giving adequate stability to the ankle. The athlete stated that she had been compliant with icing her ankle, but not totally compliant with the use of anti-inflammatory medication or remaining nonweightbearing. The physical findings by the team physician for the follow-up evaluation are given in Table 28-1. The team physi-

Table 28-1

FOLLOW-UP EVALUATION FINDINGS BY THE TEAM PHYSICIAN

Significant swelling about the ankle and dorsum of the foot

Ecchymosis at the base of the digits, as well as the perimalleolar area

Less tenderness in the tarsal sinus and anterior talofibular ligament but remains tender with swelling overlying the lateral malleolus

Improved dorsiflexion and plantarflexion

Neurologic exam remains intact with adequate strength with resisted dorsiflexion and eversion, though painful

Intact sensation

No proximal fibular sensation

cian outlined all treatment options to the athlete, her parents, the head athletic trainer at her high school. All involved parties decided that the athlete should begin an aggressive rehabilitation/reconditioning program at the high school under the direct supervision of the head athletic trainer. The athlete was seen 5 days a week for approximately 60 minutes per session.

FUNCTIONAL PROGRESSION

After 2 weeks of the initial rehabilitation program, the athlete began a gradual increase of functional activities with the goal of returning to volleyball. The functional progression of activities is outlined in Table 28-2. This functional rehabilitation period lasted for 4 weeks. The athlete was seen 4 to 5 days per week for 60 to 75 minutes per day. At the end of each session, the athlete elevated her ankle and placed it in the AirCast ankle unit. She iced her ankle for 15 minutes and the AirCast unit applied intermittent compression.

Medical Follow-up

After 6 weeks of dedicated rehabilitation, the athlete returned to the team physician with her parents. Her chief complaints at this time were persistent left ankle pain, both medially and laterally, as well as pain involving the dorsum of the foot. In addition to returning to interscholastic volleyball, the athlete also returned to marching band. The physical findings of this medical follow-up appointment are outlined in Table 28-1. The athlete experienced some discomfort while playing volleyball and there was increased discomfort while marching in the band, especially when moving backward. After conferring with one of his fellow colleagues, the team physician recommended a bone scan to rule out osteochondritis dissecans (OCD) of the left ankle. The athlete and her parents were in complete agreement with this recommendation. The bone scan was performed 7 days later. The results of the bone scan revealed that there was increased tracer activity within the left ankle, which may be related to ligamentous injury, although the possibility of fracture could not be excluded. Further evaluation with magnetic resonance imaging (MRI) was considered. After conferring with the radiologist and in light of two normal sets of x-rays, the findings were thought to be more consistent with a more diffuse injury to an ankle sprain rather than a fracture or bony trauma. With all of the parties present including the athlete, parents, and head athletic trainer, the team physician outlined a plan that was agreed upon by all. The plan was to continue with the functional rehabilitation/reconditioning program and continued use of anti-inflammatory medication. Activities such as marching band and volleyball were eliminated to allow for a complete recovery for basketball season.

SUMMARY

Of the 23,000 ankle sprains that occur each day, the majority of these injuries are classified as "simple sprains" requiring short-term immobilization followed by a rehabilitation/reconditioning program. However, it is imperative that sports medicine clinicians are able to recognize the syndesmotic or "high" ankle sprain. Timely recognition, proper diagnosis, and a period of immobilization followed by a complete rehabilitation/reconditioning functional program is the key to returning the athlete to competition. In retrospect, a longer period of immobilization along with better compliance during the early phases of the injury would have benefitted this athlete. The initial treatment and the functional rehabilitation program were beneficial to the athlete in preparing her to return to interscholastic sports. She was able to return to pre-injury status, but 16 weeks later. Upon her return to interscholastic sports, the athlete wore a laced ankle orthosis for both practice and games.

REFERENCES

1.   University of Pennsylvania Health System. Diagnosis and treatment. *Complex Ankle Sprain.* 1998;9(Fall):2.

2.   Garrick JB, and Schelkins PH. Managing ankle sprain: keys to preserving motion and strength. *The Physician and Sportsmedicine.* 1997;25(3):56-58.

3.   The First Aider. *The High Ankle Sprain: Deceptive and Dangerous.* Cramer Products, Incorporated. 1990;59(Spring):3.

4.   Liu SH, Jason WJ. Lateral ankle sprains and instability problems. *Clin Sports Med.* 1994;13(4):793-809.

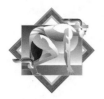

Index

BUILD *Your Library*

This book and many others on numerous different topics are available from SLACK Incorporated. For further information or a copy of our latest catalog, contact us at:

Professional Book Division
SLACK Incorporated
6900 Grove Road
Thorofare, NJ 08086 USA
Telephone: 1-856-848-1000
1-800-257-8290
Fax: 1-856-853-5991
E-mail: orders@slackinc.com
www.slackbooks.com

We accept most major credit cards and checks or money orders in US dollars drawn on a US bank. Most orders are shipped within 72 hours.

Contact us for information on recent releases, forthcoming titles, and bestsellers. If you have a comment about this title or see a need for a new book, direct your correspondence to the Editorial Director at the above address.

Thank you for your interest and we hope you found this work beneficial.

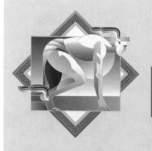

Expand Your Library
With These Exceptional Texts!

Other Exciting Books in the Athletic Training Library *Include:*

Title	Author	Book #	Price
❑ Professional Behaviors in Athletic Training	Hannam	44094	$24.00
❑ The Athletic Trainer's Guide to Strength and Endurance Training	Wiksten	44310	$24.00
❑ Current Topics in Musculoskeletal Approach: A Case Study Approach	DeCarlo	44345	$24.00
❑ Research in Athletic Training	Ingersoll	44396	$24.00

Subtotal $____

NJ and CA Sales Tax* $____

Handling Charge $ 4.50

Total $____

Name: _____

Address: _____

City: _____ State: _____ Zip Code: _____

Phone: _____ Fax: _____

Charge my: ❑ AMERICAN EXPRESS   ❑ MasterCard   ❑ VISA   Account#:_____

Exp. date: _____ Signature: _____

Prices are subject to change. Shipping charges may apply.
*Purchases in NJ and CA are subject to tax. Please add applicable state and local taxes.

CODE:4A687

Mail Order Form To: SLACK Incorporated
Professional Book Division
6900 Grove Road
Thorofare, NJ 08086-9864

Call: 800-257-8290 or 856-848-1000
Fax: 856-853-5991
Email: Orders@slackinc.com

Visit Our World Wide Web: www.slackbooks.com